The EHRA Book of

Pacemaker, ICD, and CRT Troubleshooting

European Society of Cardiology publications

The ESC Textbook of Cardiovascular Medicine (Second Edition)
Edited by A. John Camm, Thomas F. Lüscher, and Patrick W. Serruys

The EAE Textbook of Echocardiography
Editor-in-Chief: Leda Galiuto, with Co-editors: Luigi Badano, Kevin Fox, Rosa Sicari, and José Luis Zamorano

The ESC Textbook of Intensive and Acute Cardiovascular Care (Second Edition)
Edited by Marco Tubaro, Pascal Vranckx, Susanna Price, and Christiaan Vrints

The ESC Textbook of Cardiovascular Imaging (Second Edition)
Edited by José Luis Zamorano, Jeroen Bax, Juhani Knuuti, Patrizio Lancellotti, Luigi Badano, and Udo Sechtem

The ESC Textbook of Preventive Cardiology
Edited by Stephan Gielen, Guy De Backer, Massimo Piepoli, and David Wood

The EHRA Book of Pacemaker, ICD, and CRT Troubleshooting: Case-based learning with multiple choice questions
Edited by Haran Burri, Jean-Claude Deharo, and Carsten Israel

Forthcoming
The EACVI Echo Handbook
Edited by Patrizio Lancellotti and Bernard Cosyns

The ESC Handbook of Preventive Cardiology: Putting prevention into practice
Edited by Catriona Jennings, Ian Graham, and Stephan Gielen

The EHRA Book of

Pacemaker, ICD, and CRT Troubleshooting

Case-based learning with multiple choice questions

Edited by

Haran Burri MD
EHRA Education Committee Chairman
Assistant Professor
Electrophysiology Unit
Cardiology Service
University Hospital of Geneva
Geneva, Switzerland

Co-editors

Jean-Claude Deharo MD
EHRA Accreditation Committee Member
Professor
Rhythmology Department
Timone Hospital
Marseilles, France

Carsten Israel MD
EHRA Education Committee Member
Associate Professor
Evangelical Hospital
Bielefeld, Germany

OXFORD
UNIVERSITY PRESS

EUROPEAN Heart Rhythm ASSOCIATION
A Registered Branch of the ESC

EUROPEAN SOCIETY OF CARDIOLOGY®

OXFORD
UNIVERSITY PRESS

Great Clarendon Street, Oxford, OX2 6DP,
United Kingdom

Oxford University Press is a department of the University of Oxford. It furthers the University's objective of excellence in research, scholarship, and education by publishing worldwide. Oxford is a registered trade mark of Oxford University Press in the UK and in certain other countries

Published in the United States of America by Oxford University Press
198 Madison Avenue, New York, NY 10016, United States of America

British Library Cataloguing in Publication Data
Data available

Library of Congress Control Number: 2015934017

ISBN 978–0–19–872777–4

Printed and bound by CPI Group (UK) Ltd, Croydon, CR0 4YY

To our teachers, who have shown us that knowledge is a gift that should be shared with generosity, and, most of all, to our loved ones.

Endorsements

Pacemakers, ICDs, and CRT devices are used increasingly in the management of arrhythmias and a number of different cardiac conditions. Specialists, general cardiologists, and general physicians are now closely involved in managing patients with these devices. *The EHRA Book of Pacemaker, ICD, and CRT Troubleshooting* is written by leading specialists from Europe and is designed for all physicians looking for a clear and comprehensive introduction to the troubleshooting management of these devices. Designed to bring you from your current level of knowledge to a level of fully advanced troubleshooting manager, this book features 70 real-life IPG, ICD, and CRT cases, accompanied by thorough explanations and analyses. Presented in a clear and casual writing style, the book's levelled approach takes a complex subject and makes it simple. Whether you are an EMT, nurse, medical student, or physician wanting to learn or brush up on your knowledge of pacemaker, ICD, or CRT troubleshooting, this text will meet your needs. The text has been created to be continuously useful during your development and is intended to be read and reread, as you advance in your knowledge and comfort level with the material.

Angelo Auricchio, MD, PHD, FESC

Director Clinical Electrophysiology Programme, Division of Cardiology,
Fondazione Cardiocentro Ticino, Lugano, Switzerland
Co-Director, Center of Computational Medicine in Cardiology,
Università della Svizzera Italiana, Lugano, Switzerland
Scientific Director, Fondazione Ticino Cuore, Lugano, Switzerland
Professor of Cardiology, University of Magdeburg, Magdeburg, Germany
Immediate Past-President of the European Heart Rhythm Association

The book by Dr Burri, Dr Israel, and Dr Deharo is a godsend, because troubleshooting of complicated contemporary heart rhythm devices is difficult. Only very few recent books have addressed this complex subject comprehensively. The book describes the timing cycles involved in the various cases in a clear way, so that they can be more easily understood and remembered. The book is ideally suited for workers preparing for an examination given by the European Heart Rhythm Association and the Heart Rhythm Society. It will also be useful to all health care workers dealing with heart rhythm devices.

S Serge Barold, MD

Clinical Professor of Medicine Emeritus,
University of Rochester,
Rochester, New York, USA

The authors, all noted cardiologists with a special expertise in device management, have prepared a unique volume of device (pacemakers, ICDs, and CRT devices)-based cases that test the clinician's ability to interpret multiple facets of device-based therapy. This book is the perfect volume for examination preparation. Many practitioners (cardiac electrophysiologists, cardiologists, nurses, device technicians, cardiac technologists), at all levels of experience and knowledge, will find this volume invaluable for improving their ability to analyse device function and malfunction. The bottom line is this book is a 'must have' for any clinician who cares for cardiac patients with implantable devices.

Kenneth A Ellenbogen, MD, FAHA, FACC, FHRS

Kontos Professor of Cardiology
Chairman of Cardiology
VCU School of Medicine, Richmond, VA, USA

Foreword

I am very pleased to have been asked to provide a foreword to this first of several specialist "handbooks", commissioned by the European Heart Rhythm Association (EHRA), and written and overseen by the Education Committee of EHRA. The project was originally conceived by Panos Vardas, then the President of the EHRA. The subjects are highly technical and very practical. They are specifically designed as teaching aids to assist practitioners to become and remain truly expert in their role. This particular volume concerns the troubleshooting of cardiovascular implantable electronic devices (CIEDs), specifically pacemakers, implantable cardioverter defibrillators and cardiac re-synchronisation therapy.

The book is authored by three true experts in their field. The concept is to provide a highly illustrated volume of real cases with technical challenges drawn from clinical practice. The format is to provide a minimum of technical information and to present ECG recordings, chest X-rays, echocardiograms, pacemaker log data, stored or real time electrograms with the manufacturers' annotations and other technical outputs in order to challenge the reader. The test comes in the form of multi-choice questions. The correct answer is given and the explanations are provided in a few sentences relating to specific annotations added to each trace. There are three sections in the book, going from relatively easy and straightforward examples to much more difficult and puzzling cases. References for further reading are provided for those who want to dig more deeply.

This type of educational aid is very well suited to preparing those who would like to take formal assessments of their skills, at national or international levels. In this case the handbook is very useful for those intending to take the EHRA accreditation examinations. However, the study of this practical book should be of very great value to all technicians, physiologists, nurses and doctors who have the responsibility to follow patients fitted with CIEDs.

A. John Camm, MD, FESC

Professor of Clinical Cardiology, St. George's University of London,
Professor of Cardiac Electrophysiology, Imperial College, London, United Kingdom, and
Editor-in-Chief of EP-Europace, the official journal of EHRA

Preface

As the complexity of cardiac rhythm devices grows, so does the necessity to understand device behaviour, in order to perform proper follow-up of device patients. Case-based teaching is an effective way to learn device function. This book is a collection of teaching cases that have been gathered for over more than a decade. The cases presented here serve to illustrate common problems that the device specialist may be faced with, or uncommon situations for which structured and logical reasoning paves the path to elucidation.

This book is not a technical manual of device algorithms. Algorithms of the different device manufacturers are almost impossible to memorize and may be outdated as soon as new models are introduced. However, understanding the general principles of device function and being able to reason in a structured and logical manner when interpreting device tracings is of timeless value. The material provided here will assist those studying for the European Heart Rhythm Association (EHRA) accreditation exam in cardiac pacing, even if the level of complexity of some of the cases may exceed that which is expected of them to pass the exam. It is also intended to be of use to cardiologists and technical consultants who do not intend to pass the exam but deal with device patients.

The book is divided into three sections: pacemakers, implantable cardioverter–defibrillators (ICDs), and cardiac resynchronization therapy (CRT). Each of these sections comprises cases that are of increasing levels of difficulty. The questions are also structured to build upon the knowledge acquired from previous cases, so it is recommended to work through them in their given order. The names of device manufacturers are seldom indicated in the cases, as this information is usually irrelevant, and it is our wish to transmit principles that are applicable across device companies.

The aim of this book is to consolidate technical knowledge, sharpen skills of observation, and train logical reasoning to be able to tackle device troubleshooting. Most of all, we wish to stimulate the reader's interest in the field of cardiac pacing and give the sense of satisfaction that comes with understanding.

Haran Burri

Jean-Claude Deharo

Carsten Israel

Acknowledgements

The cases in this book are all from Dr Haran Burri's clinical practice, unless mentioned otherwise. We wish to thank the following colleagues who let us use their cases for this book:

Dr Michael Anelli-Monti
(Medical University of Graz, Graz, Austria):
Case 21

Mr Thomas Bruggemann
(Biotronik, Berlin, Germany):
Cases 7 and 17

Mr Henny Leersen
(St-Jude Medical, St Paul, MN, USA):
Case 29

Dr Andrea Menafoglio
(San Giovanni Hospital, Bellinzona, Switzerland):
Case 18

Dr Sergey Moiseenko
(Minsk, Belarus):
Case 33

Dr Cédric Vuille
(Nyon, Switzerland):
Cases 25 and 31

We also wish to thank Mrs Marta Roca (Medtronic) for proofreading the manuscript, and Mr Martin Dummann (Biotronik), Mrs Sofia Gago (Sorin), and Mr Ed Van der Veen (Boston Scientific) for their technical advice.

Contents

Symbols and abbreviations

=	equal to
≥	equal to or greater than
>	greater than
<	less than
%	per cent
+	plus
±	plus or minus
AF	atrial fibrillation
a.m.	*ante meridiem* (before noon)
AP	atrial pacing
AR	atrial refractory
AS	atrial sensed
ATP	antitachycardia pacing
AV	atrioventricular
AVI	atrioventricular interval
AVNRT	atrioventricular nodal re-entrant tachycardia
AVRT	atrioventricular re-entrant tachycardia
bpm	beat per minute
CRT	cardiac resynchronization therapy
CRT-D	cardiac resynchronization therapy defibrillator
CS	coronary sinus
ECG	electrocardiogram
EGM	electrogram
ER	evoked response
FFRW	far-field R-wave
Hz	hertz
ICD	implantable cardioverter–defibrillator
J	joule
LOC	loss of capture
LV	left ventricular
LVEF	left ventricular ejection fraction
min	minute
mm	millimetre
ms	millisecond
MTR	maximum tracking rate
mV	millivolt
NIPS	non-invasive pacing study
PAVB	post-atrial ventricular blanking
PVAB	post-ventricular atrial blanking
PVARP	post-ventricular atrial refractory period
PVC	premature ventricular contraction
RBBB	right bundle branch block
RNRVAS	repetitive non-re-entrant ventriculoatrial synchrony
RV	right ventricular/right ventricle
SVT	supraventricular tachycardia
TARP	total atrial refractory period
TOE	transoesophageal echocardiogram
UTR	upper tracking rate
V	volt
VA	ventriculoatrial
VF	ventricular fibrillation
VP	ventricular pacing
VPB	ventricular premature beat
VRP	ventricular refractory period
VS	ventricular sensed
VT	ventricular tachycardia

Introduction

A systematic approach to device electrocardiogram (ECG)/electrogram (EGM) tracings is proposed as a ten-step process, which will allow the reader to troubleshoot cases in a structured manner.

Systematic device ECG/EGM analysis

1. Which ECG leads/EGM channels (chamber, polarity) are displayed, and what is the scale?
2. What is the baseline rhythm?
3. Is there evidence of intrinsic atrial activity, sensing, pacing, and capture?
4. Is there evidence of intrinsic ventricular activity, sensing, pacing, and capture?
5. Are the intervals between the spikes and P/QRS complexes constant?
6. What is the morphology of the paced QRS complex?
7. Evaluation of timing and intervals (AA, VV, AV, VA, etc.).
8. What is the likely pacing mode?
9. Is there evidence of malfunction (undersensing, oversensing, non-pacing, non-capture)?
10. Is there evidence of pseudomalfunction (device algorithm, functional undersensing, etc.)?

Basics of pacemaker troubleshooting

Non-pacing (lack of a spike)

Pseudomalfunction: hysteresis, night rate, device algorithm
Oversensing
Battery/circuit problem
Lead connection problem

Non-capture (lack of entrainment of a P-wave or QRS)

Threshold rise: infarction, drugs (flecainide)
Lead problem (insulation defect, fracture, displacement, perforation)
Battery end of life
Programming error

Undersensing

Lead displacement
New bundle branch block, infarction
Premature beat with perpendicular electrogram vector
Programming error
'Physiological undersensing' during refractory period

Oversensing

Ventricular far-field/T-wave/P- or R-wave double-counting
Lead problem (fracture, connection problem)
Electromagnetic interference
Myopotentials (pectoral/diaphragmatic)

VVI timing cycles and refractory periods

Timing cycles of the VVI pacing mode are shown in the figure.

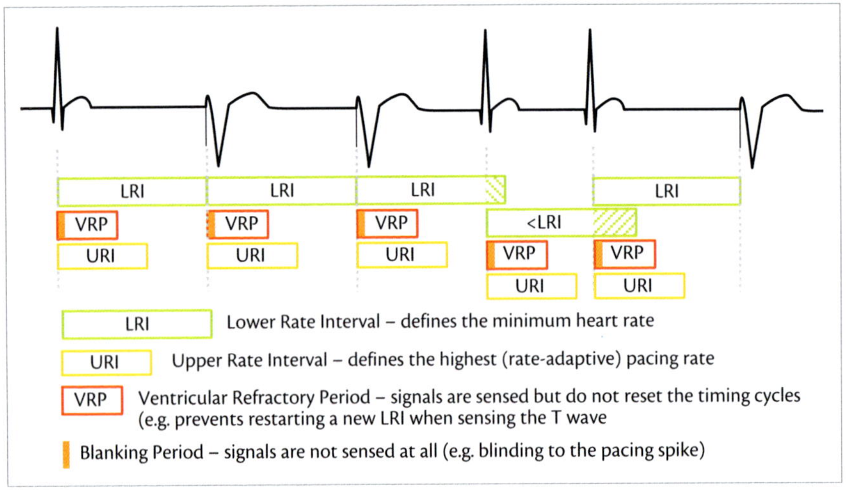

DDD timing cycles and refractory periods

Timing cycles of the DDD pacing mode are shown in the figure.

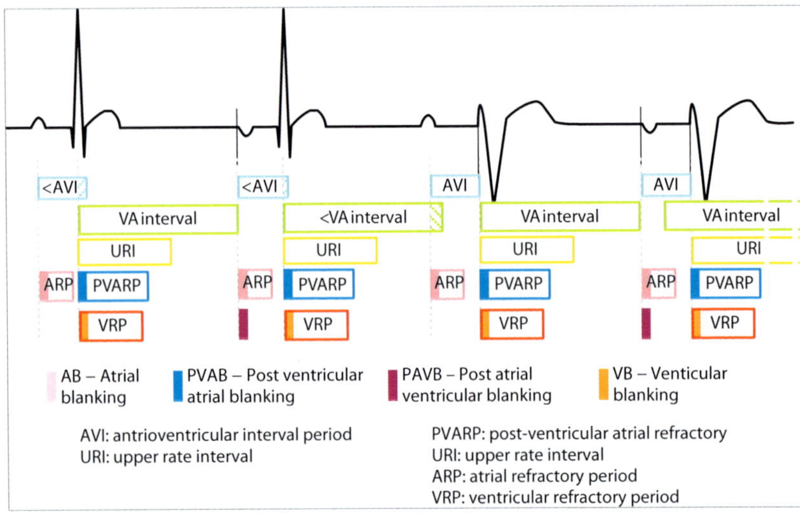

Summary of DDD timing cycles

A summary of the DDD pacing mode timing cycle triggers and their typical durations is shown in the table.

	AS	AP	VS	VP	Typical duration (ms)
A Blanking	✔	✔	✔	✔	50–200
A Refractory	✔	✔	✔	✔	120–150 (post-AP); 250–400 (post-VP)
V Blanking		✔	✔	✔	20–50 (post-AP); 150–250 (post-VP)
V Refractory			✔	✔	150–300

Definitions:

Blanking: signals are not at all detected, independent of their amplitude and the programming of sensitivity.

Refractory: signals are detected but will be ignored for pacing cycles (i.e. the next scheduled pace will not be reset) and only used for calculation of rate, detection of tachyarrhythmias, and mode switching.

Blanking and refractory periods may vary, according to:

- manufacturer
- model
- paced or sensed event
- programmed pacing polarity.

Main marker channel annotations of the different device manufacturers (the list is not exhaustive)

Boston Scientific

AS	Atrial Sense - After Refractory and AFR window
AS–Hy	Atrial Sense - In Hysteresis Offset
AS–Fl	Atrial Sense - In AFR window
(AS)	Atrial Sense - During TARP
AP	Atrial Pace - Lower Rate
AP↓	Atrial Pace - Rate Smoothing Down
AP↑	Atrial Pace - Rate Smoothing Up
AP–FB	Atrial Pace - Fallback (in ATR)
AP–Hy	Atrial Pace - At Hysteres is Rate
AP–Sr	Atrial Pace - Sensor Rate
AP→	Atrial Pace - Inserted after AFR
AP–Ns	Atrial Pace - Noise (asynchronous pacing)
AP–Tr	Atrial Pace - Trigger Mode
RVS	Right Vent Sense - After Refractory
[RVS]	Right Vent Sense - During Blanking
RVP	Right Vent Pace - Lower Rate or Atrial Tracked
RVP↓	Right Vent Pace - Rate Smoothing Down
RVP↑	Right Vent Pace - Rate Smoothing Up
RVP–FB	Right Vent Pace - Fallback (in ATR)
RVP–Hy	Right Vent Pace - At Hysteresis Rate
RVP–Sr	Right Vent Pace - Sensor Rate
RVP–MT	Right Vent Pace - Atrial Tracked at MTR
RVP–Ns	Right Vent Pace - Atrial Tracked at MTR
RVP–Tr	Right Vent Pace - Trigger Mode
RVP–VRR	Right Vent Pace - Ventricular Rate Regulation
LVS	Left Vent Sense - After Refractory
[LVS]	Left Vent Sense - During Blanking
LVP	Left Vent Pace - Lower Rate or Atrial Tracked
LVP↓	Left Vent Pace - Rate Smoothing Down
LVP↑	Left Vent Pace - Rate Smoothing Up
LVP–Hy	Left Vent Pace - At Hysteresis Rate
LVP–Sr	Left Vent Pace - Sensor Rate
LVP–MT	Left Vent Pace - Atrial Tracked at MTR
LVP–Ns	Left Vent Pace - Noice (asynchronous pacing)
LVP–Tr	Left Vent Pace - Trigger Mode
LVP–VRR	Left Vent Pace - Ventricular Rate Regulation
Inh–LVP	Left Vent Pace - Inhibited Due to LVPP
PVC	PVC after Refractory

VT–1	VT–1 Zone Sense
VT	VT Zone Sense
VF	VF Zone Sense
AN	Atrial Rate Noise
RVN	Right Ventricular Rate Noise
LVN	Left Ventricular Rate Noise
ATR↓	Atrial Tachycardia Sense - Count Down
ATR↑	Atrial Tachycardia Sense - Count Up
ATR–Dur	ATR Duration Started
ATR–FB	ATR Fallback Started
ATR–End	ATR Fallback Ended
FB	ATR in Progress
RID–TU	Rhythm ID Template Update
RID+	Rhythm ID Correlated
RID–	Rhythm ID Uncorrelated
C––	RhythmMatch™ Correlated without percentage
U––	RhythmMatch™ Uncorrelated without percentage
PVP→	PVARP after PVC
PMT–B	PMT Termination
AF–Rhythm	AFib Rhythm
V–Epsd	Ventricular Tachy Start Episode
V–EpsdEnd	Ventricular Tachy End Episode
V>A	Ventricular Rate Faster than Atrial Rate
AFibV	V AFib Criteria Met
V–Dur	Duration Met
Stb	Stable
Unstb	Unstable
Suddn	Sudden Onset
Gradl	Gradual Onset
V–Detect	Ventricular Detection Met
Chrg	Start/End Charge
Dvrt	Therapy Diverted
Shock	Shock Delivered
SRD	Sustained Rate Duration Expired

Biotronik

As/Ap	Atrial sensing/pacing
Vs/Vp	Ventricular sensing/pacing
LVp/LVs	Left ventricular pacing/sensing
RVp/RVs	Right ventricular pacing/sensing
Ars	Atrial refractory sensing
Ars (FFP)	Ars in far-field protection window
Vrs	Ventricular refractory sensing
Aflut	Atrial flutter detected
Afib	Atrial fibrillation detected
Msw.DDI	Modeswitch to DDI
Det. VF	VF detected
Rdt.	Redetection criteria are fulfilled
1:1	1:1 A:V ratio
———	Charging of the capacitors
Term.	Tachycardia episode has terminated
Psh. VVI	Post shock pacing mode is VVI

Medtronic

AS/AP	Atrial sensing/pacing
AR	Atrial refractory sense
Ab	Atrial event in blanking period
VS/VP	Ventricular sensing pacing
BV	Biventricular pace
VR	Ventricular refractory sense
TS	Sense in (slow) VT zone
T•F	Sense in fast VT zone via VT
TF•	Sense in fast VT zone via VF
FS	Sense in VF zone
TDI	VT detected
TFI	FVT detected
FDI	VF dected
TP	Tachy pace (ATP)
CE	Charge end
CD	Charge delivered

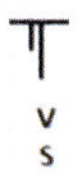

Ventricular safety pacing

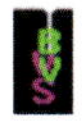
Triggered biventricular pacing

Sorin

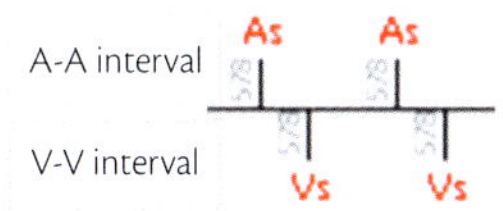

Ap/A	Atrial pacing
As/P	Atrial sensing
Ar	Atrial refractory sensing
Vs/R	Ventricular sensing
Vp	Ventricular pacing
Vr	Ventricular refractory sensing
bV	Biventricular pacing

St-Jude Medical

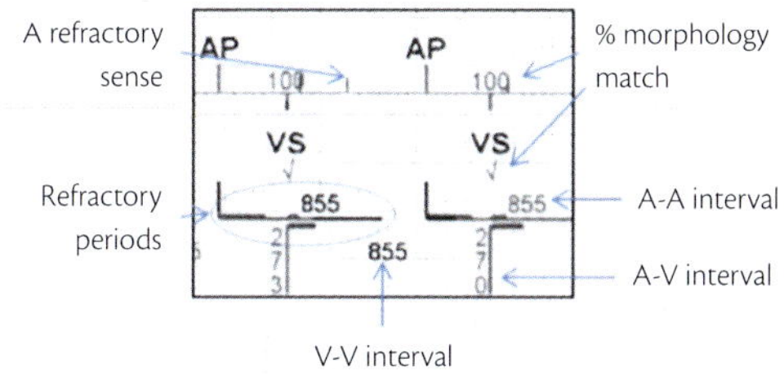

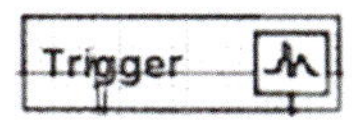

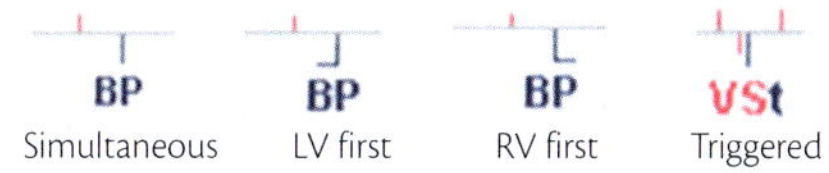

AMS	Modeswitch
LOC	Loss of capture
VPP	Ventricular backup pacing
–	Interval that is not binned
VS	Binning of interval in Sinus zone
T1	Binning of interval in VT1 zone
T2	Binning of interval in VT2 zone
F	Binning of VF interval
F̲	Reconfirmation of VF

FURTHER INFORMATION

Section 1

PACEMAKERS

Cases 1–35

Introduction to the case

A patient with paroxysmal complete atrioventricular (AV) block was implanted with a dual-chamber pacemaker. At follow-up, the real-time electrogram (EGM) strip, shown in Figure 1.1, was recorded.

Question

Figure 1.1 Real-time EGM recording

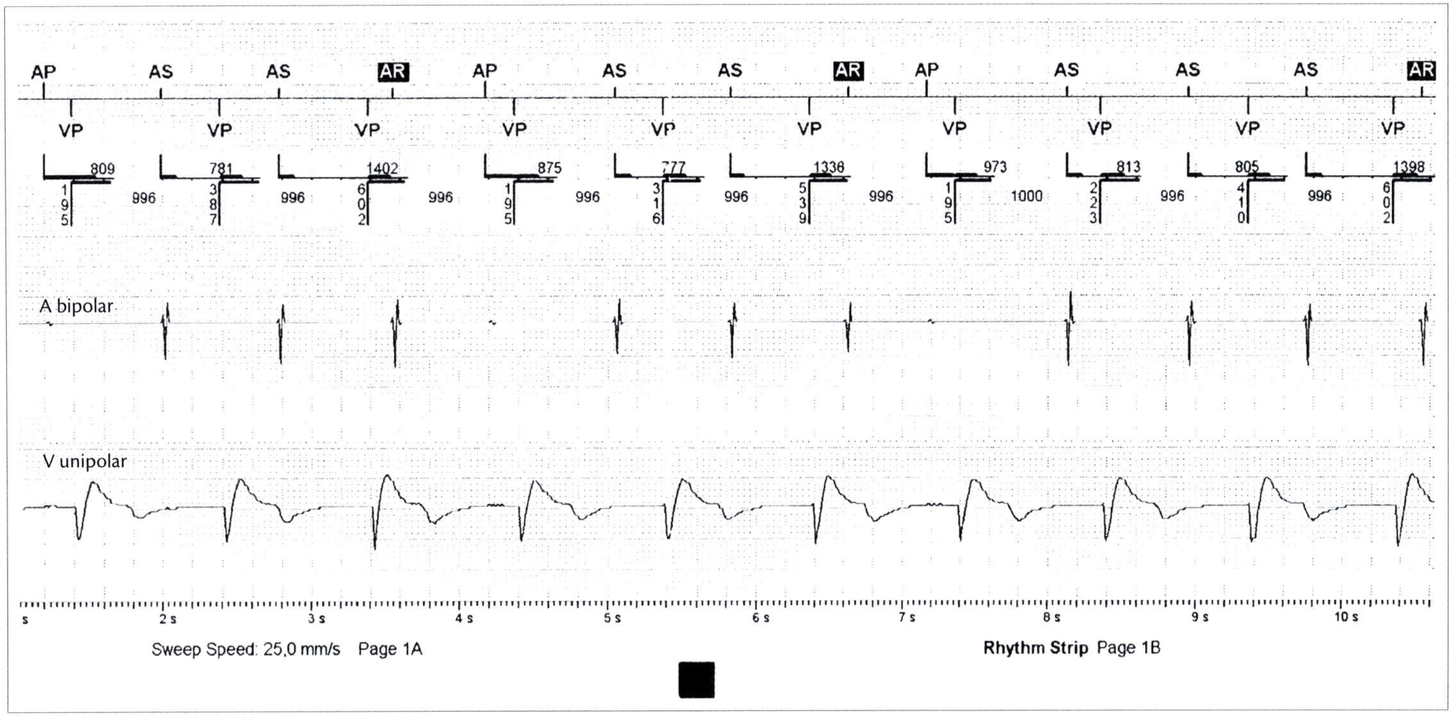

In what pacing mode is the device programmed?

A VDI

B DDI

C VDD

D DDD

Answer

B DDI

Figure 1.2 Annotated real-time EGM recording

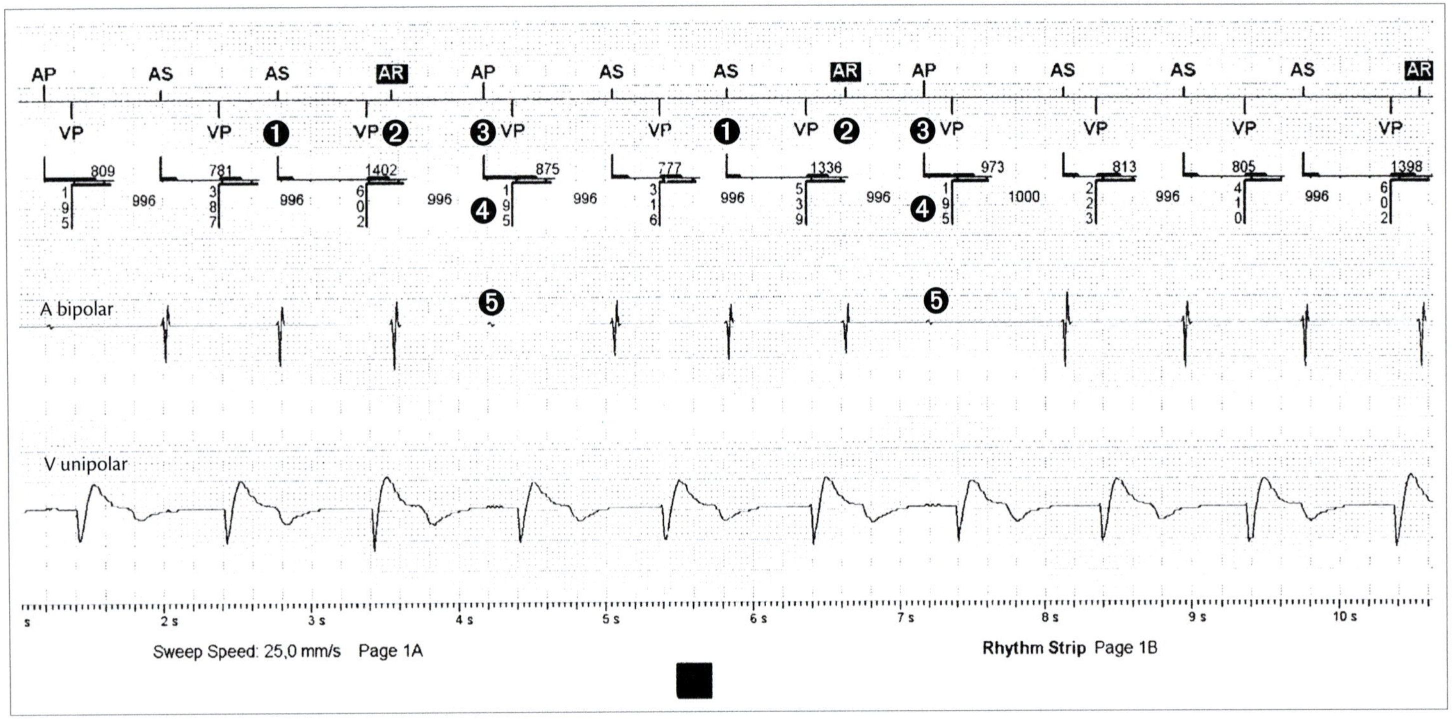

The baseline rhythm is sinus with complete AV block (Figure 1.2). Atrial pacing (AP) is occurring, so the VDI and VDD modes can be excluded. The device was programmed in the DDI mode with a baseline rate of 60bpm.

❶ There is loss of AV synchrony with atrial sensed events (AS) at a constant ventricular pacing (VP) rate of 60bpm (the VP–VP intervals are labelled at 996–1000ms, due to cycles of the device clock). This excludes DDD and VDD pacing modes, which track sensed atrial activity.

❷ In the DDI mode, a ventriculoatrial (VA) interval is triggered after a VP or ventricular sensed (VS) event. Atrial refractory sensed events (AR) that fall within the post-ventricular atrial refractory period (PVARP) do not inhibit AP.

❸ AP occurs at the end of the VA interval (800ms in this example, which corresponds to the programmed lower ventricular rate interval of 1000ms–the paced AV interval (AVI) of 200ms).

❹ AV synchrony is maintained after AP events (the paced AVI was programmed at 200ms but is labelled here as 195ms, due to the device clock cycles).

❺ The EGM amplitude of AP events is low, due to the autogain function.

Comments

The DDI(R) pacing mode

This patient had paroxysmal AV block, with long AS–VS intervals detected by the device during 1:1 AV conduction. This was, in part, due to first-degree AV block and partly due to right bundle branch block (RBBB) (resulting in late sensing of the ventricular EGM by the right ventricular (RV) lead). In order to avoid having to programme very long AV delays in the DDD mode, to avoid unnecessary RV pacing*, the device was programmed in the DDI mode.

This non-tracking mode, shown in Figure 1.2, is most often used with automatic mode switch during atrial tachyarrhythmias, in order to avoid rapid ventricular pacing. It may also be used in patients with paroxysmal AV block, but AV synchrony will be lost in case of AV block with AS events (as in this example). AV synchrony is, however, maintained in the case of AP such as in patients with sinus dysfunction. The DDI(R) pacing mode with a long paced AV delay (there is no programmed sensed AV delay) may be considered, if the device does not have specialized algorithms to avoid ventricular pacing.

* This may be ineffective in reducing ventricular pacing, may favour endless-loop tachycardia, and may result in pacing on the T-wave in case of ventricular premature beats (VPBs) falling in the post-atrial ventricular blanking (PAVB)—see future cases in this book.

Introduction to the case

An 82-year-old woman had been implanted with a single-chamber ventricular pacemaker 6 years ago for atrial fibrillation (AF) with symptomatic bradycardia. She presented to the hospital with shortness of breath and twitching of the left pectoral region. Her pacemaker follow-up, performed 6 months ago, had been completely normal. The results of the device follow-up performed at that time are shown in Table 2.1, and the electrocardiogram (ECG) recorded at admission is shown in Figure 2.1.

Table 2.1 Device settings and tested parameters

Programming	
Mode	VVIR
Rate	60–110bpm
Pacing output (bipolar)	2.5V/0.4ms
Sensitivity setting (bipolar)	2.8mV
Tests	
Battery voltage	2.71V
Battery impedance	1200 ohms
Lead impedance (bipolar)	625 ohms
Capture threshold (bipolar)	1.2V/0.4ms
Sensing threshold (bipolar)	6.8mV

Question

Figure 2.1 ECG recorded at admission

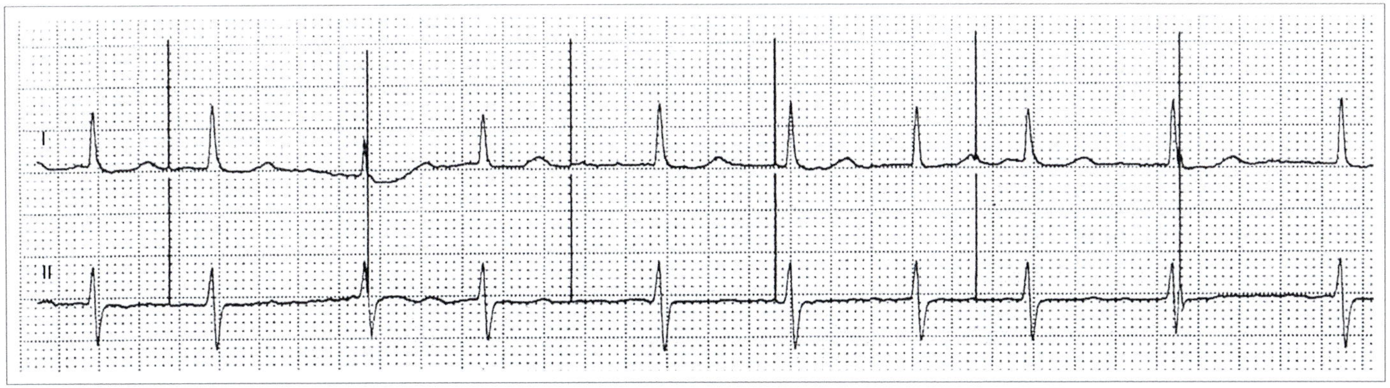

What do you observe?

A Ventricular undersensing

B Ventricular oversensing

C Ventricular non-pacing

D Both A and C are correct

Answer

A **Ventricular undersensing**

Figure 2.2 Annotated ECG recorded at admission

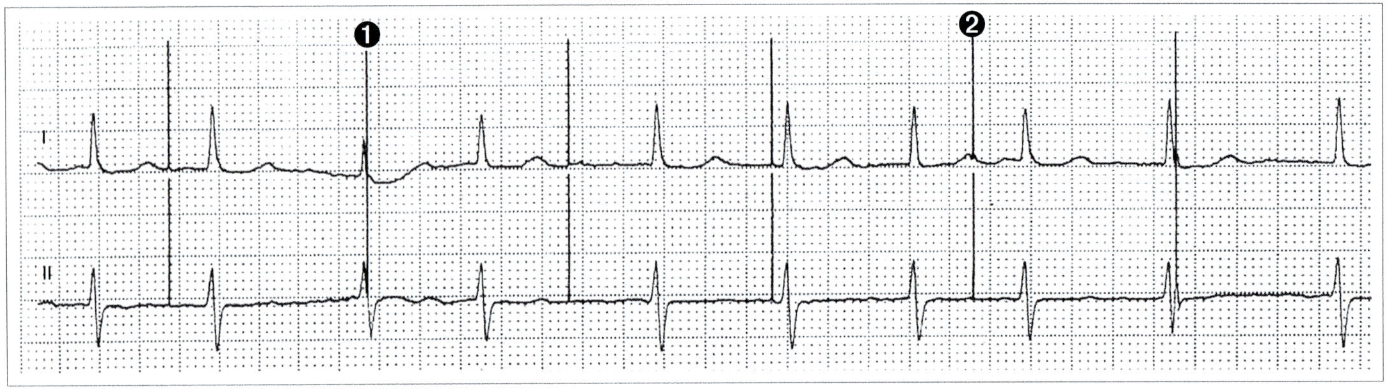

The pacing spikes in Figure 2.2 occur at exactly 60bpm (the baseline rate), with all spikes showing ventricular undersensing and non-capture. This should not be confused with non-pacing, which refers to the lack of delivery of a pacing spike where one is expected.

❶ This beat could be interpreted as normal device function with pseudofusion, as the spike occurs almost simultaneously with the QRS complex. With pseudofusion, the pacing spike occurs at, or shortly after, QRS onset, but before the depolarization wavefront has reached the lead dipole. The pacing spike occurs during the myocardial refractory period and therefore does not capture the ventricle.

❷ The ventricular spike occurs on the T-wave which may be potentially pro-arrhythmic, but this is not the case here, as there is no capture.

Comments

Subclavian crush

A chest X-ray showed complete lead section due to subclavian crush (Figure 2.3A). A chest X-ray had been performed shortly before the previous device follow-up by the patient's general practitioner for cough and already showed signs of lead damage (Figure 2.3B).

This case illustrates how normal parameters (including impedance) do not rule out damage to a lead. This is of particular relevance in pacemaker-dependent patients who may be experiencing symptoms compatible with device dysfunction and in whom a chest X-ray and Holter recording should be performed if device interrogation does not elucidate the problem.

Subclavian crush may result from medial subclavian puncture and may be avoided by favouring axillary vein puncture or cephalic vein cutdown for lead implantation.

Figure 2.3 Chest X-rays showing complete lead section due to subclavian crush (a) and evidence of lead damage 7 months ago, when device parameters were normal (b).

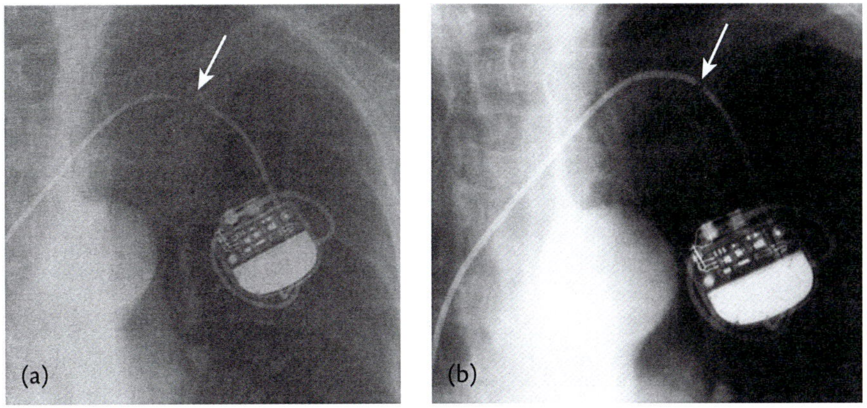

Introduction to the case

An 82-year-old patient with ischaemic heart disease and mildly reduced left ventricular ejection fraction (LVEF) was implanted, 1 month ago, with a St-Jude Medical single-chamber pacemaker for AF and symptomatic bradycardia.

The pacemaker was programmed to VVIR 60–110bpm.

The presenting EGM at follow-up is shown in Figure 3.1.

Question

Figure 3.1 Real-time EGM recorded at 1-month follow-up

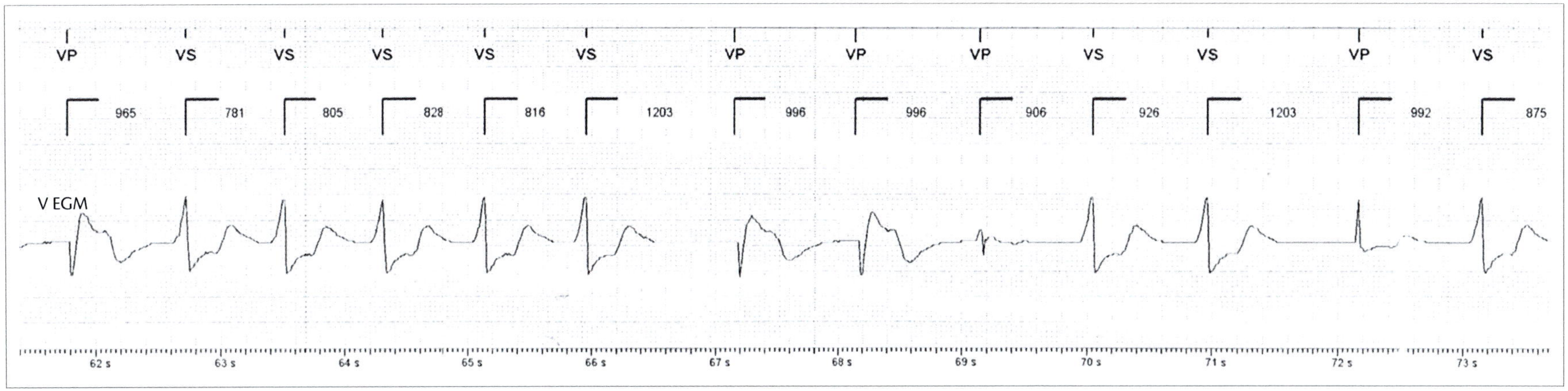

How do you explain pacing below the baseline rate?

A Ventricular oversensing

B Rate hysteresis

C Programming error

D Loss of capture

Answer

B **Rate hysteresis**

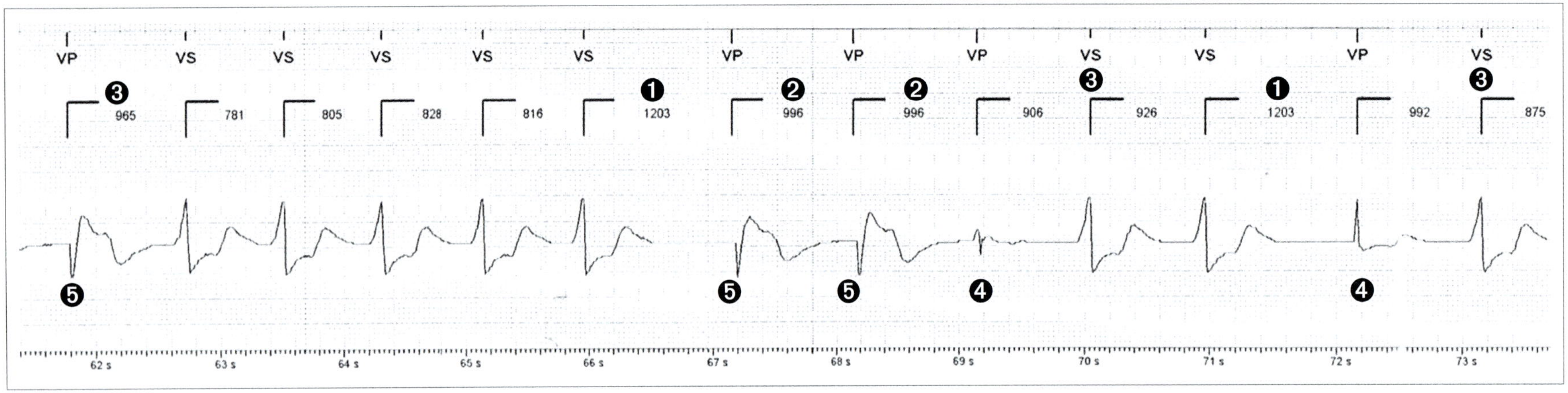

Figure 3.2 Annotated real-time EGM recorded at 1-month follow-up

The device was programmed at a baseline rate of 60bpm and with a hysteresis of 50bpm (Figure 3.2).

❶ The VS–VP interval is 1203ms, corresponding to the rate of hysteresis (the interval should be theoretically 1200ms but is slightly different, due to processing by the internal clock).

❷ The VP–VP interval is 996ms (should theoretically be 1000ms; see (1)), corresponding to the baseline rate (the patient is at rest, so the rate is not sensor-driven).

❸ As soon as there is a VS event, the hysteresis rate is reactivated.

❹ These two beats with different EGM morphologies correspond to varying degrees of fusion between ventricular capture and intrinsic conduction. Pseudofusion would have resulted in the same morphology as the intrinsic ventricular EGM.

❺ These three beats correspond to full ventricular capture.

Comments

Rate hysteresis

Hysteresis is useful to avoid unnecessary pacing and is available for single-chamber, as well as dual-chamber devices. In this case, it was used to minimize ventricular pacing at rest, in order to avoid an adverse effect on cardiac pump function.

With hysteresis, the intrinsic heart rate is allowed to fall below the baseline rate, as long as it is above the hysteresis rate. As soon as the hysteresis rate is reached, the device paces at the baseline rate, until a ventricular event is sensed (i.e. that occurs faster than the baseline rate) (Figure 3.3).

Some devices allow programming additional hysteresis parameters, e.g. the number of cycles at which pacing occurs at the hysteresis rate before switching to the baseline rate.

Figure 3.3 Rate hysteresis

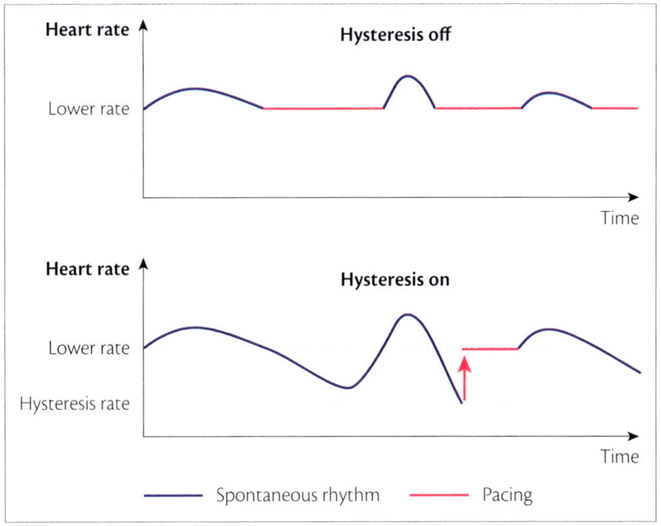

Introduction to the case

A 76-year-old man with symptomatic sinus node dysfunction and no other cardiovascular history, was implanted with a single-chamber pacemaker. At the 1-month follow-up visit, he complained of worsening dyspnoea, fatigue, and orthostatic dizziness. Device interrogation showed normal parameters. The presenting ECG is shown in Figure 4.1.

Question

Figure 4.1 Presenting ECG at 1-month follow-up

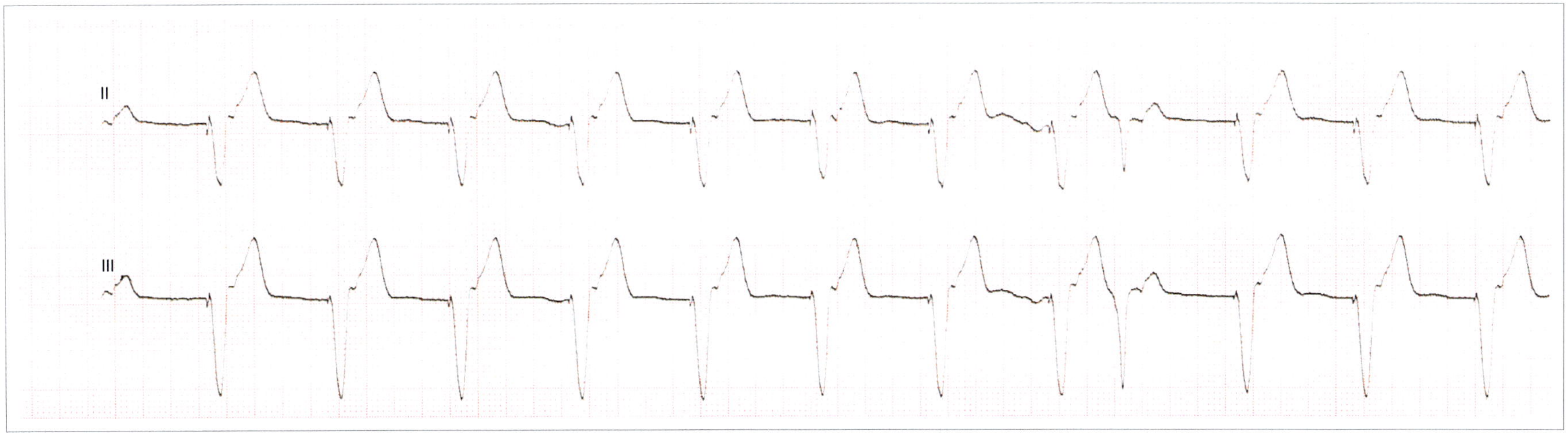

What is the cause of the patient's symptoms?

A Pacemaker syndrome

B Inadequate rate response

C AF

D Ventricular systolic dysfunction

Answer

A **Pacemaker syndrome**

Figure 4.2 Annotated presenting ECG at 1-month follow-up

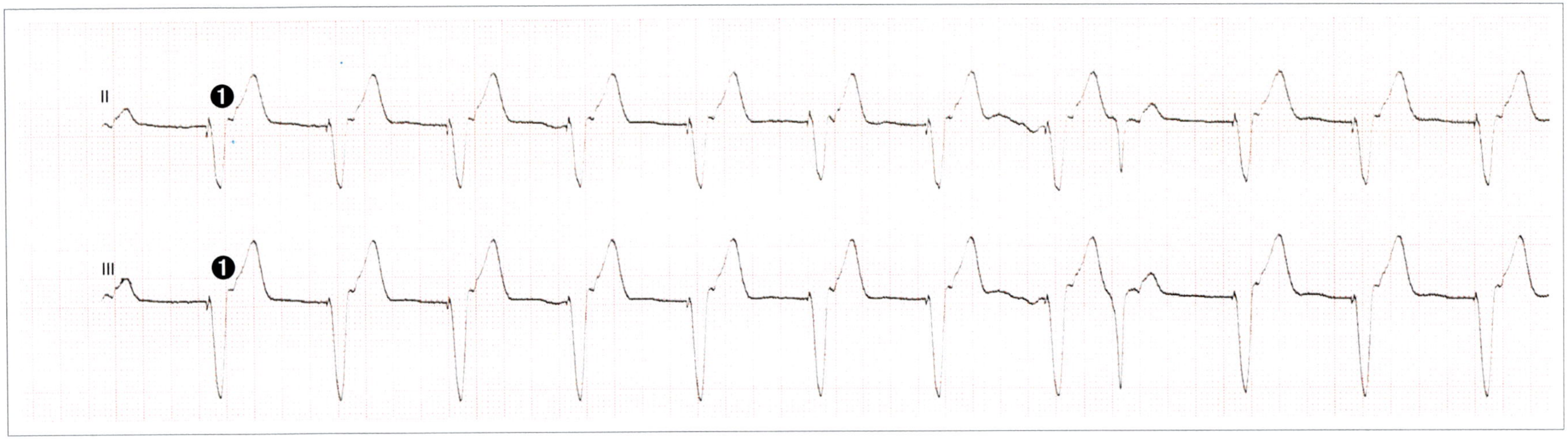

This patient is in sinus rhythm, with VP and 1:1 retrograde VA conduction (Figure 4.2).

❶ Retrograde P-waves can be visualized after each paced QRS complex.

Comments

Pacemaker syndrome

Although there is no universal definition for pacemaker syndrome, it manifests itself by a variety of symptoms (fatigue, dyspnoea, dizziness, orthopnoea, fullness in the neck, etc.). It is believed to be due to AV dyssynchrony in patients with a VVI(R) device in sinus rhythm, with or without retrograde conduction.[1] It may be encountered in up to 26% of these patients[1–3] and usually occurs during the first months following implantation.[1,3] Changing to dual-chamber pacing significantly improves symptoms in these patients.[3] In this example the ventricular lead was repositioned in the atrium to provide AAIR pacing, after having tested for normal AV conduction. DDDR pacing is the first choice in case of sick sinus syndrome[4] and is preferable to AAIR pacing.[5] However, AAIR pacing is still an option[4] and, in this case, was chosen, in order to be able to use the same generator.

References

1. Link MS, Hellkamp AS, Estes NAM 3rd, *et al.* High incidence of pacemaker syndrome in patients with sinus node dysfunction treated with ventricular-based pacing in the Mode Selection Trial (MOST). *J Am Coll Cardiol* 2004; **43**: 2066–71.
2. Lamas GA, Lee KL, Sweeney MO, *et al.* Ventricular pacing or dual-chamber pacing for sinus-node dysfunction. *N Engl J Med* 2002; **346**: 1854–62.
3. Lamas GA, Orav EJ, Stambler BS, *et al.* Quality of life and clinical outcomes in elderly patients treated with ventricular pacing as compared with dual-chamber pacing. Pacemaker Selection in the Elderly Investigators. *N Engl J Med* 1998; **338**: 1097–104.
4. Brignole M, Auricchio A, Baron-Esquivias G, *et al.* 2013 ESC guidelines on cardiac pacing and cardiac resynchronization therapy: the task force on cardiac pacing and resynchronization therapy of the European Society of Cardiology (ESC). Developed in collaboration with the European Heart Rhythm Association (EHRA). *Europace* 2013; **15**: 1070–118.
5. Nielsen JC, Thomsen PE, Højberg S, *et al.* A comparison of single-lead atrial pacing with dual-chamber pacing in sick sinus syndrome. *Eur Heart J* 2011; **32**: 686–96.

Introduction to the case

A 72-year-old patient was admitted for stroke. He had been implanted with a dual-chamber pacemaker 2 months ago for sinus dysfunction. Interrogation of the pacemaker was normal and did not disclose any atrial arrhythmias that may have explained the neurological event. A chest X-ray was performed and is shown in Figure 5.1.

Question

Figure 5.1 Postero-anterior (a) and lateral (b) chest X-rays

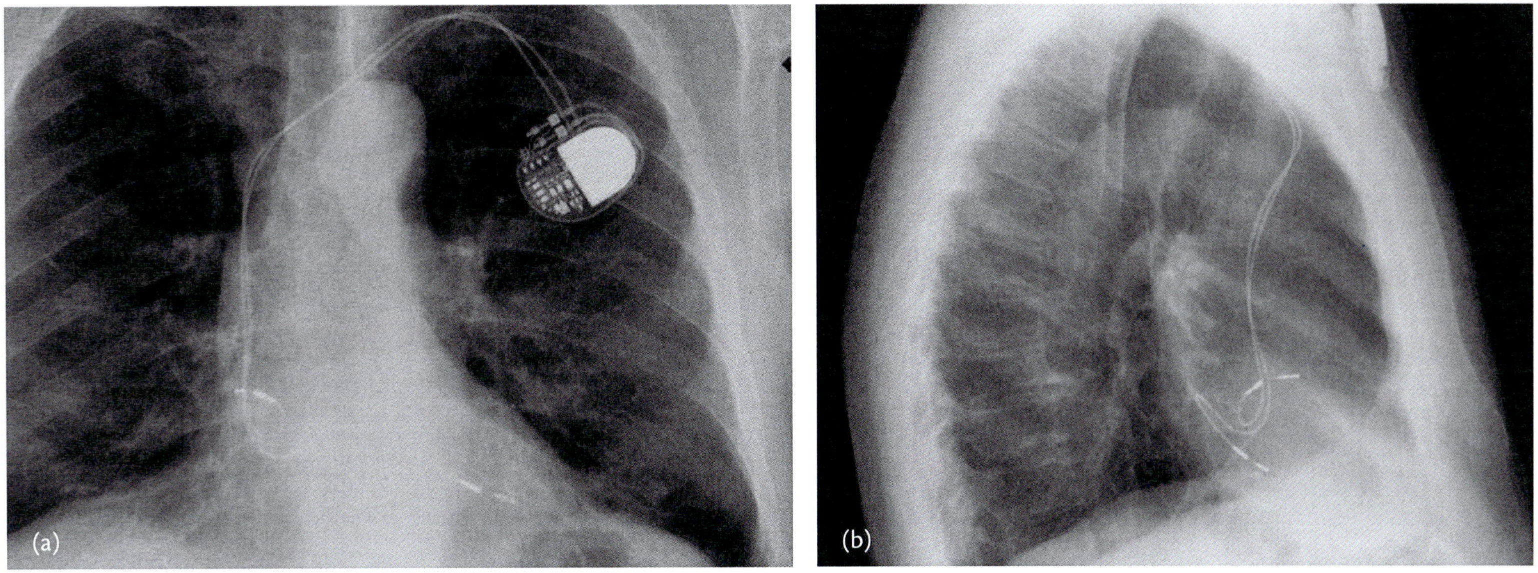

Where is the ventricular lead positioned?

A RV apex

B Coronary sinus (CS) tributary

C Right ventricle (RV) with situs inversus

D Left ventricle via a patent foramen ovale

Answer

D **Left ventricle via a patent foramen ovale**

Figure 5.2 Annotated postero-anterior (a) and lateral (b) chest X-rays (c) transthoracic echocardiogram

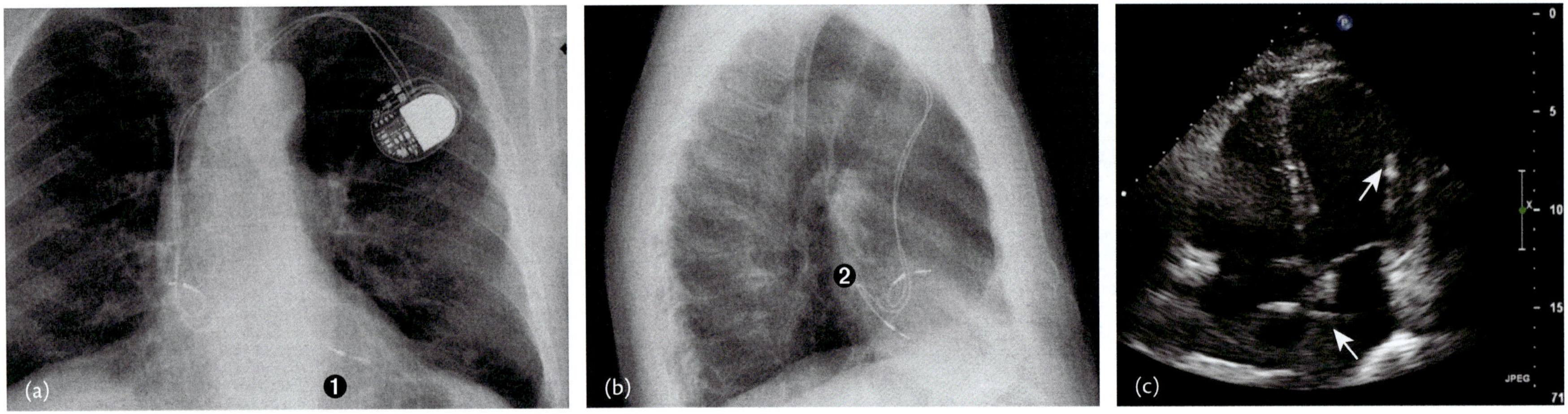

An echocardiogram confirmed that the lead was positioned via a patent foramen ovale in the left ventricle (Figure 5.2 c, arrows).

❶ An apical RV lead would be expected to be situated in a lower position than this.

❷ The lateral chest X-ray shows the ventricular lead to be posterior, whereas an RV lead would be anteriorly located (Figure 5.3) in a patient implanted with an apical RV lead. An endocardial left ventricular (LV) lead does not course at the border of the cardiac silhouette, contrary to a CS lead which is epicardial (Figure 5.3).

Comments

Recognizing ventricular lead position

This case illustrates the utility of performing multiple fluoroscopic views at implantation to rule out malposition of pacing leads. The patient was anticoagulated, and, because the lead had been very recently implanted, it was repositioned in the RV after a transoesophageal echocardiogram ruled out residual thrombi.

LV capture results in a negative QRS in lead I (which may be observed occasionally also with RV pacing)[1] and an RBBB QRS morphology. The differential diagnosis of an RBBB pattern of a paced QRS complex is:

1 LV endocardial pacing via a patent foramen ovale, an atrial/ventricular septal defect, or an arterial puncture
2 LV epicardial pacing via a CS tributary
3 ventricular perforation
4 ventricular fusion/pseudofusion in a patient with pre-existing RBBB and intrinsic AV conduction
5 'pseudo-RBBB' pattern due to misplacement of V1 and V2 electrodes above the 4th intercostal space. This is probably the commonest cause of an RBBB-like pattern of the paced QRS complex.

Figure 5.3 Lateral chest X-ray of a patient with an apical RV lead and a CS lead (a). Morphologies of paced QRS complexes at different sites are shown in (b)

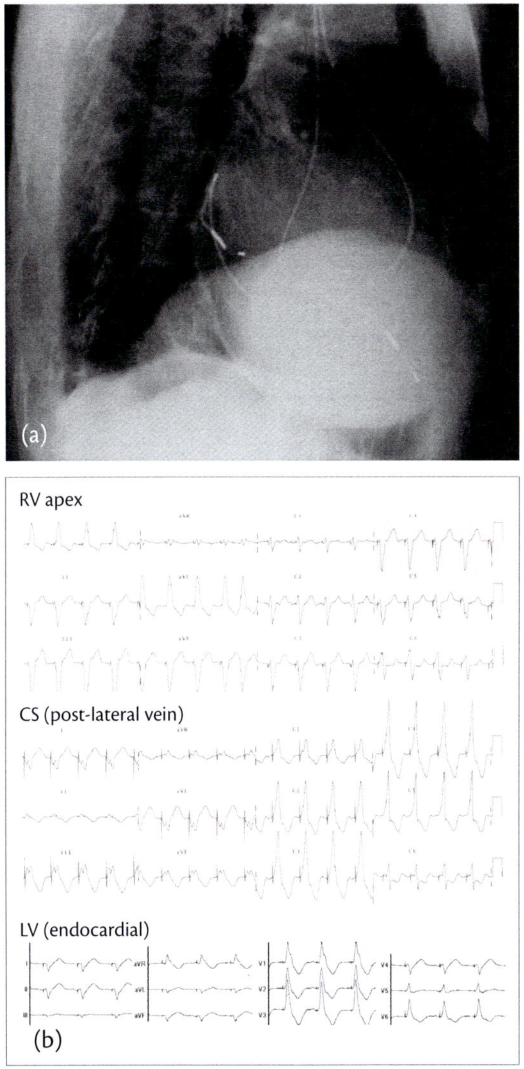

Reference

1. Burri H, Park C, Zimmermann M, *et al.* Utility of the surface electrocardiogram for confirming right ventricular septal pacing: validation using electroanatomical mapping. *Europace* 2011; **13**: 82–6.

Introduction to the case

An atrial threshold test was performed in a patient with sinus node dysfunction and normal AV conduction. The test was performed by pacing in the AAI mode and decrementing the atrial voltage amplitude at a pulse duration of 0.4ms.

The real-time EGM tracing recorded during the threshold test is shown in Figure 6.1.

Question

Figure 6.1 Real-time EGM recorded during the atrial threshold test

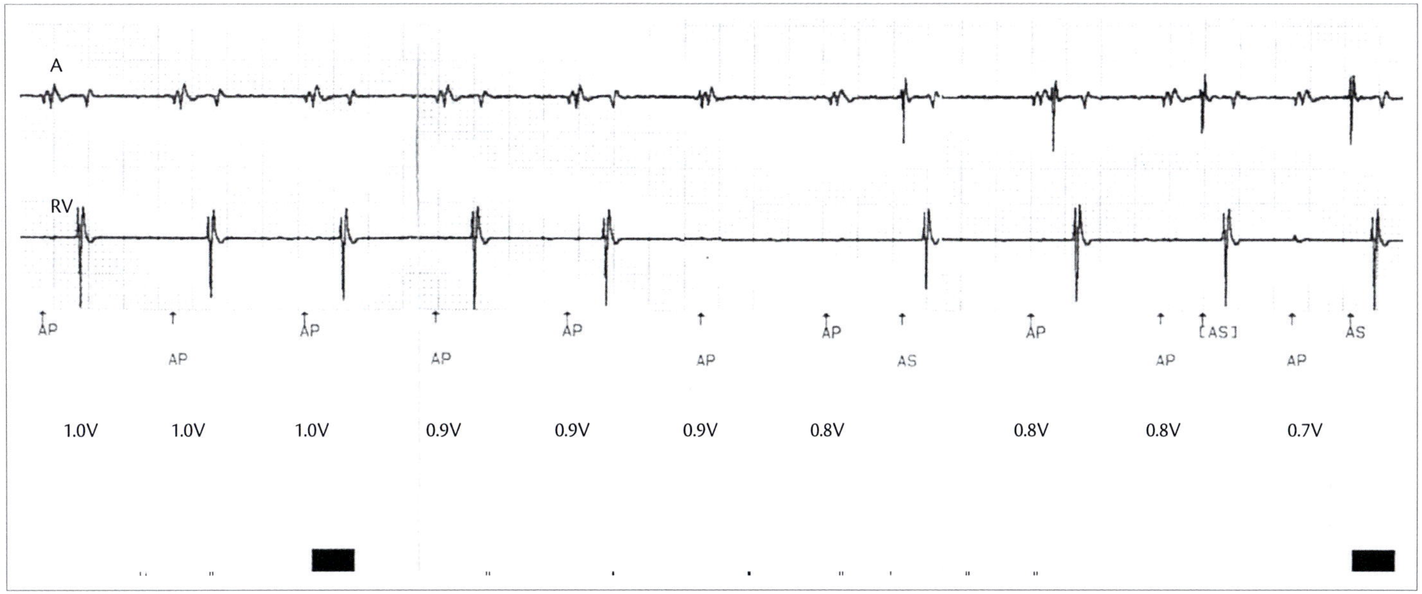

What is the atrial capture threshold amplitude?

A 1.0V

B 0.9V

C 0.8V

D 0.7V

Answer

A **1.0V**

Figure 6.2 Annotated real-time EGM recorded during the atrial threshold test

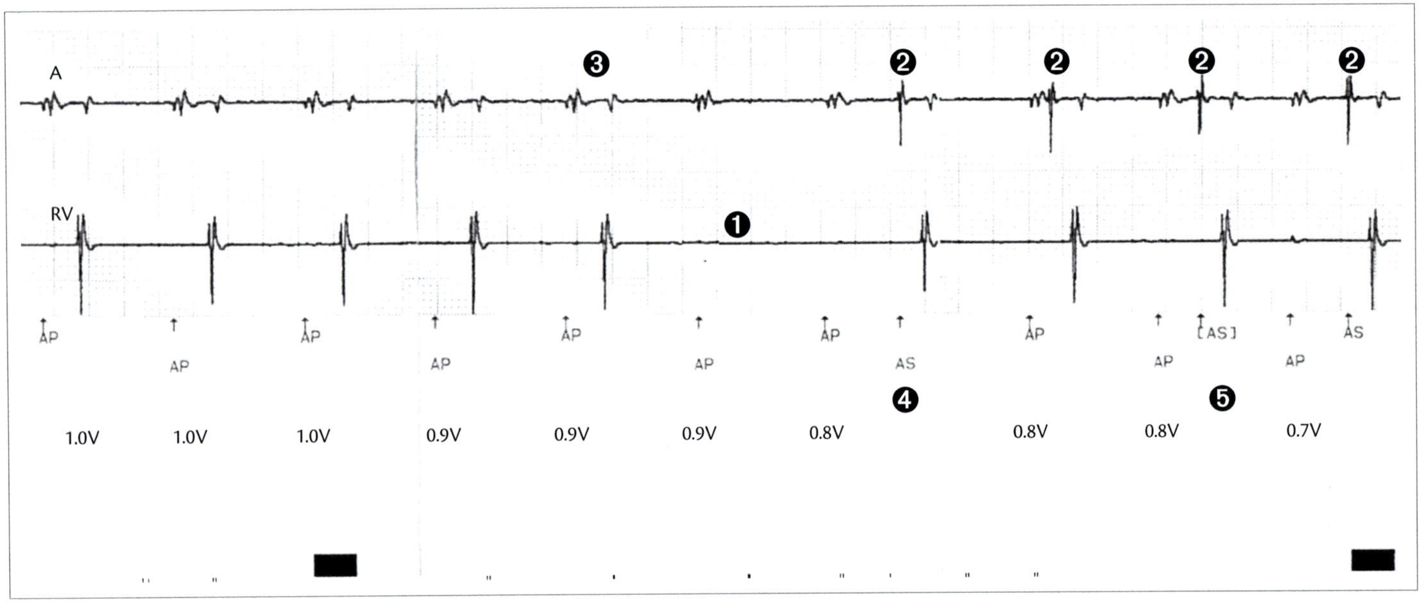

Capture threshold refers to the output which results in *consistent* capture (Figure 6.2).

❶ The absence of a conducted R-wave suggests the loss of atrial capture for the 3rd paced beat at 0.9V (the previous beats show consistent AV conduction).

❷ Sinus rhythm resumes after loss of atrial capture.

❸ Note that, in this case, the local atrial EGMs, with and without capture, look similar (apart from the presence or absence of the far-field R-wave (FFRW)).

❹ The AS event resets the A–A timing cycle.

❺ The AS event falls in the refractory period (depicted by [AS]) and therefore does not reset the A–A timing cycle.

Comments

Atrial capture threshold testing

Techniques for performing atrial threshold testing are:

1 evaluation of the surface ECG P-wave (which is, however, not always well visualized)
2 testing in the AAI or AOO mode in case of 1:1 AV conduction, as in this example
3 evaluation of the atrial EGM for a change in near-field morphology (depicted by * in Figure 6.3). However, this may not always be reliable (compare with Figures 6.2 and 6.4).
4 in case of 1:1 retrograde VA conduction, atrial threshold testing with DDD pacing will yield a retrograde P-wave after loss of atrial capture (Figure 6.4).
5 Pace slightly faster than the sinus rate, and look for intrinsic atrial rhythm at loss of atrial capture (such as in the present case example). This will, however, give a slightly inaccurate result if the sinus node recovery time is long.

Figure 6.3 Change in atrial EGM morphology with loss of capture

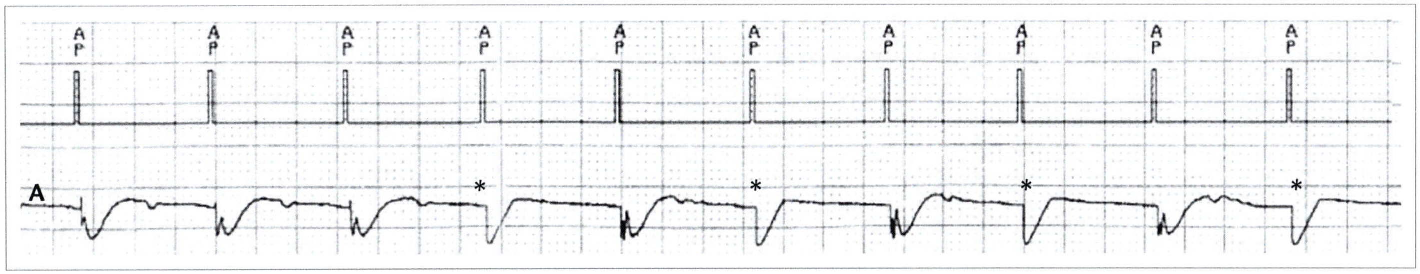

Figure 6.4 Atrial threshold test performed with DDD pacing, showing 1:1 retrograde VA conduction (*) at loss of atrial capture (LOC). Note that, in this case, the atrial EGM looks identical, with or without atrial capture (circles)

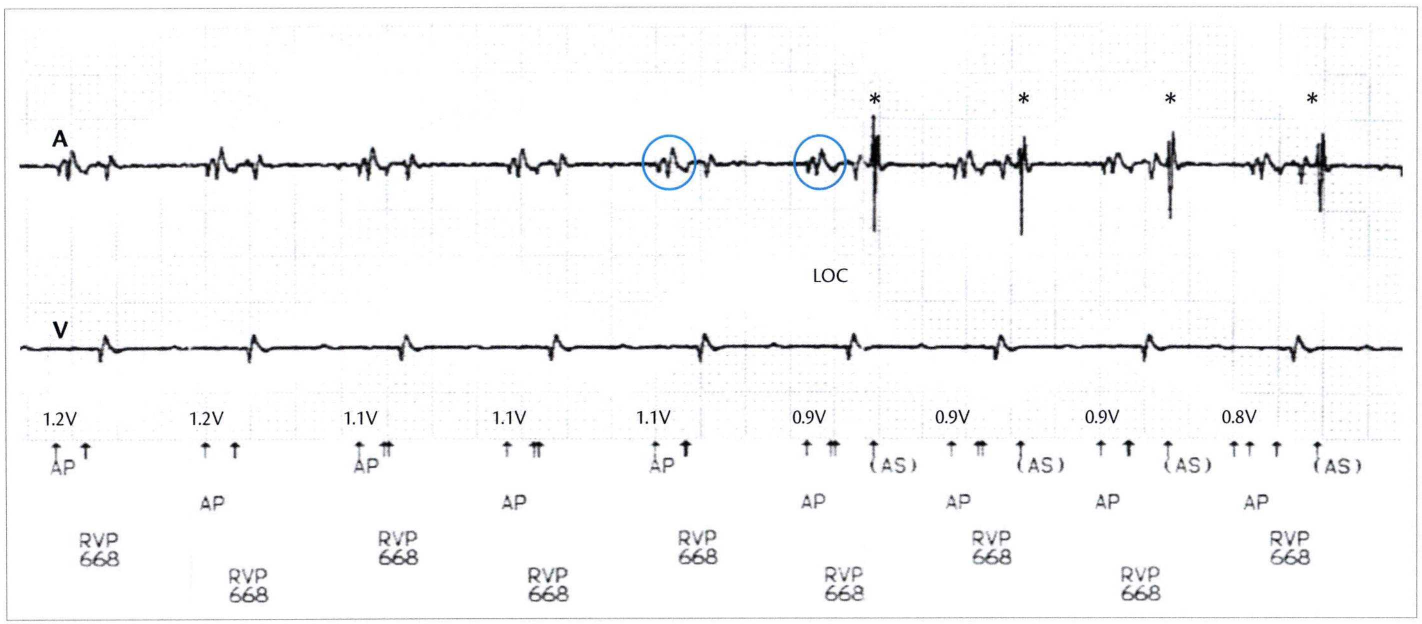

Introduction to the case

A 56-year-old patient was implanted with a dual-chamber pacemaker for complete heart block. He complained of dyspnoea upon exertion. Device settings are listed in Table 7.1. Device interrogation during a bicycle exercise test is shown in Figure 7.1.

Table 7.1 Device settings

Pacing mode	DDD
Baseline rate	60bpm
Upper tracking rate (UTR)	120bpm
Paced AV delay (adaptive)	170-120ms
AV delay sense offset	–30ms
PVARP	250ms

Question

Figure 7.1 Real-time EGM recorded during a bicycle exercise test

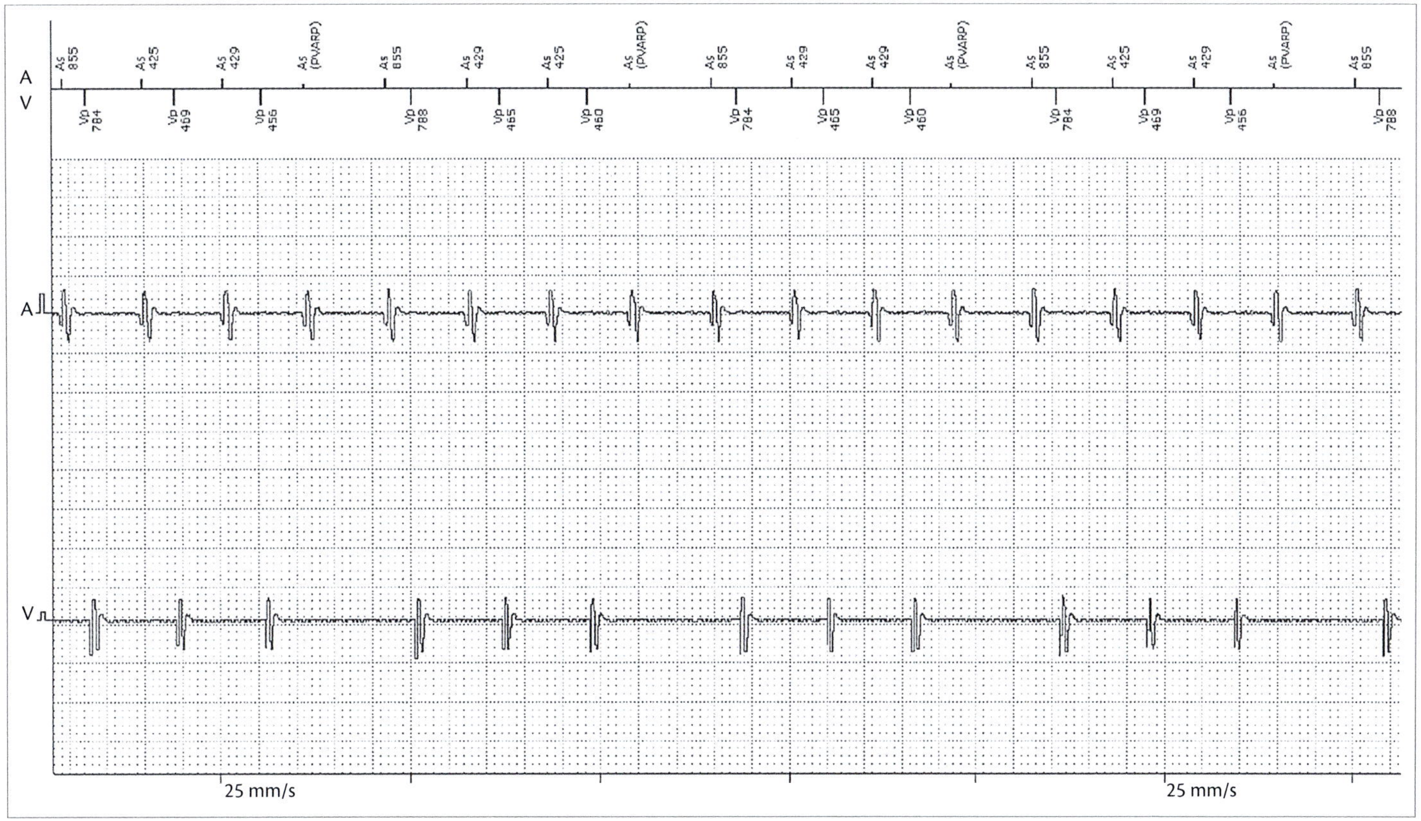

Courtesy of Mr T Bruggemann

What can be observed?

A Wenckebach behaviour

B Atrial undersensing

C Mode switch

D Ventricular non-capture

Answer

A Wenckebach behaviour

Figure 7.2 Annotated real-time EGM recorded during a bicycle exercise test

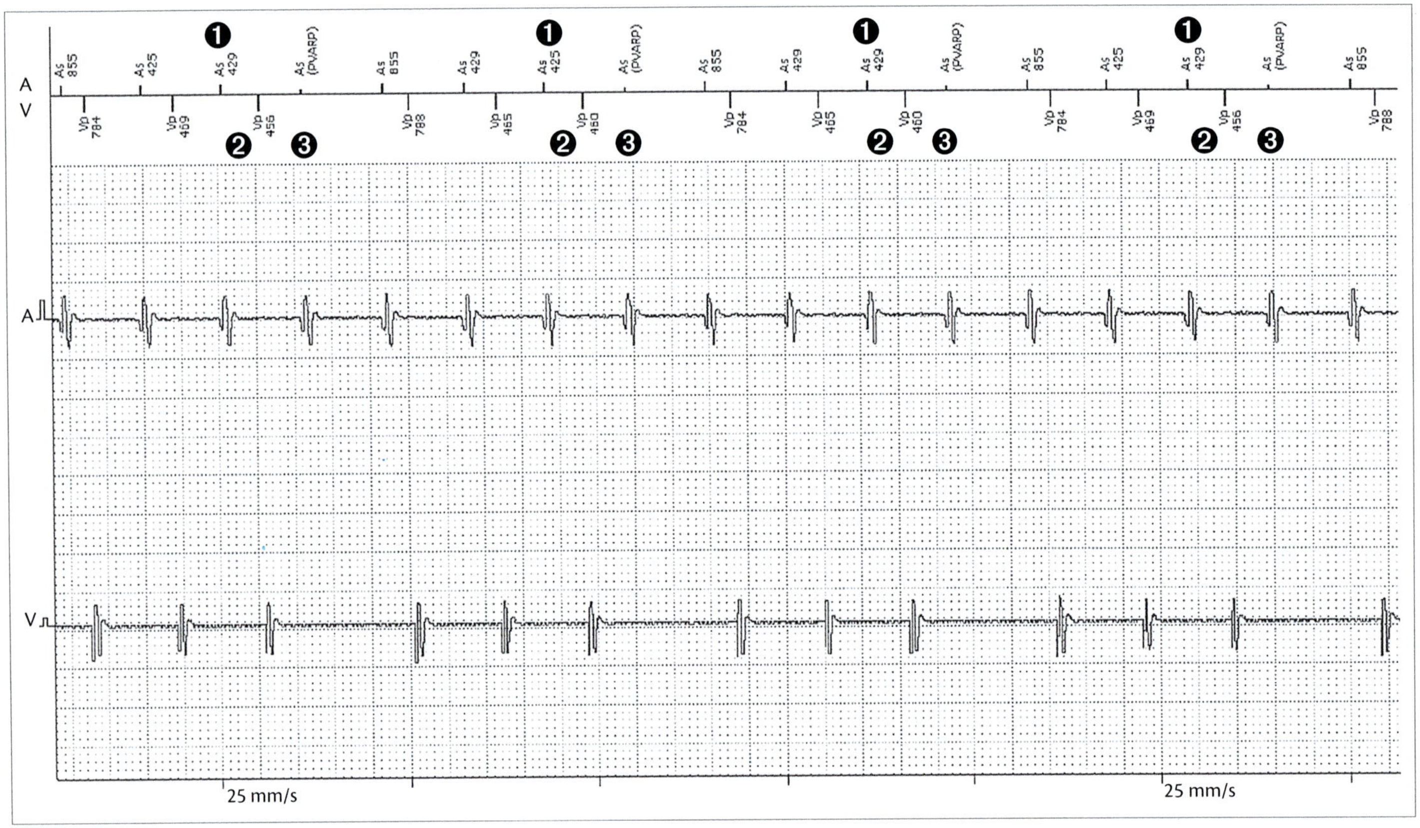

Courtesy of Mr T Bruggemann

A 4:3 Wenckebach response can be observed in Figure 7.2.

❶ The sinus rate is about 140bpm (P–P interval of 425ms), which exceeds the programmed UTR of 120bpm.

❷ Progressive lengthening of the AVI can be observed. This occurs until . . .

❸ . . . the AS event falls into the PVARP, resulting in a refractory AS event. This event does not trigger an AVI, resulting in a non-tracked P-wave and Wenckebach behaviour.

Comments

Pacemaker upper rate behaviour

Wenckebach response occurs when the atrial rate exceeds the programmed UTR, and up to the functional upper limit of 1:1 tracking (Figure 7.3). Wenckebach response occurs progressively (e.g. with a 5:4, then 4:3 then 3:2 response), and is similar to AV Wenckebach block other than the fact that the RR intervals do not progressively decrease (Figure 7.4). Ventricular pacing is delivered constantly at the upper rate interval (URI), but the *average* heart rate decreases step-wise as the ratio of non-tracked atrial events (i.e. pauses) increases. Wenckebach response therefore avoids a sudden drop in heart rate once the programmed UTR has been reached. Once the atrial rate exceeds the TARP interval (which is the AVI+PVARP), 2:1 response occurs (the rate at which this is observed can be calculated by 60,000/TARP). This is why the UTR should always be programmed below the 2:1 response rate (the dotted red line in Figure 7.3 shows rate behaviour in case the UTR is programmed up to the upper limit of 1:1 tracking). If modeswitch is enabled, the device reverts to a non-tracking mode with ventricular pacing at the lower rate (LR) as shown in Figure 7.3, or a sensor-driven rate. The fall in heart rate to the LR at onset of modeswitch is usually gradual thanks to rate-smoothing algorithms present in most modern devices. If modeswitch is not enabled, a 3:1, 4:1 etc. response will occur as atrial rate increases (Figure 7.4).

Figure 7.3 Upper rate behaviour

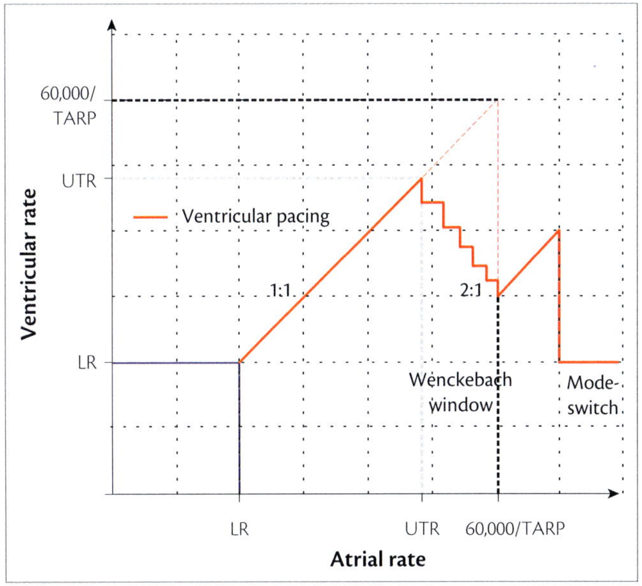

Figure 7.4 Diagram of tracking response at different atrial rates
The device is programmed with a fixed AVI and PVARP. Note the prolongation of the AVI to avoid violating the programmed maximum ventricular pacing rate (defined by the URI)

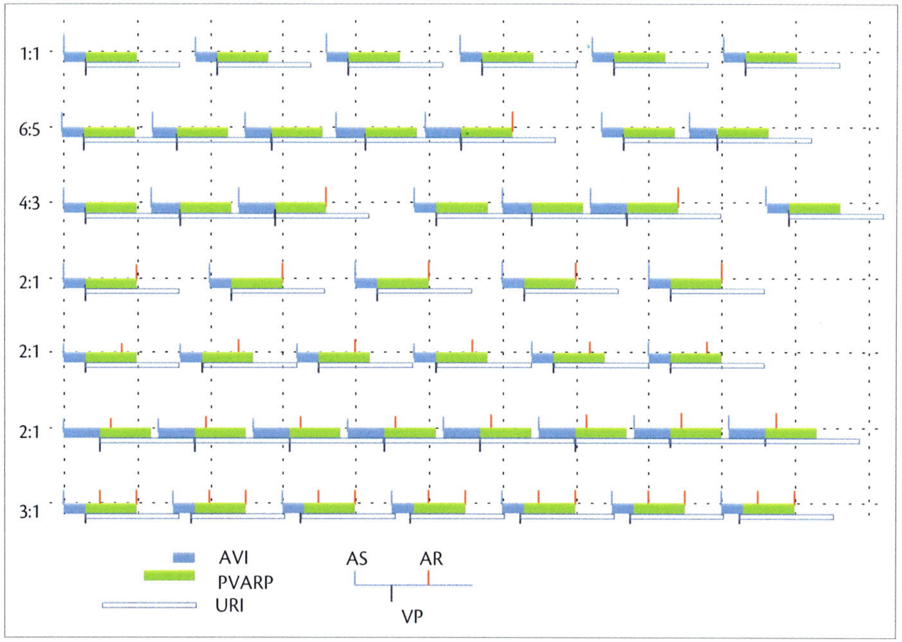

Introduction to the case

A 72-year-old patient with permanent AF and bradycardia had a single-chamber pacemaker implanted. The device was programmed to VVIR 60–120bpm. The rate response parameters were modified at follow-up, due to persistent breathlessness. She presented again, due to breathlessness and palpitations. Her rate histograms are shown in Figure 8.1.

Question

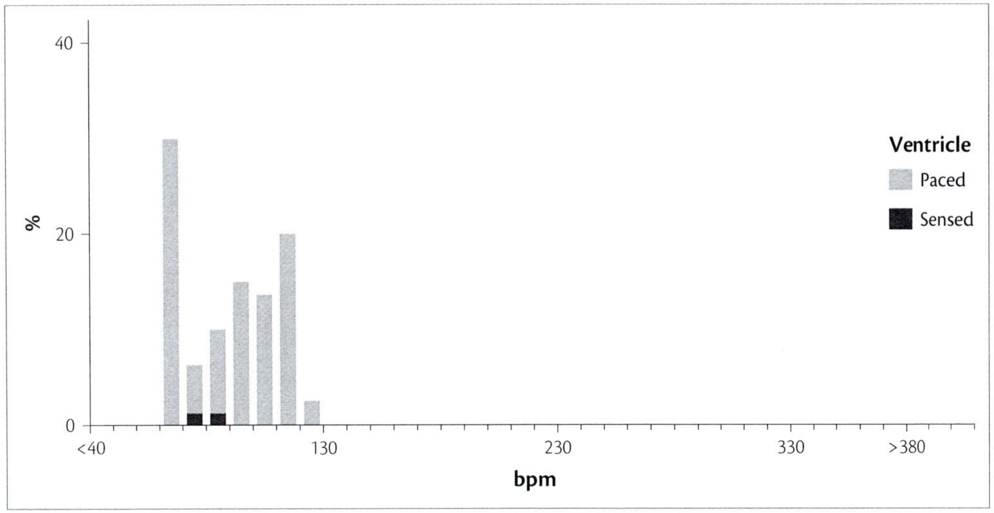

Figure 8.1 Ventricular rate histogram

What is the problem with the sensor settings?

A No problem, the rate histogram is satisfactory

B The sensor threshold is too low, and the slope too steep

C The sensor threshold is too high, and the slope too steep

D The sensor threshold is too high, and the slope is not steep enough

Answer

B The sensor threshold is too low, and the slope too steep

Figure 8.2 Annotated ventricular rate histogram

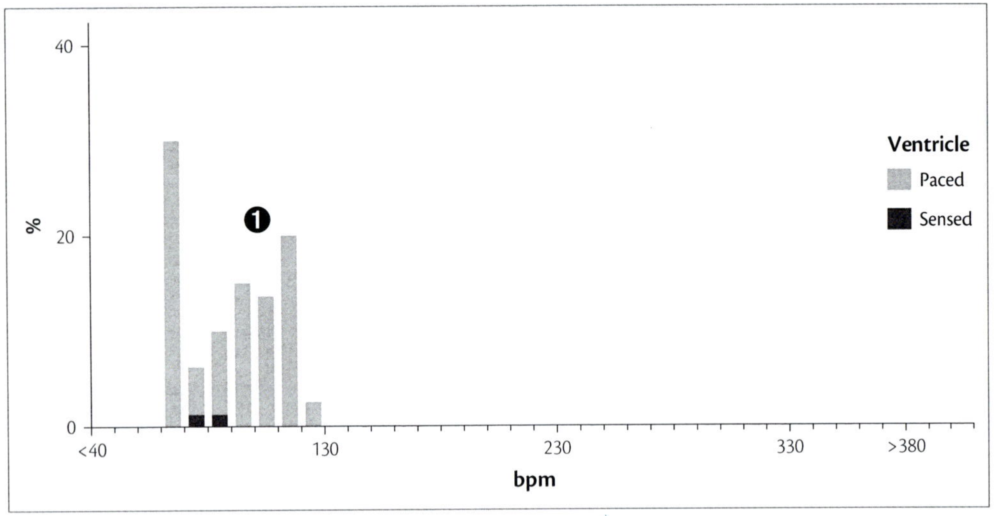

❶ In Figure 8.2, the rate histogram shows a large proportion of sensor-driven events, i.e. at a rate above the baseline (resting) rate of 60bpm. This proportion is too high for a patient of this age, implying that the sensor threshold is too low (i.e. too sensitive). The profile of the histogram shows an increasing proportion of events at an increasing heart rate, indicating that the sensor slope is too steep.

Comments

Rate response

Basic parameters of sensor settings include the threshold and slope, the functions of which are displayed in Figure 8.3.

The threshold sensitivity setting determines the activity level required to trigger rate response. The programmed slope will then determine the increase in heart rate for a given level of activity. Figure 8.4 shows a case that required lowering the threshold (i.e. making it more sensitive).

It is usually better to change one single parameter at a time, unless the rate histograms clearly indicate otherwise, or the device has a modelling feature that allows a simulating rate response at different settings for recorded sensor data. Patient history is of course essential, as modifying sensor settings is only warranted in case of symptoms.

Figure 8.4 Example of sensor threshold programmed too high (i.e. not sensitive enough)

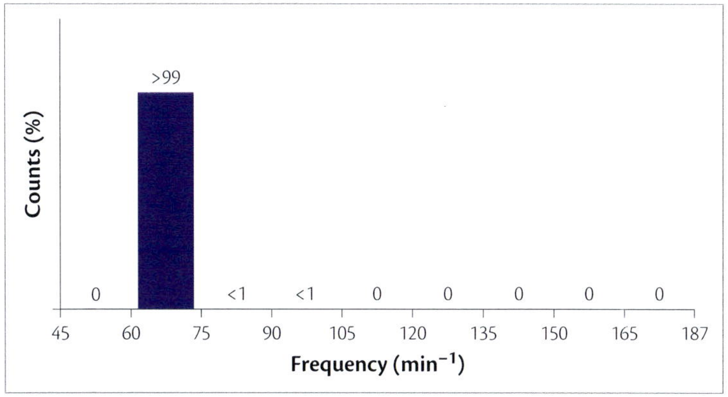

Figure 8.3 Rate response parameters

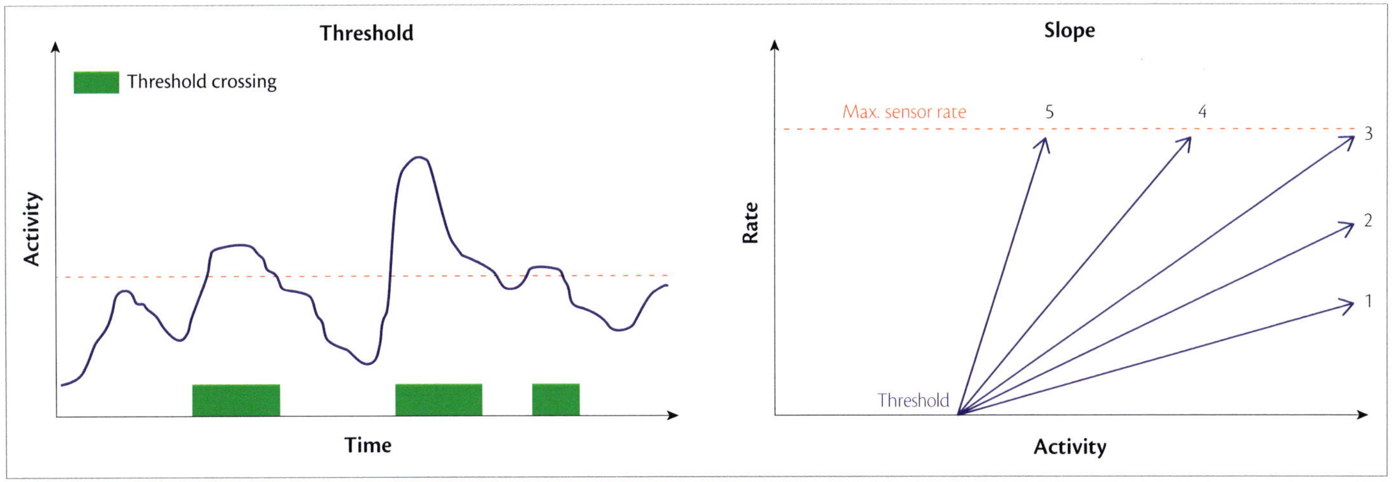

Introduction to the case

An 80-year-old woman implanted with a VDD pacemaker for complete AV block had recently undergone a generator replacement. She reported malaise, while carrying her shopping. The device settings are shown in Table 9.1.

Table 9.1 Device settings

Mode	VDD
Baseline rate	50bpm
UTR	120bpm
Atrial sensing (bipolar)	0.2mV
Ventricular sensing (unipolar)	2.5mV
VP (bipolar)	2.5V at 0.35ms
AV delay (adaptive)	80–125ms
Post-ventricular atrial blanking (PVAB)	150ms

Upon device interrogation, multiple ventricular high-rate episodes were retrieved from the device memory, one of which (lasting 10s) is shown in Figure 9.1.

Question

Figure 9.1 Ventricular high-rate episode retrieved from the device memory (the atrial and ventricular EGMs are displayed on a single channel)

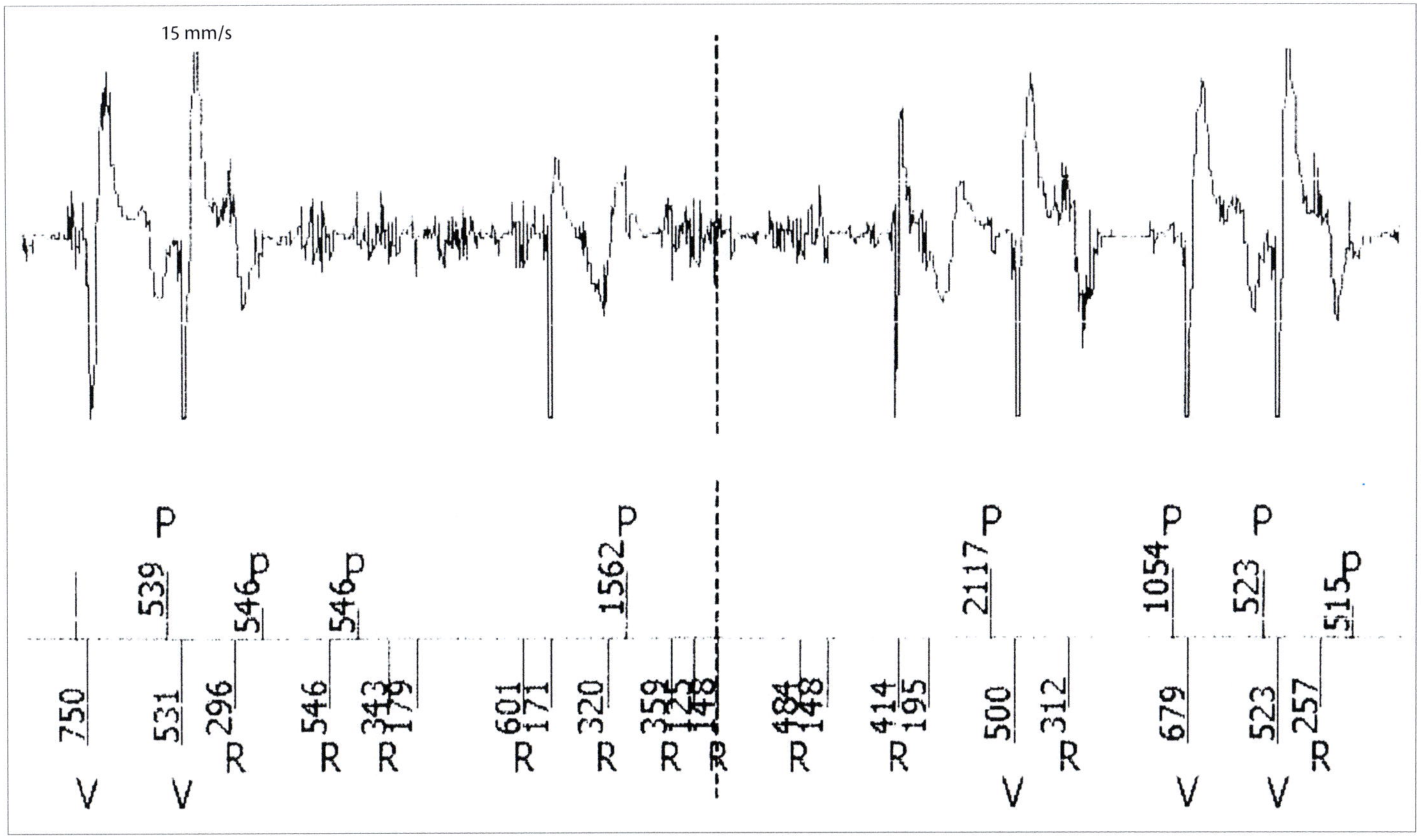

What is the cause of the patient's symptoms?

A Ventricular tachycardia (VT)

B AF

C Ventricular non-capture

D Ventricular oversensing

Answer

D Ventricular oversensing

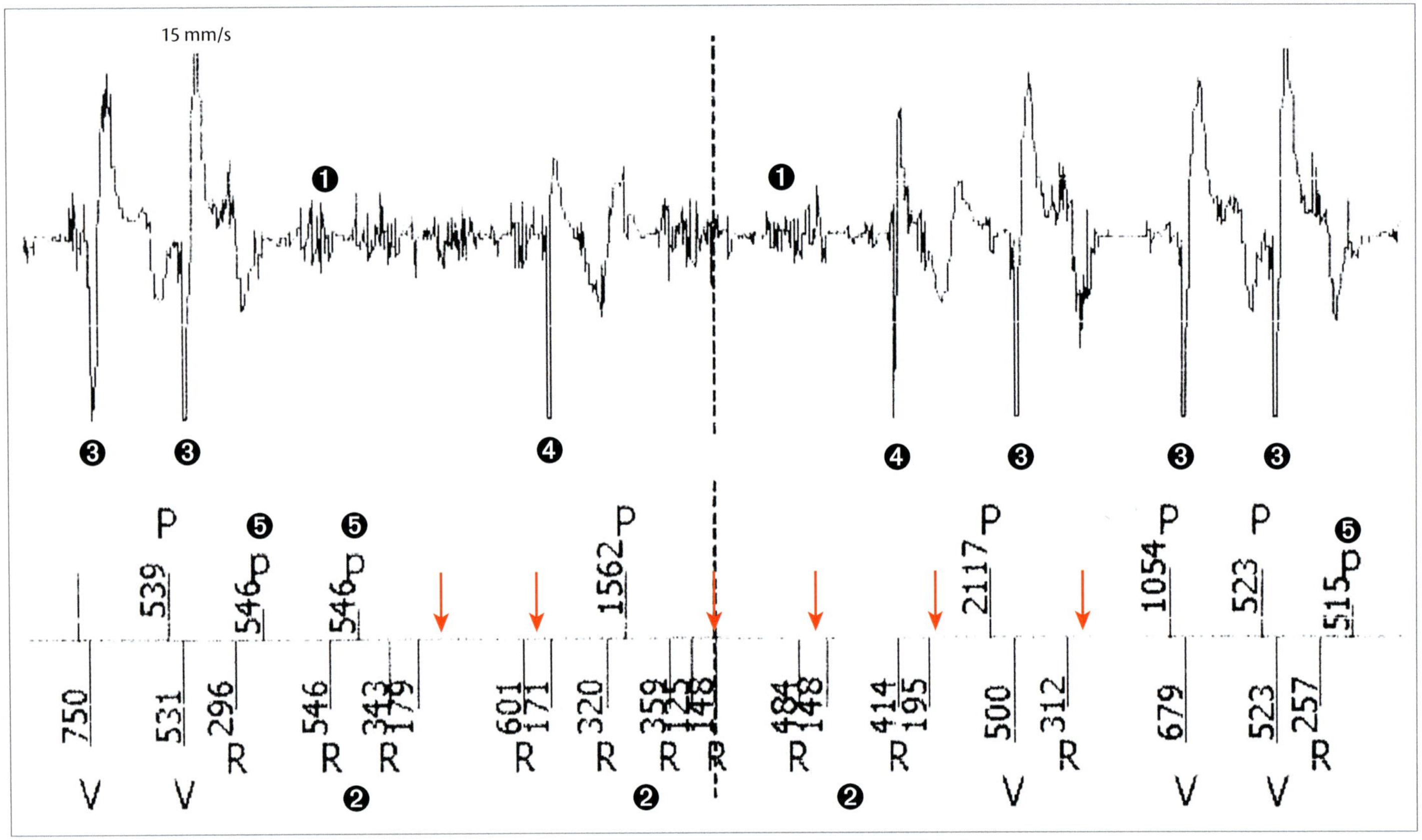

Figure 9.2 Annotated ventricular high-rate episode retrieved from the device memory

❶ High-rate signals can be observed on the EGM channel (Figure 9.2).

❷ The markers indicate that the high-rate signals are sensed by the ventricular channel only. The signals correspond to pectoral myopotentials, resulting from the unipolar sensing configuration (that had been programmed by mistake at generator replacement). This results in ventricular oversensing which inhibits pacing.

❸ These EGM signals correspond to ventricular capture.

❹ These EGM signals correspond to a ventricular escape rhythm at about 30bpm.

❺ These AS events fall in the PVARP and are depicted by a short bar (the event sensed outside the PVARP are indicated by a long bar).

↓ Note that there are only few AS events during ventricular oversensing. This is due to the P-waves falling in the PVAB period or possibly also due to atrial undersensing (which is relatively frequent with VDD devices due to the floating atrial dipole). The atrial signals are hidden by the myopotentials, but their likely timing is indicated by the interpolated arrows.

Comments

Pectoral myopotential oversensing

Pectoral myopotential oversensing resulted from the unipolar sensing configuration and was confirmed by asking the patient to press her hands together (prayer manoeuvre; Figure 9.3), which reproduced the myopotential artefacts on the real-time EGM.

Ventricular oversensing is a potentially lethal condition in pacemaker-dependent patients (as it may lead to asystole). The problem was corrected in this case by setting the ventricular sensing to a bipolar configuration.

Figure 9.3 Prayer manoeuvre to reproduce pectoral muscle oversensing

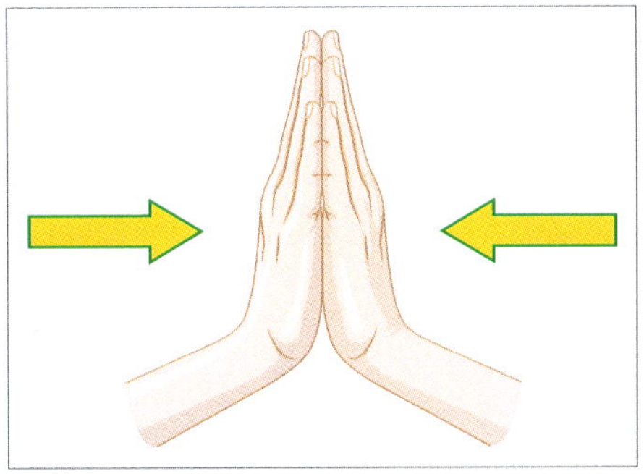

CASE 10

Introduction to the case

A 72-year-old patient with complete AV block was followed by remote monitoring. The device settings are shown in Table 10.1, and the atrial rate histogram is shown in Figure 10.1. High-rate atrial episodes were recorded, and the EGMs of two such episodes are shown in Figure 10.2.

Figure 10.1 Atrial rate histogram. The atrium was paced in 4%, and the ventricle in 100%, of the time

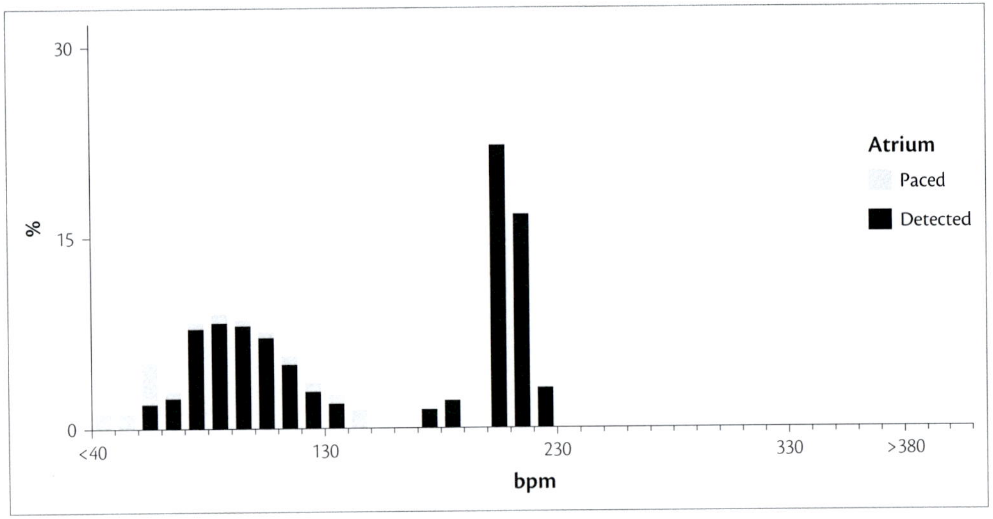

Table 10.1 Device settings

Pacing mode	DDDR
Lower rate	50bpm
Upper rate	130bpm
Atrial output (bipolar)	2.4V@0.4ms
Ventricular output (bipolar)	2.4V@0.4ms
Atrial sensitivity (bipolar)	0.2mV
Ventricular sensitivity (bipolar)	2.5mV
Paced AV delay	180–140ms
Sense compensation	−45ms
PVAB after ventricular sense	100ms
PVAB after ventricular pace	150ms
PVARP	325ms
Post-PVC PVARP extension	400ms
Ventricular blanking after atrial pace	30ms
Ventricular refractory period (VRP)	250ms

Question

Figure 10.2 Atrial high-rate episode EGMs retrieved from the device memory

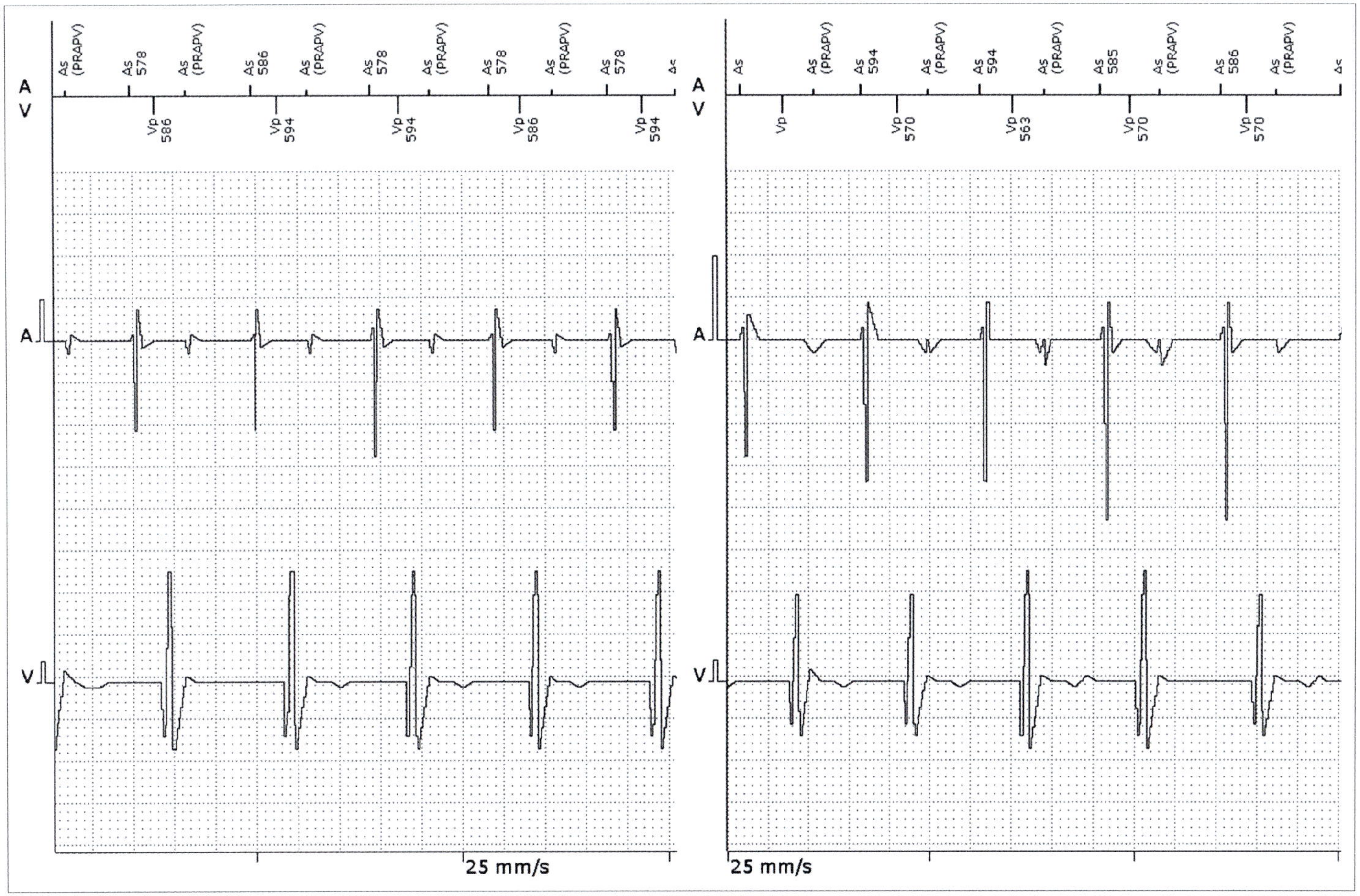

What is the cause of the atrial high-rate episodes?

A Atrial bigeminy

B Atrial tachycardia

C AV crosstalk

D Far-field R-wave (FFRW) oversensing

Answer

D Far-field R-wave (FFRW) oversensing

Figure 10.3 Annotated atrial high-rate episode EGMs retrieved from the device memory

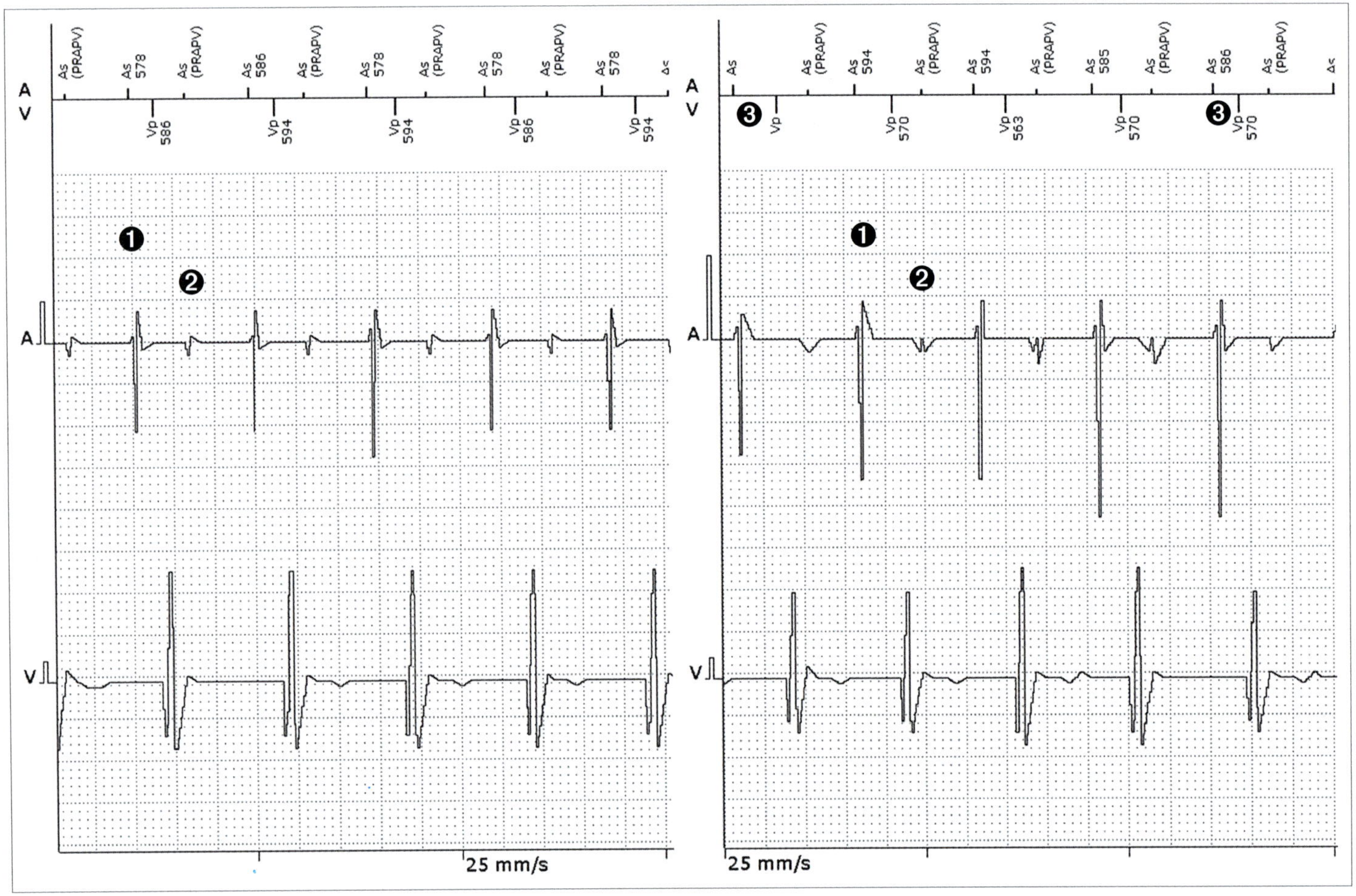

This is an example of FFRW oversensing that may cause erroneous diagnosis of atrial high-rate episodes (Figure 10.3).

❶ The sharp signals are the near-field atrial EGM. Note the cyclic variation in amplitude, due to changes in lead orientation as a result of respiration.

❷ The smaller signals are FFRWs that occur at just under 160ms after VP and fall within the PVARP (but after atrial blanking of 150ms).

❸ Note the variable AVIs, due to the device function in a non-tracking (DDIR) mode as a result of inappropriate mode switch caused by the FFRW oversensing.

Comments

Far-field R-wave oversensing

A number of factors may favour FFRW oversensing:

- proximity of the atrial lead to the ventricle
- unipolar sensing configuration
- programming a high sensitivity
- short PVAB
- inter-electrode spacing of the lead (with closer spacing, resulting in less FFRW oversensing).

It also depends upon the orientation of the vector of the QRS complex, with respect to the electrodes of the atrial lead (therefore, amplitudes of the FFRW of paced and sensed QRS complexes may differ). FFRW oversensing may cause inappropriate mode switch, as in this example. The easiest way to correct the problem is to lengthen the PVAB, as was done in this case, from 150ms to 180ms. A more difficult issue to deal with is sensing of FFRW when it occurs *before* ventricular sensing (Figure 10.4). This occurs in about 25% of patients,[1] especially in the setting of RBBB where the depolarization wavefront is sensed late into the QRS complex by the RV lead.

Reference

1. Lewalter T, Tuininga Y, Frohlig G, *et al*. Morphology-enhanced atrial event classification improves sensing in pacemakers. *Pacing Clin Electrophysiol* 2007; **30**: 1455–63.

Figure 10.4 FFRW oversensing occurring before sensing by the RV lead

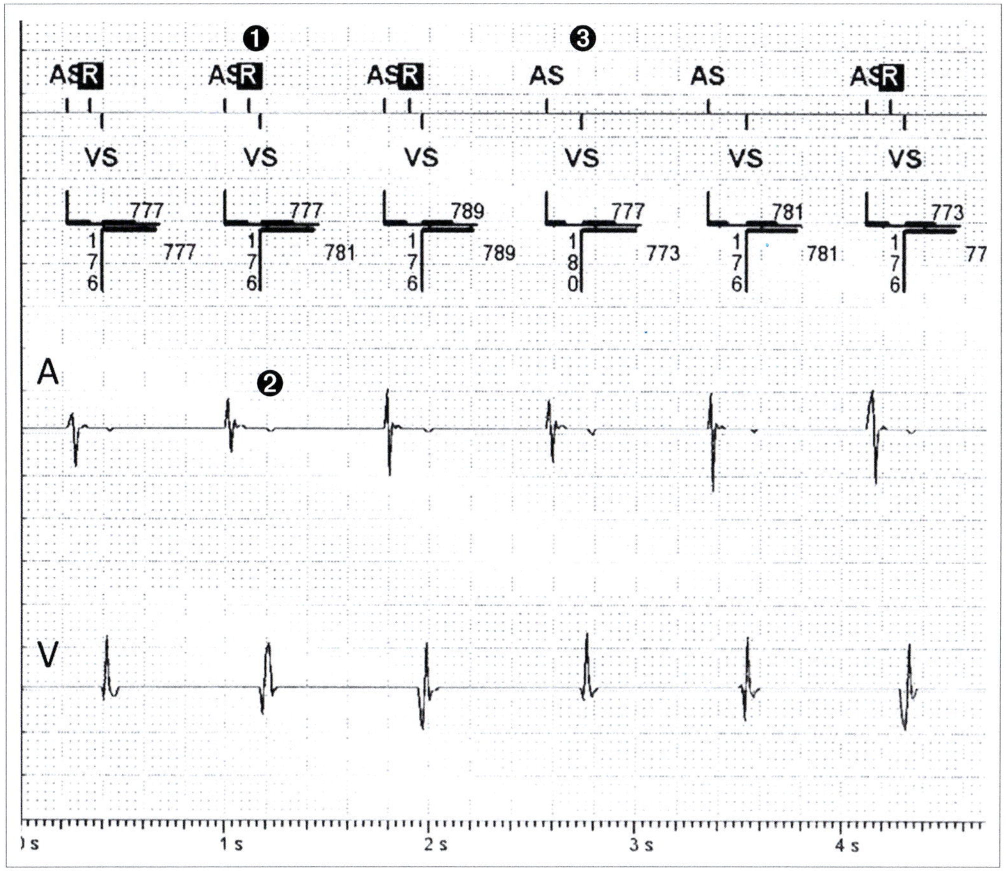

❶ The FFRW is being sensed before the VS event. It is labelled as a refractory event, as it falls within the AVI.

❷ The FFRW is observed to be of low amplitude.

❸ FFRW oversensing is intermittent. Changing the sensitivity level from 0.1mV to 0.4mV corrected the problem (but changing the PVAB would not have changed anything).

CASE 11

Introduction to the case

A 76-year-old woman with ischaemic heart disease and 45% LVEF, implanted with a dual-chamber pacemaker for sinus dysfunction, was admitted with decompensated heart failure. The pacemaker was interrogated, and the real-time EGM is shown in Figure 11.1. The device settings are shown in Table 11.1.

Table 11.1 Device settings

Mode	DDDR
Baseline rate	60bpm
UTR	130bpm
Paced AV delay	300ms
Sense compensation	−20ms
AP output (bipolar)	2.5V/0.4ms
Ventricular output (bipolar)	2.5V/0.4ms
Atrial sensitivity (bipolar)	0.3mV
Ventricular sensitivity (bipolar)	2.5mV
PVARP	Auto

Question

Figure 11.1 Real-time EGM at device interrogation

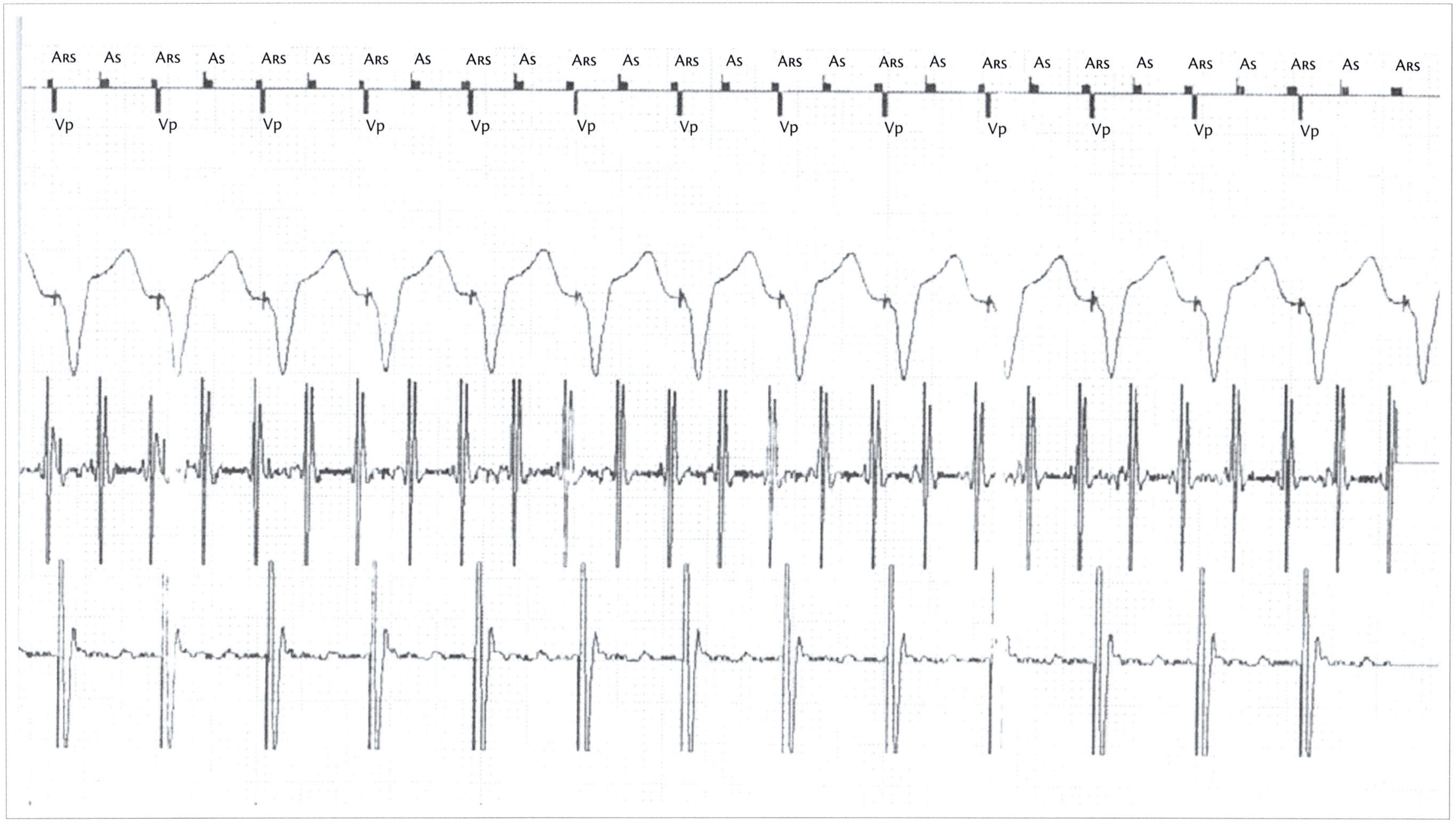

What is the most likely reason for the pacing rate?

A Runaway pacemaker

B Inactivated mode switch

C Rate-adaptive pacing

D 2:1 locked-in atrial flutter

Answer

B Inactivation of mode switch

Figure 11.2 Annotated real-time EGM at device interrogation

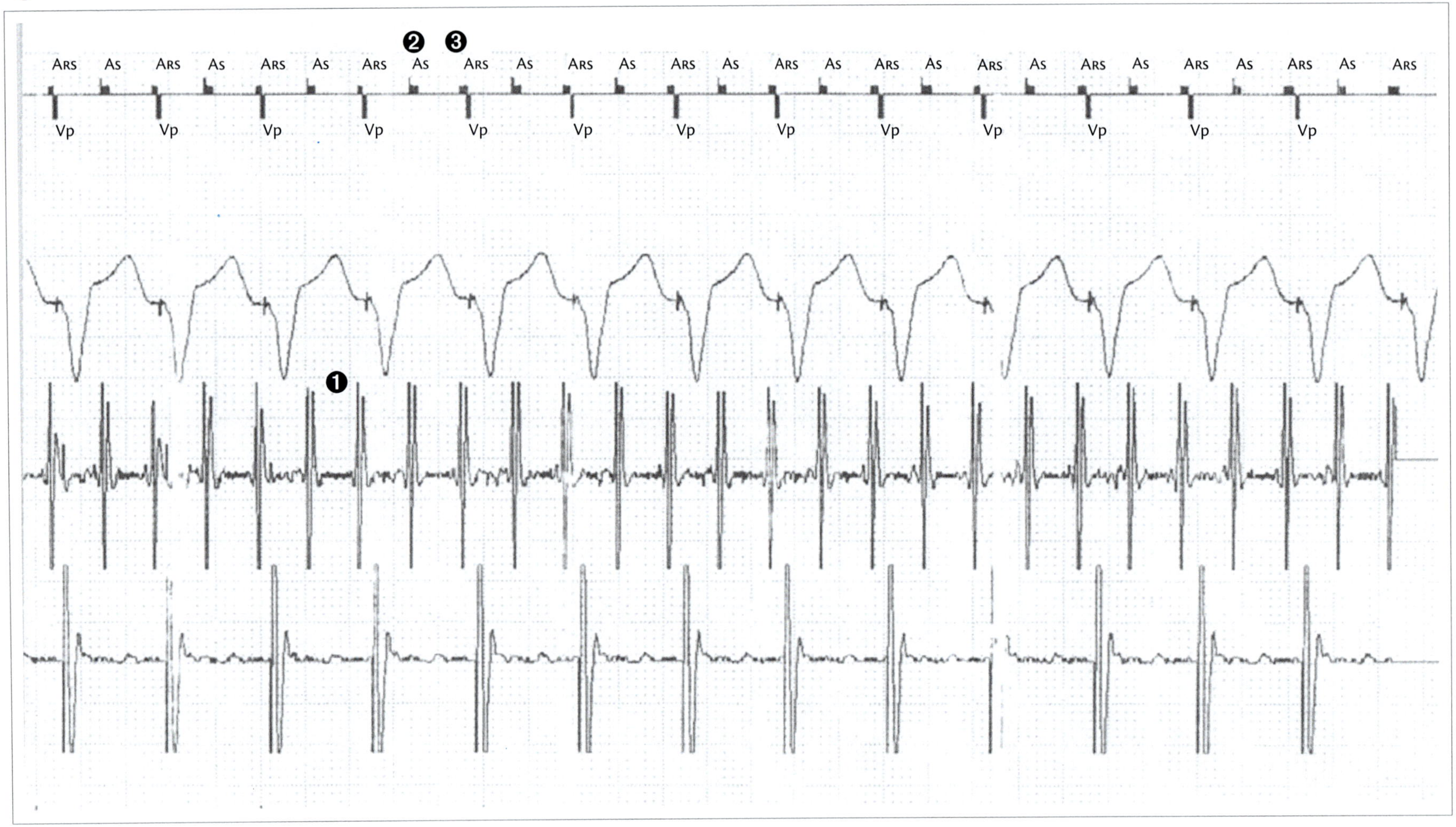

In Figure 11.2, The pacemaker is pacing close to the UTR, due to inactivation of mode switch.

❶ The atrial EGM shows flutter at a cycle length of 230ms (260bpm).

❷ The AS events (falling outside the PVARP) triggers an AVI with VP. The AVIs had been programmed long, in order to favour intrinsic AV conduction.

❸ This atrial event is classified as refractory (ARS), as it falls within the AVI and does not reset the AV timer. The fact that all atrial events are sensed indicates that this is not 2:1 locked-in atrial flutter (where every 2nd atrial event falls into the PVAB period and is not sensed).

Comment

Mode switch

Mode switch should be routinely activated in all pacemakers and ICDs, even if the patients do not have a history of atrial arrhythmias, as they are prevalent in this population. The mode switch function reprogrammes the pacing mode into a non-tracking mode, i.e. DDI(R) or VDI(R), when the atrial rate crosses a predefined threshold (e.g. 175bpm) for a given period of time or a specific number of beats.

In this patient, mode switch had been unintentionally deactivated, leading to the tracking of atrial flutter and rapid VP with decompensated heart failure. Mode switch was reactivated, with resumption of intrinsic ventricular rhythm (Figure 11.3).

Figure 11.3 Real-time EGM after reactivation of mode switch

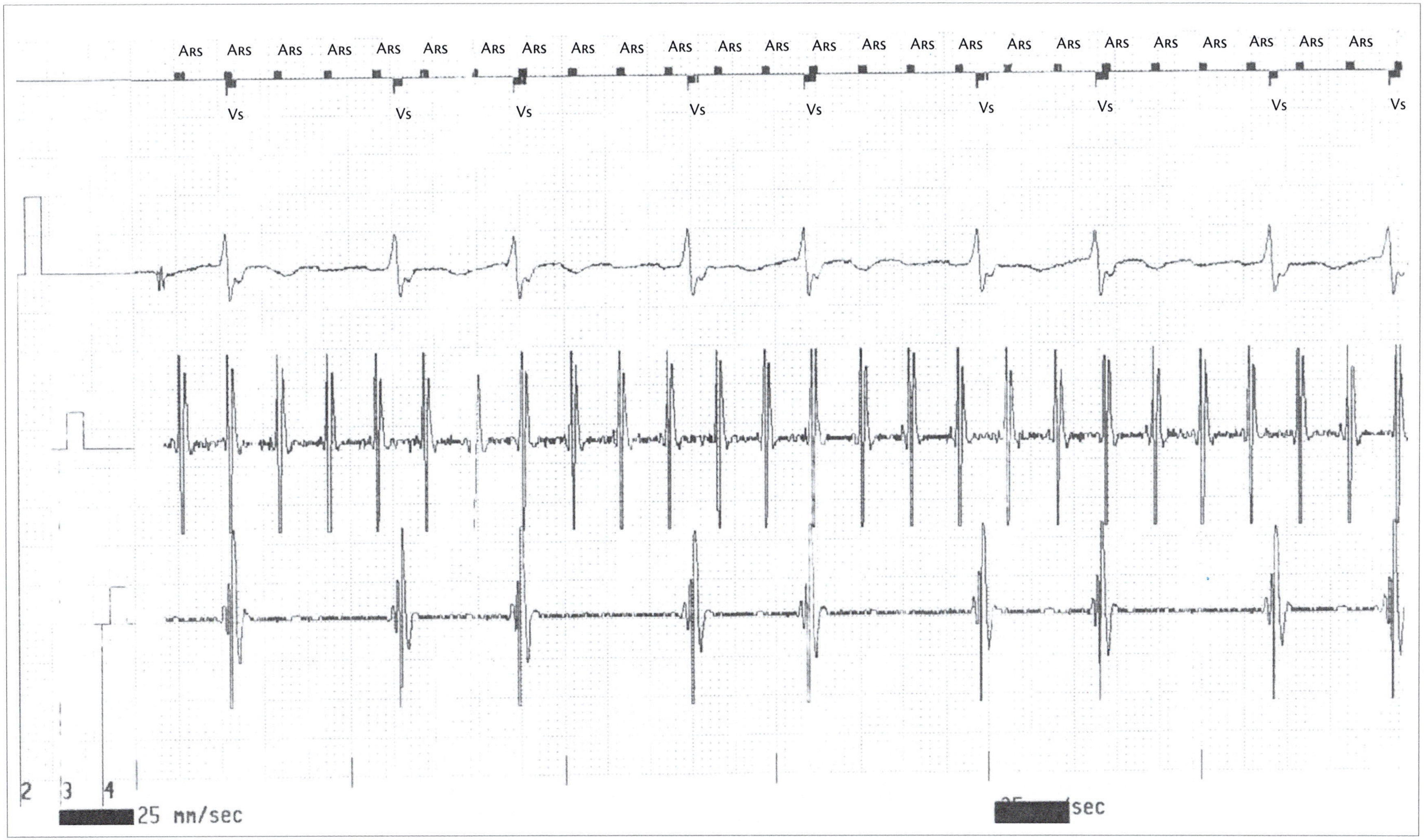

Introduction to the case

A Holter recording was performed due to dizziness in a patient with a dual-chamber pacemaker, implanted for symptomatic paroxysmal AV block. The device settings are shown in Table 12.1.

Table 12.1 Device settings

Pacing mode	DDD
Baseline rate	50bpm
UTR	130bpm
Sensed AV delay	170ms
Paced AV delay	200ms

Question

Figure 12.1 Holter recording

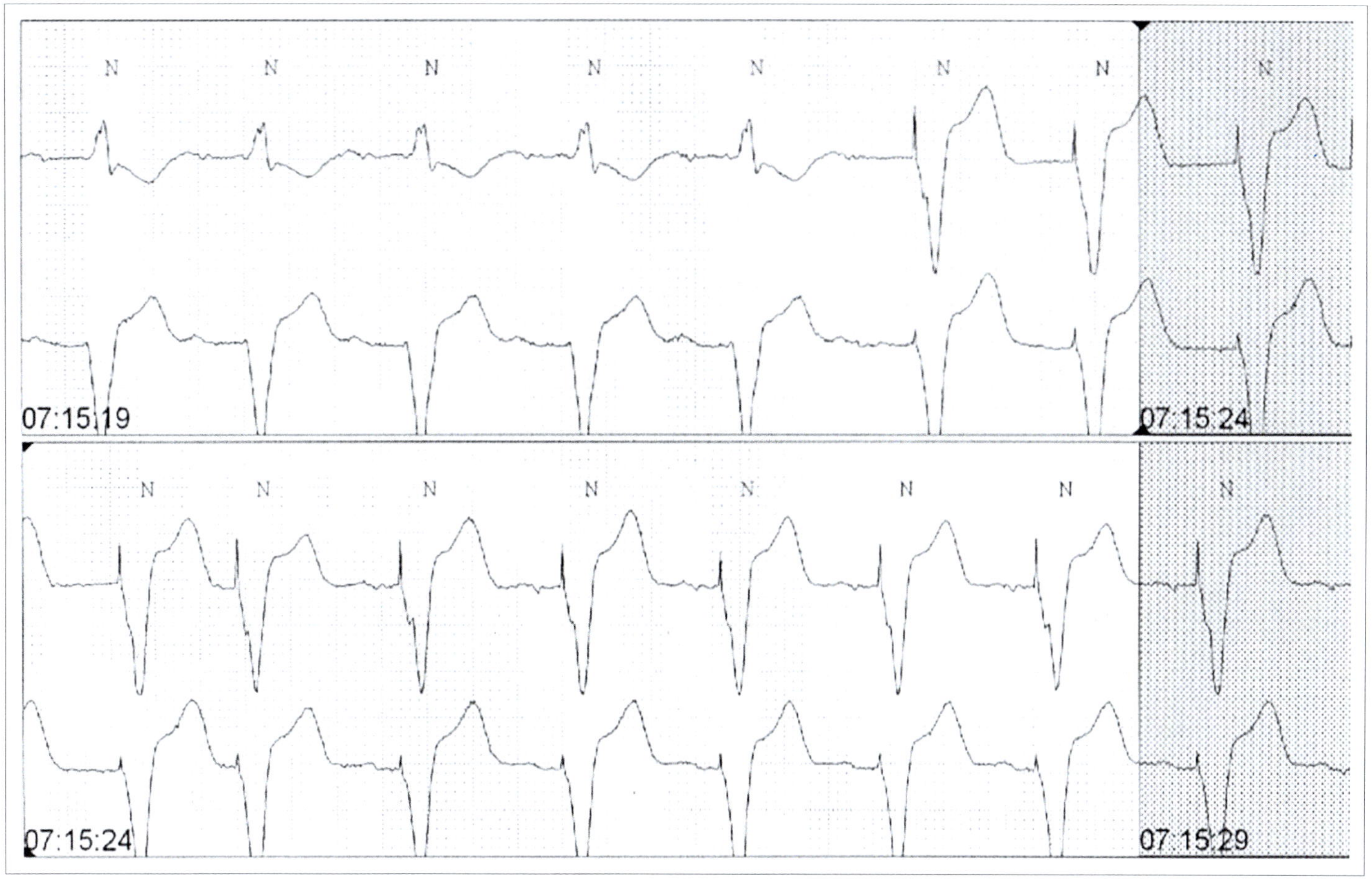

What do you observe in Figure 12.1?

A Intermittent atrial undersensing

B AV hysteresis

C Atrial non-capture

D ADI pacing mode

Answer

B AV hysteresis

Figure 12.2 Annotated Holter recording

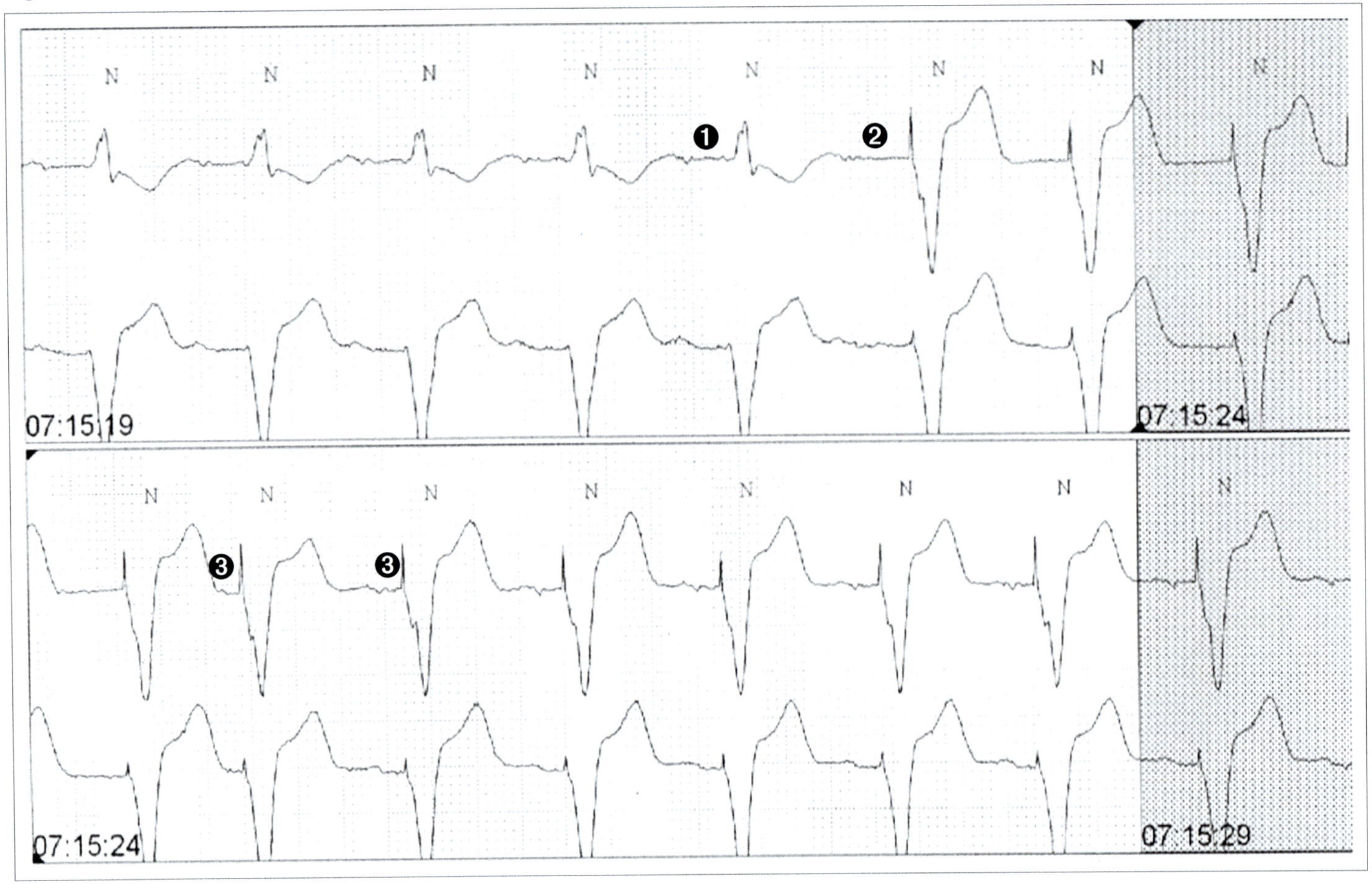

Dizziness was attributed to low blood pressure and was unrelated to the phenomenon seen here in Figure 12.2, which is normal pacemaker behaviour.

❶ The 1st five beats show sinus rhythm with intrinsic AV conduction, with first-degree AV block and bundle branch block.

❷ The following four beats show sinus rhythm with ventricular pacing and an extended AVI, due to repetitive AV hysteresis of 200ms (the sensed AV delay amounts to 370ms). The P-waves are not always visible, as they fall in the preceding T-wave, but are tracked by the pacemaker.

❸ The sensed AVI reverts to the programmed value of 170ms, due to the absence of AV conduction.

Comments

Atrioventricular hysteresis

The AV hysteresis algorithm is designed to avoid unnecessary ventricular pacing. An AV delay extension is programmed for a defined number of beats (200ms for four beats in this example). If ventricular sensing does not occur, the device reverts to the programmed AV delay for a defined period of time, at the end of which the AV delay is extended again to test for resumption of intrinsic AV conduction (Figure 12.3; recorded in another patient).

Figure 12.3 AVI extension with resumption of AV conduction

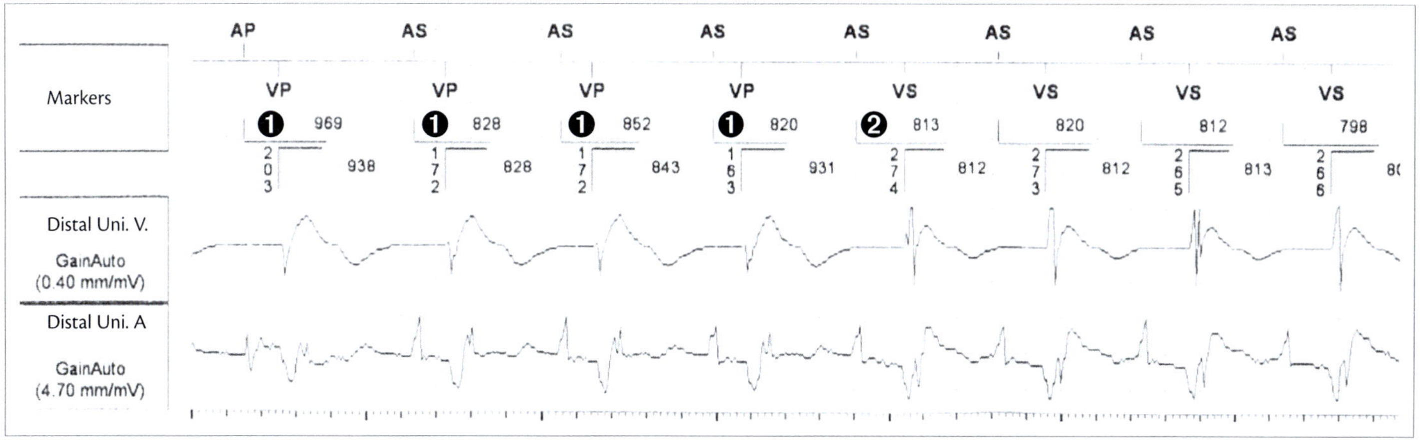

❶ The 1st four beats show DDD pacing, with paced and sensed AV delays of 200ms and 170ms, respectively.

❷ An AV delay extension of 200ms is activated, revealing intrinsic AV conduction, perpetuating the AV delay extension for the following beats.

Introduction to the case

A patient was implanted with a dual-chamber pacemaker for symptomatic Wenckebach AV block. A Holter was performed and is shown in Figure 13.1.

Question

Figure 13.1 Holter recording

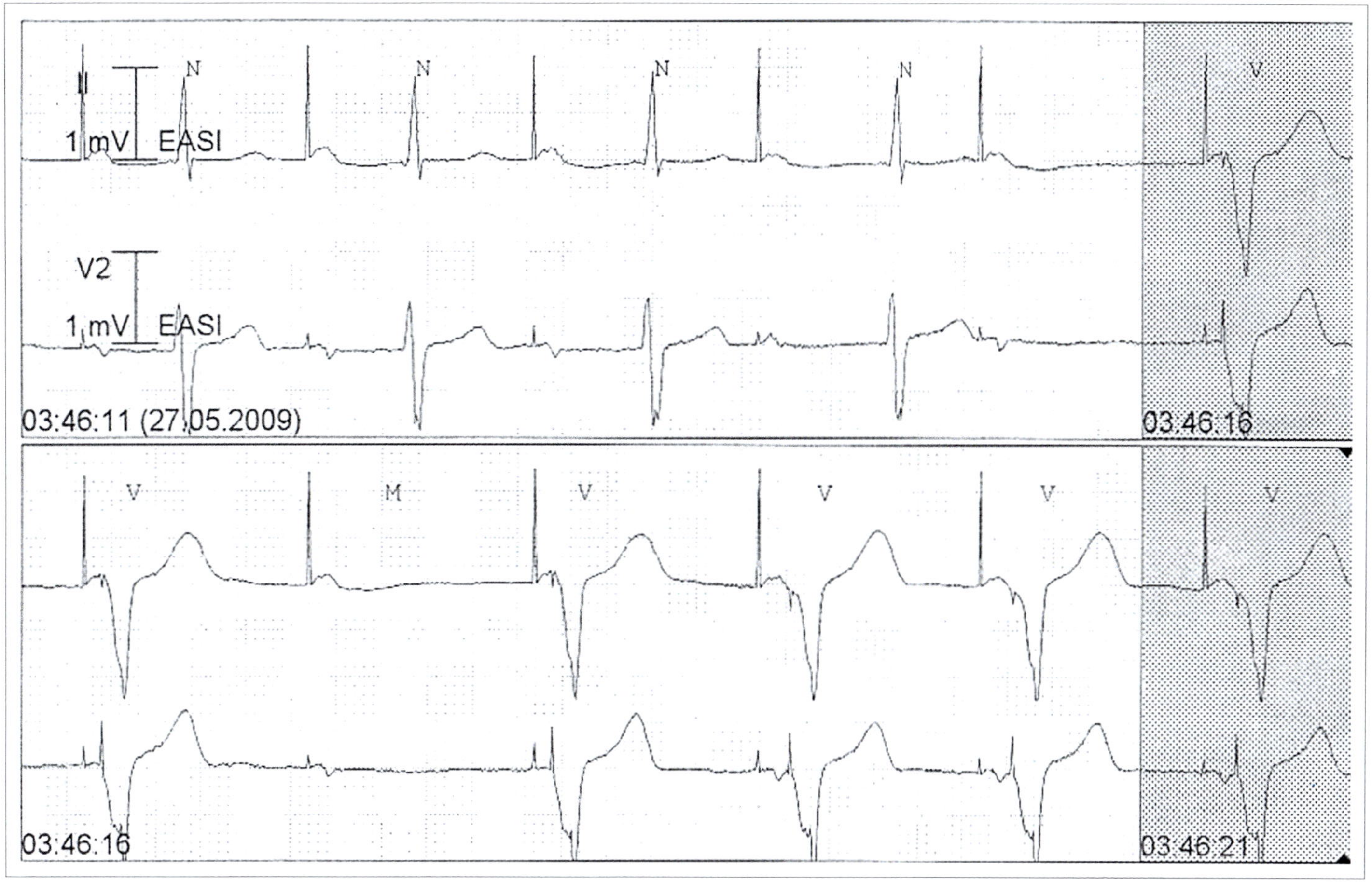

How can you explain what is observed?

A ADI/DDD switch

B Ventricular non-capture

C Ventricular oversensing

D Both A and C

Answer

A ADI/DDD switch

Figure 13.2 ADI/DDD switch

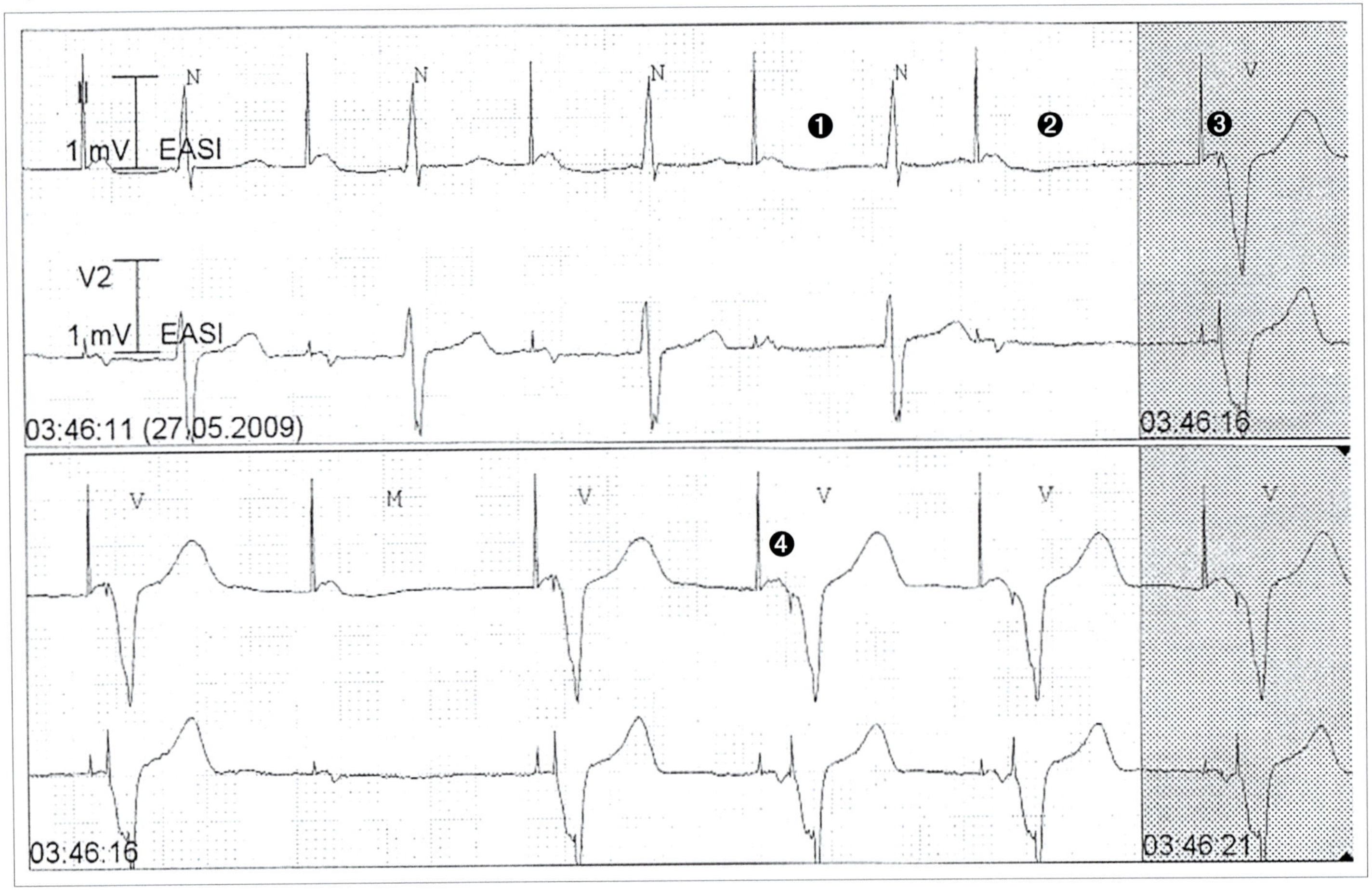

The device in Figure 13.2 is switching from an ADI mode to a DDD mode, following repetitive AV block. This is the only option that explains the shortened AVI of the cycle immediately following each non-conducted P-wave. There are no ventricular spikes that do not result in capture. Ventricular oversensing would result in resetting of the VA interval and change in the A–A timing, and does not explain the shortened AVI after the non-conducted P-waves.

❶ The device is functioning in an ADI mode. AP with intrinsic AV conduction and gradually prolonging PR intervals can be observed.

❷ Wenckebach AV block occurs.

❸ A ventricular backup pace is delivered, and the cycle repeats itself again (the shaded zone corresponds to an overlap with the following line).

❹ After blocked P-waves have been detected repeatedly, the device switches to a DDD mode.

Comments

The ADI/DDD algorithm

Several device manufacturers have introduced algorithms (with different names) that minimize ventricular pacing by allowing isolated blocked P-waves to occur intermittently. The device functions in an ADI(R) mode, until blocked P-waves occur repeatedly, resulting in a switch to a DDD mode for a specified duration, after which an AV conduction check occurs.

Algorithms of different companies have slight differences, but all allow pauses to occur, with long–short sequences. Although they reduce ventricular pacing effectively and are well tolerated by the majority of patients, it may be better to avoid this algorithm in:

1. patients with permanent complete AV block
2. patients with symptomatic first-degree AV block (as in the present case)
3. pacemaker-dependent patients who do not tolerate slow rates, and
4. in the case of a long QT interval or history of torsades de pointes (due to the pro-arythmic effect of long-short sequences in this patients).

Introduction to the case

A 72-year-old patient was implanted with a dual-chamber pacemaker for sick sinus syndrome, programmed with the ADIR/DDDR algorithm. His LVEF was normal. The device counters indicated 96% AP and 2% VP. He complained of persistent dyspnoea. A real-time EGM is shown in Figure 14.1. A transthoracic echocardiogram was performed, and the transmitral Doppler flow is shown in Figure 14.2.

Figure 14.1 Real-time EGM

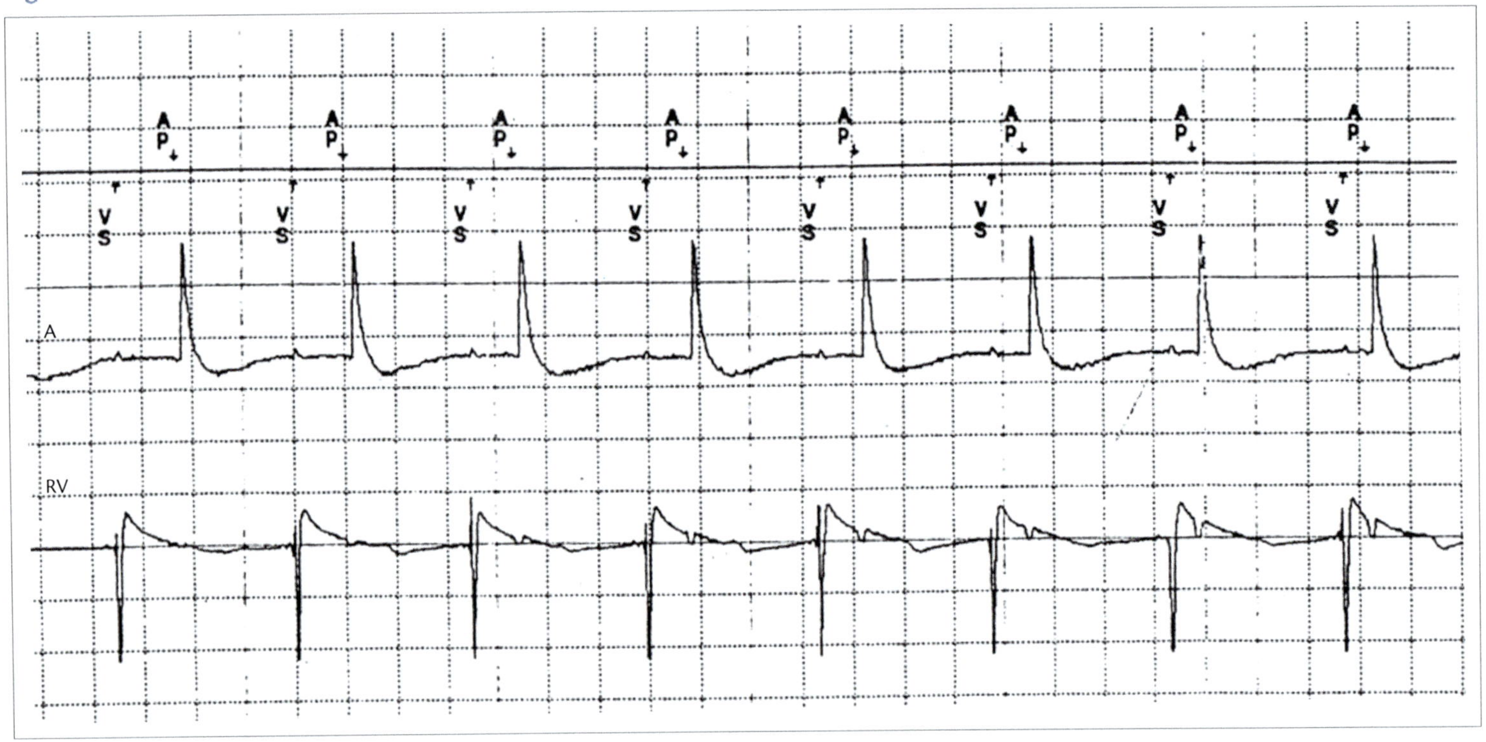

Question

Figure 14.2 Pulsed-wave (a) and continuous-wave (b) Doppler of transmitral flow

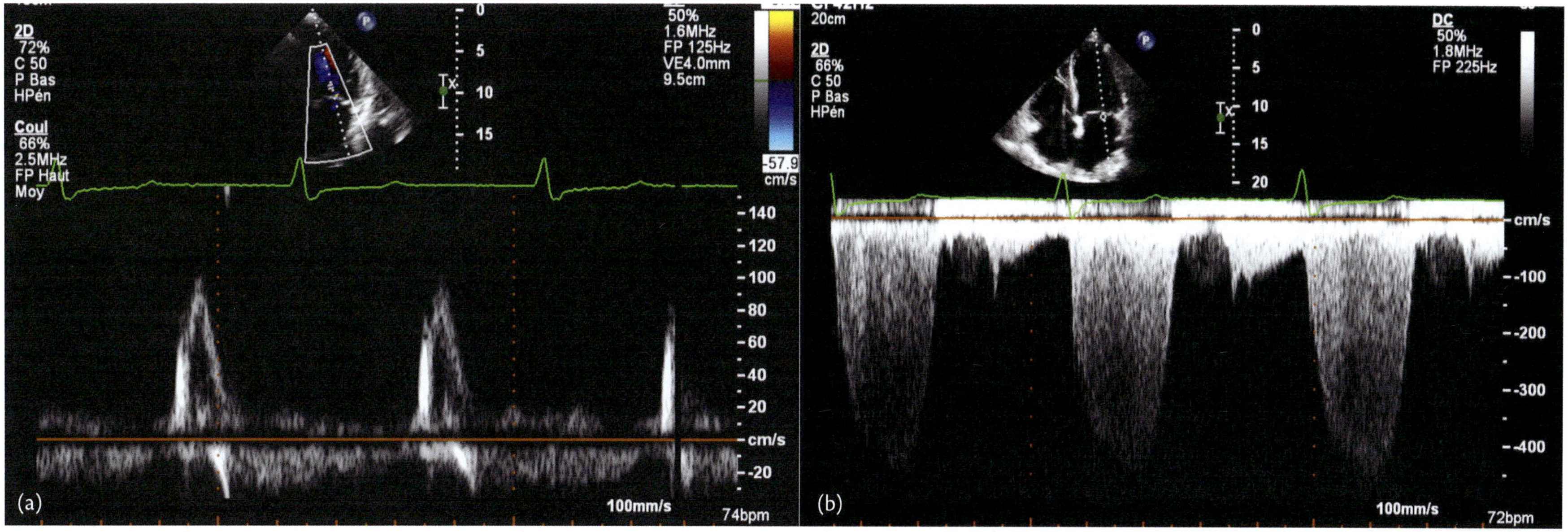

What needs to be done to improve the patient's symptoms?

A Programme in the DDDR mode

B Programme in the DDIR mode with a long AV delay

C Programme in the AAIR mode

D Implant a biventricular pacemaker

Answer

A **Programme in the DDDR mode**

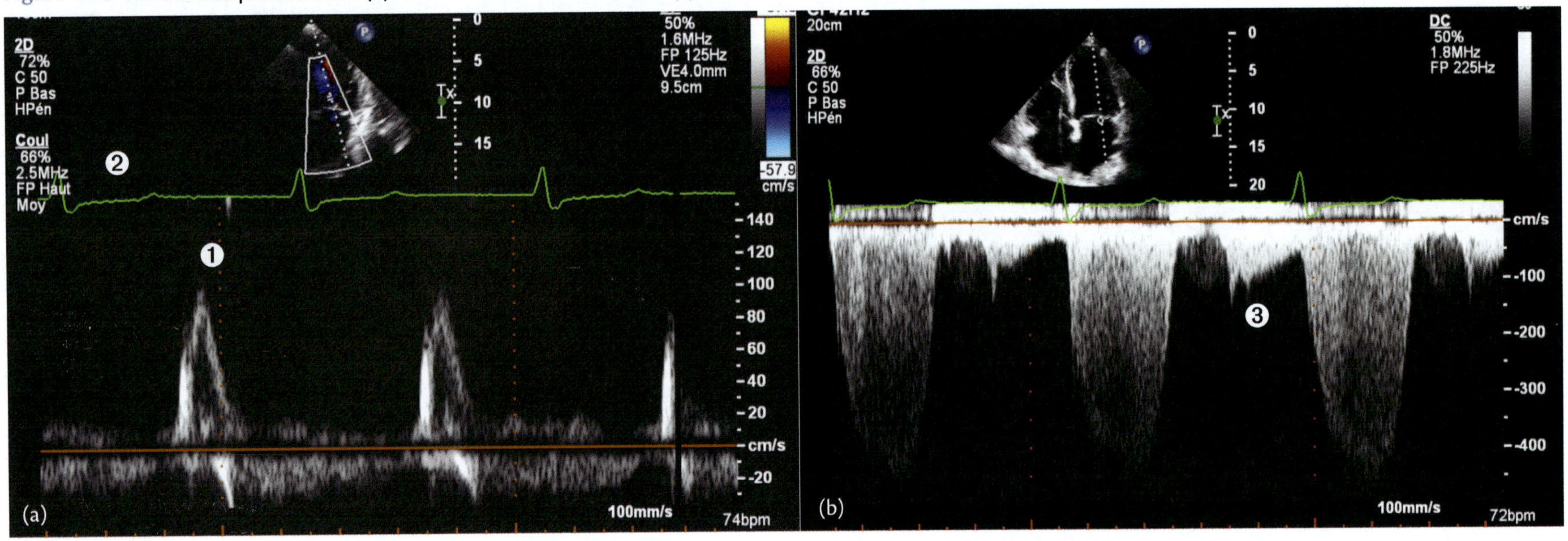

Figure 14.3 Annotated pulsed-wave (a) and continuous-wave (b) Doppler of transmitral flow

The EGM showed atrial pacing with intrinsic AV conduction and prolonged first-degree AV block, resulting in a 'P on T' phenomenon (Figure 14.3).

❶ The transmitral pulsed-wave Doppler shows an E-wave, without an A-wave.

❷ This is due to the P-wave occurring during ventricular systole.

❸ The transmitral continuous-wave Doppler shows diastolic mitral regurgitation, due to the prolonged PR interval (systolic regurgitation is also visible).

Comments

Consequences of ‘P on T’

The ADI/DDD algorithm tolerates very long AVIs, which may, as in this case, lead to ‘P on T’, with atrial contraction occurring during ventricular systole, as in the pacemaker syndrome (see Case 4). The detrimental haemodynamic effect of RV pacing in the DDD mode needs to be balanced against improved AV synchrony. In this case, programming the pacemaker to the DDD mode revealed improved ventricular filling, with the appearance of an A-wave, as seen in Figure 14.4A. Also, diastolic mitral regurgitation was eliminated, although it probably was not the main cause of the patient’s symptoms.

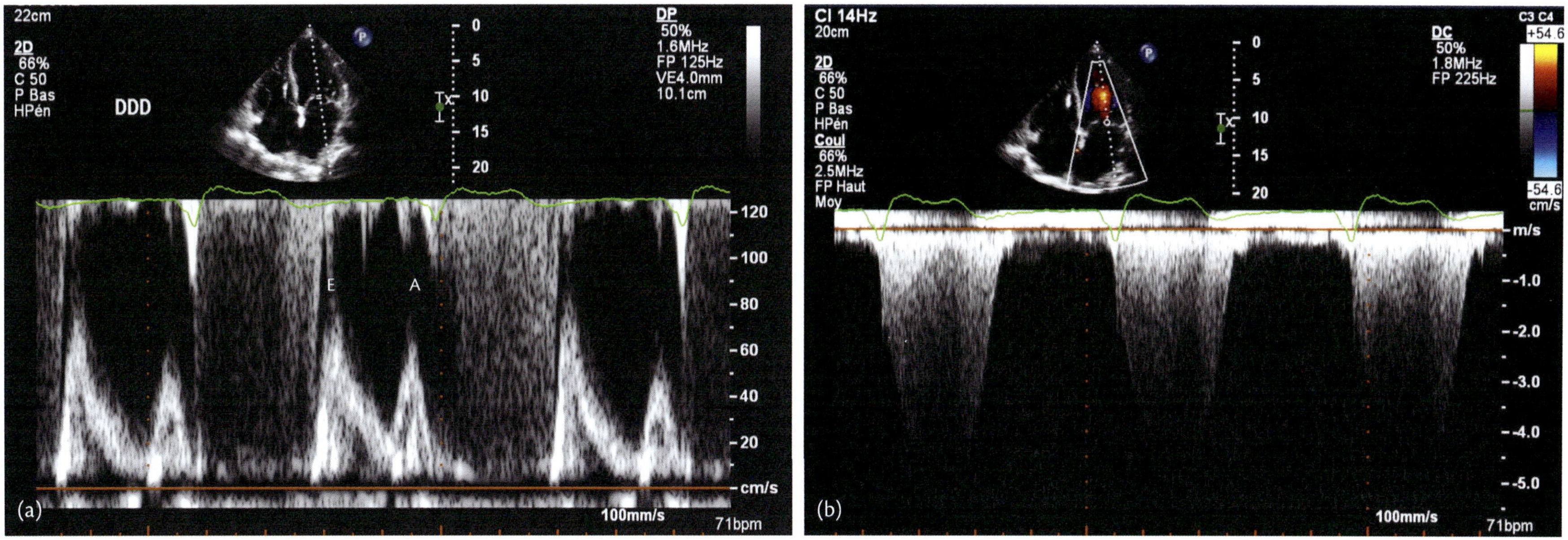

Figure 14.4 Transmitral Doppler flow, following programming to the DDD mode. Note the appearance of an A-wave (a) and disappearance of diastolic mitral regurgitation (b)

Introduction to the case

A 68-year-old patient was implanted with a DDDR pacemaker for sick sinus syndrome. He was asymptomatic. At follow-up, the episode retrieved from the device memory is shown in Figure 15.1. The device settings are shown in Table 15.1.

Table 15.1 Device settings

Mode	ADIR/DDDR
Lower rate	50bpm
Upper rate	120bpm
Adaptive AVI	140–80ms
Paced AV offset	+65ms
AVB I switch	Rest plus exercise
PR long max	350ms (AS–VS) and 450ms (AP–VS)
PR long min	250ms (AS–VS) and 350ms (AP–VS)
Pause max	3s
Atrial ouput (bipolar)	2.5V@0.35ms
Ventricular output (bipolar)	2.5V@0.35ms
Atrial sensitivity (bipolar)	0.4mV
Ventricular sensitivity (bipolar)	2.0mV
PVAB	150ms

Question

Figure 15.1 Stored EGM episode

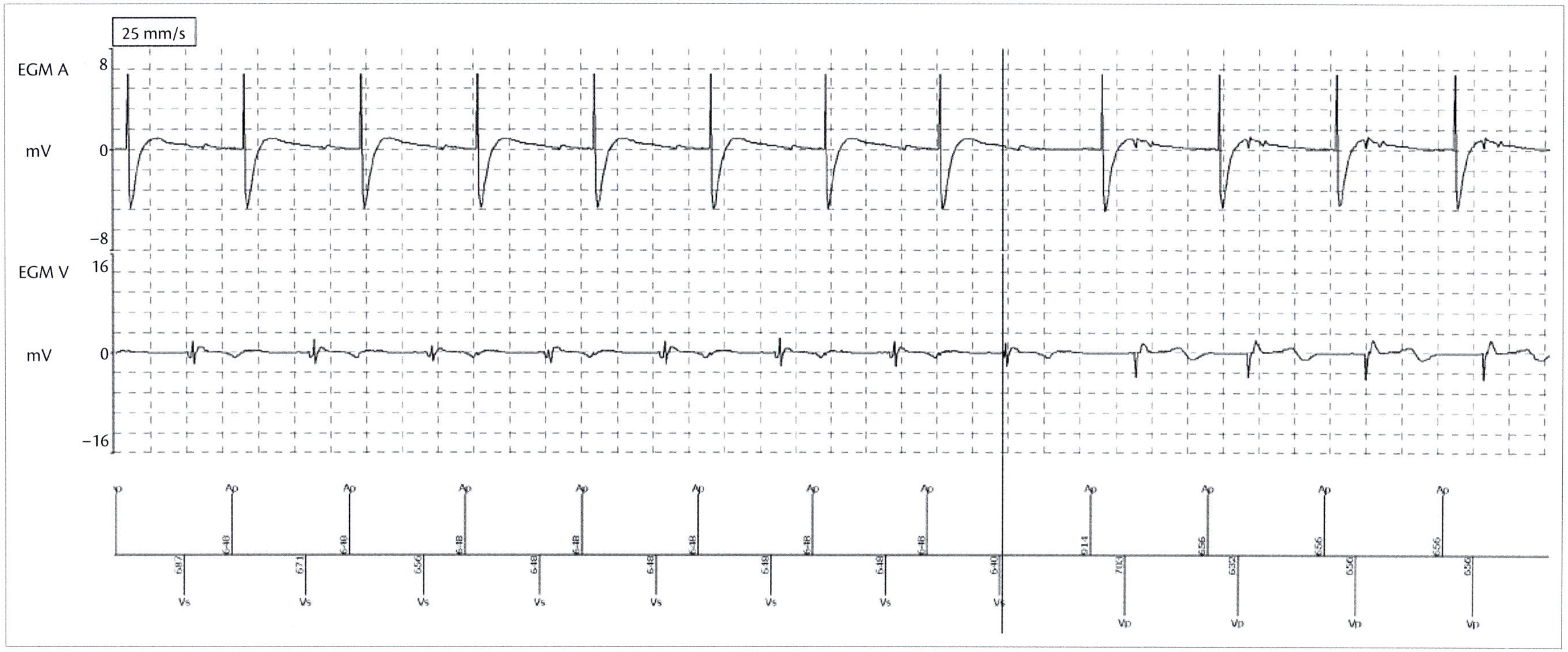

What do you observe?

A AV hysteresis

B ADIR to DDDR mode due to AVB I

C ADIR to DDDR mode due to AVB II

D ADIR to DDDR mode due to pause

Answer

B ADIR to DDDR mode due to AVB I

Figure 15.2 Annotated stored EGM episode

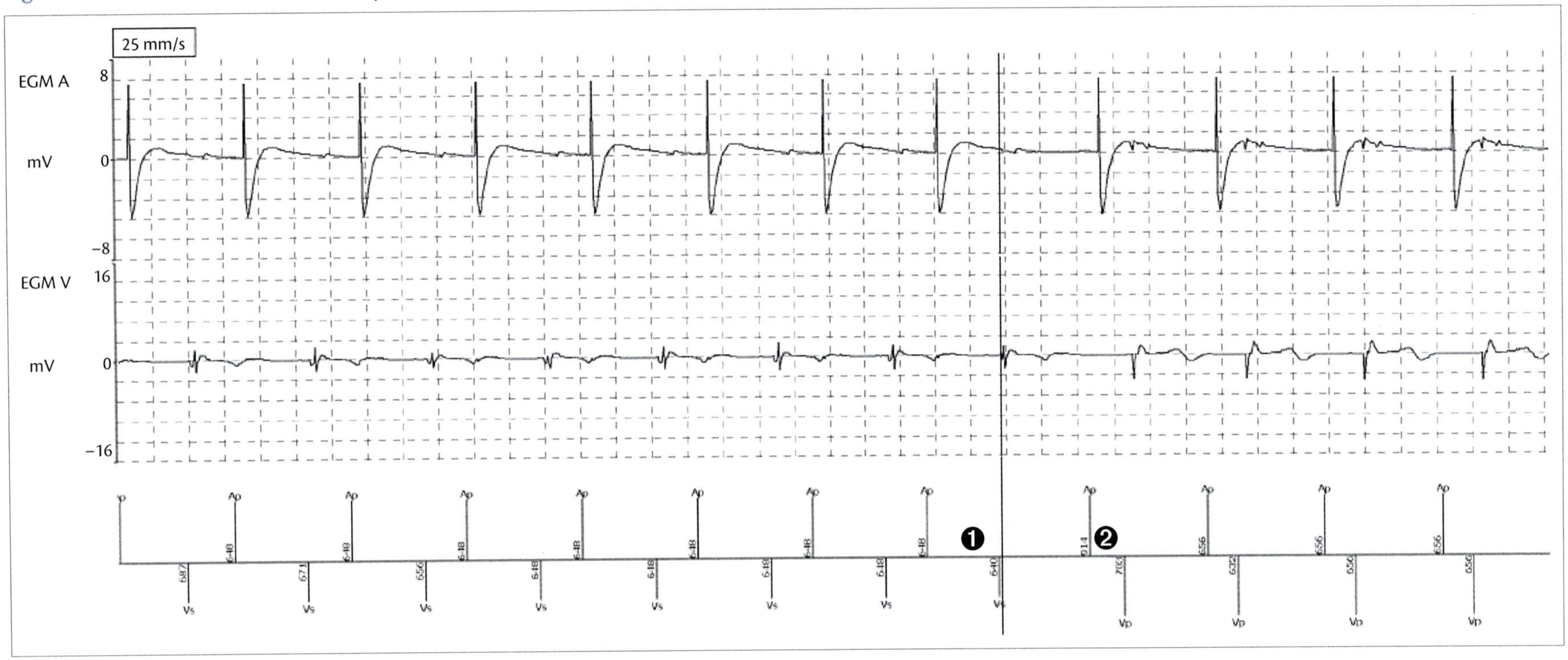

This is an example (Figure 15.2) of the first-degree AV block criterion of this Sorin device that is occurring during exercise (as the pacing rate is sensor-driven at 92bpm).

❶ The device detects long AP–VS intervals (the cut-offs are programmable and set, in this case, to >350–450ms, depending on the sensor-driven rate, and can be measured here at about 400ms).

❷ The AVI then reverts to the programmed value (which is rate-dependent and measured here at about 160ms).

Comment

Avoiding 'P on T' with the ADI(R)/DDD(R) mode

This device has an evolved AV management algorithm that switches from ADI(R) to DDD(R), based upon three criteria:

1 AV block (two consecutive or 3/12 blocked P waves)
2 ventricular pause (programmable to 2, 3, or 4s)
3 long PR intervals.

In order to avoid unduly long PR intervals that are usually allowed by the ADI(R)/DDD(R) mode, this device has a first-degree AV block criterion. A maximum PR interval can be set (200–450ms, with the default value of 350ms and an additional 100ms for AP–VS intervals, as in this case). If six consecutive cycles have intervals which are greater than these thresholds, the device switches from the ADI(R) to the DDD(R) mode, in order to avoid the 'P on T' phenomenon observed in Case 14.

Introduction to the case

The same patient, as for Case 15, had an additional episode stored in the device memory (shown in Figure 16.1). The counters indicated <1% of VP. The device settings are shown in Table 16.1.

Table 16.1 Device settings

Mode	ADIR/DDDR
Lower rate	50bpm
Upper rate	120bpm
Adaptive AVI	140–80ms
Paced AV offset	+65ms
AVB I switch	Rest plus exercise
PR long max	350ms (AS–VS) and 450ms (AP–VS)
PR long min	250ms (AS–VS) and 350ms (AP–VS)
Pause max	3s
Atrial ouput (bipolar)	2.5V@0.35ms
Ventricular output (bipolar)	2.5V@0.35ms
Atrial sensitivity (bipolar)	0.4mV
Ventricular sensitivity (bipolar)	2.0mV
PVAB	150ms

Question

Figure 16.1 EGM of stored episode

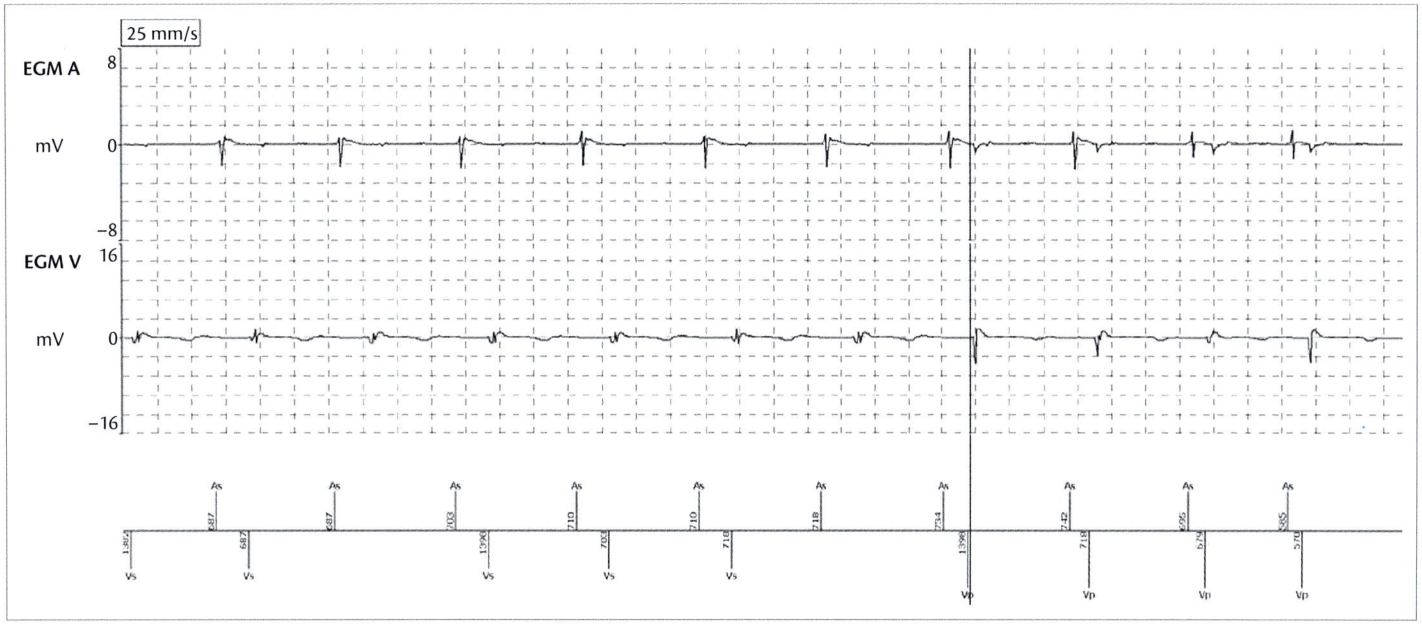

What do you observe?

A ADIR to DDDR mode due to pause

B ADIR to DDDR mode due to AVB I

C ADIR to DDDR mode due to AVB III

D ADIR to DDDR mode due to ventricular undersensing

Answer

D **ADIR to DDDR mode due to ventricular undersensing**

Figure 16.2 Annotated EGM of stored episode

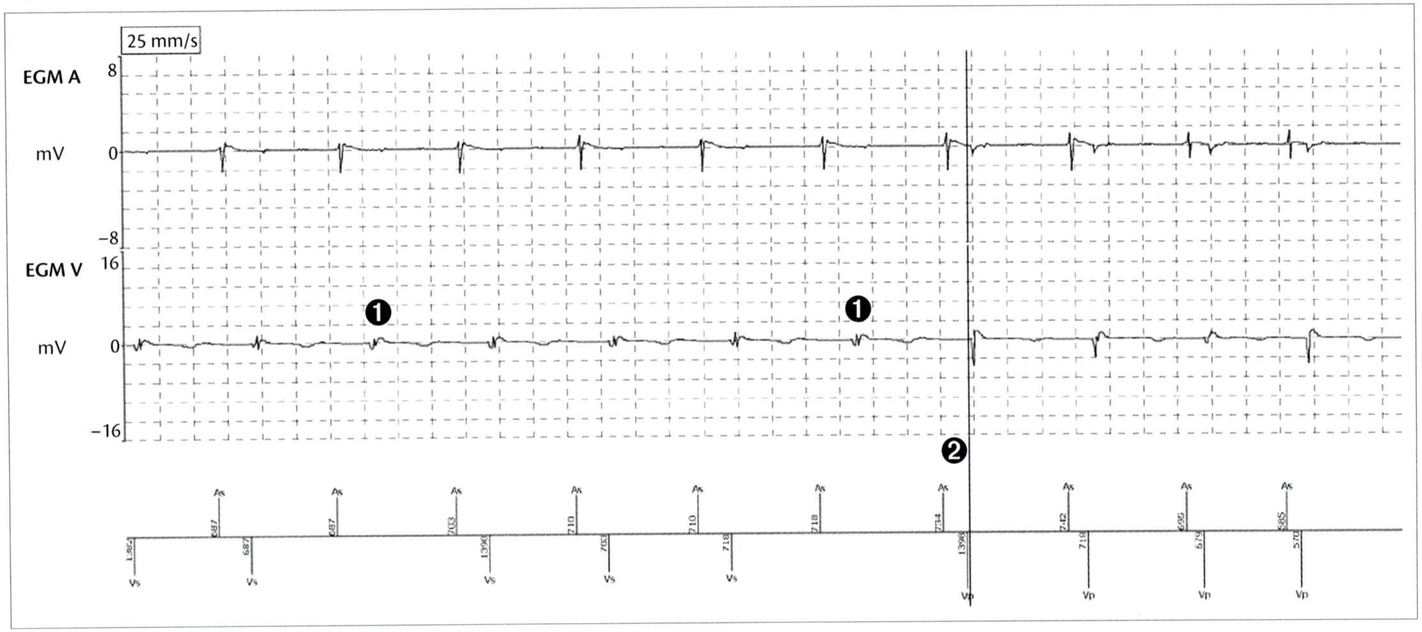

❶ A ventricular event can be observed on the EGM in these two beats but is not sensed by the device (Figure 16.2). The scale is shown on the left and confirms the low amplitude of the ventricular EGM. R-wave undersensing mimics AVB.

❷ After 3/12 undersensed R-waves (a 3rd event occurred before the EGM recording), the device switches from an ADIR to a DDDR pacing mode, based upon the AVB II criterion.

Comments

Misdiagnosis of atrioventricular block by ventricular undersensing

Ventricular undersensing occurred rarely in this patient (few ADIR/DDDR mode switches were stored in the device memory, with <1% VP), and the histograms, shown in Figure 16.3, indicated that R-wave amplitude was usually satisfactory. The R-wave amplitude during device follow-up was measured at 8.2mV, but nevertheless the sensitivity was increased slightly from 2.0mV to 1.8mV.

Figure 16.3 Histograms of sensing amplitude for conducted R-waves (a) and PVCs (b)

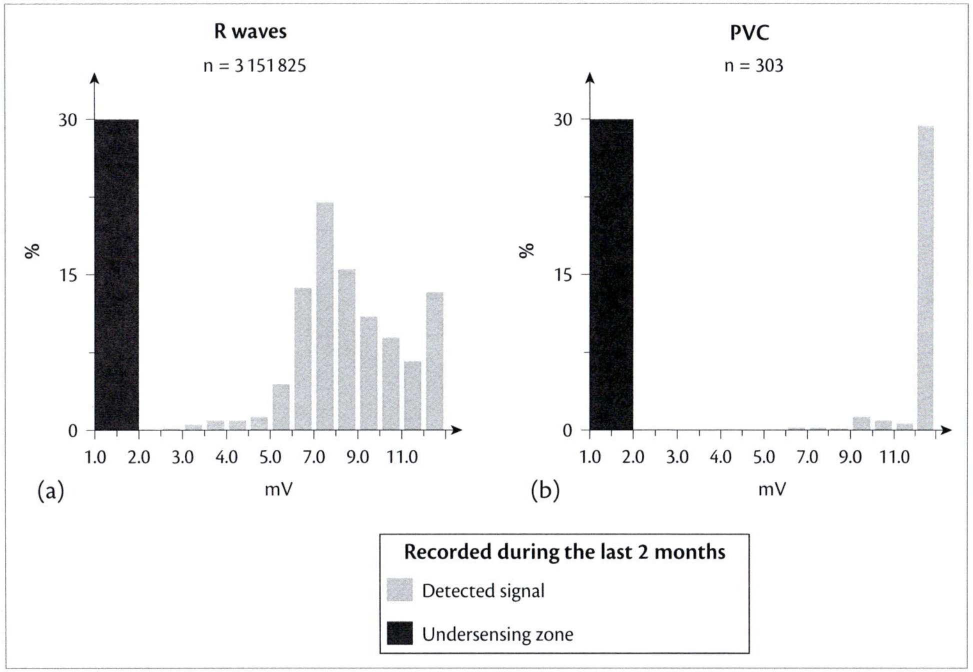

Introduction to the case

A patient was implanted with a dual-chamber pacemaker for intermittent AV block. An ECG was recorded at follow-up and is shown in Figure 17.1. The patient was asymptomatic. Device settings are shown in Table 17.1.

Table 17.1 Device settings

Mode	DDD
Lower rate	60bpm
Upper rate	120bpm
Atrial output (unipolar)	2.5V@0.4ms
Ventricular output (unipolar)	2.5V@0.4ms
Paced AVI	200ms
Sensed AVI	180ms
Atrial sensitivity (bipolar)	0.5mV
Ventricular sensitivity (bipolar)	2.5mV

Question

Figure 17.1 ECG recorded at follow-up

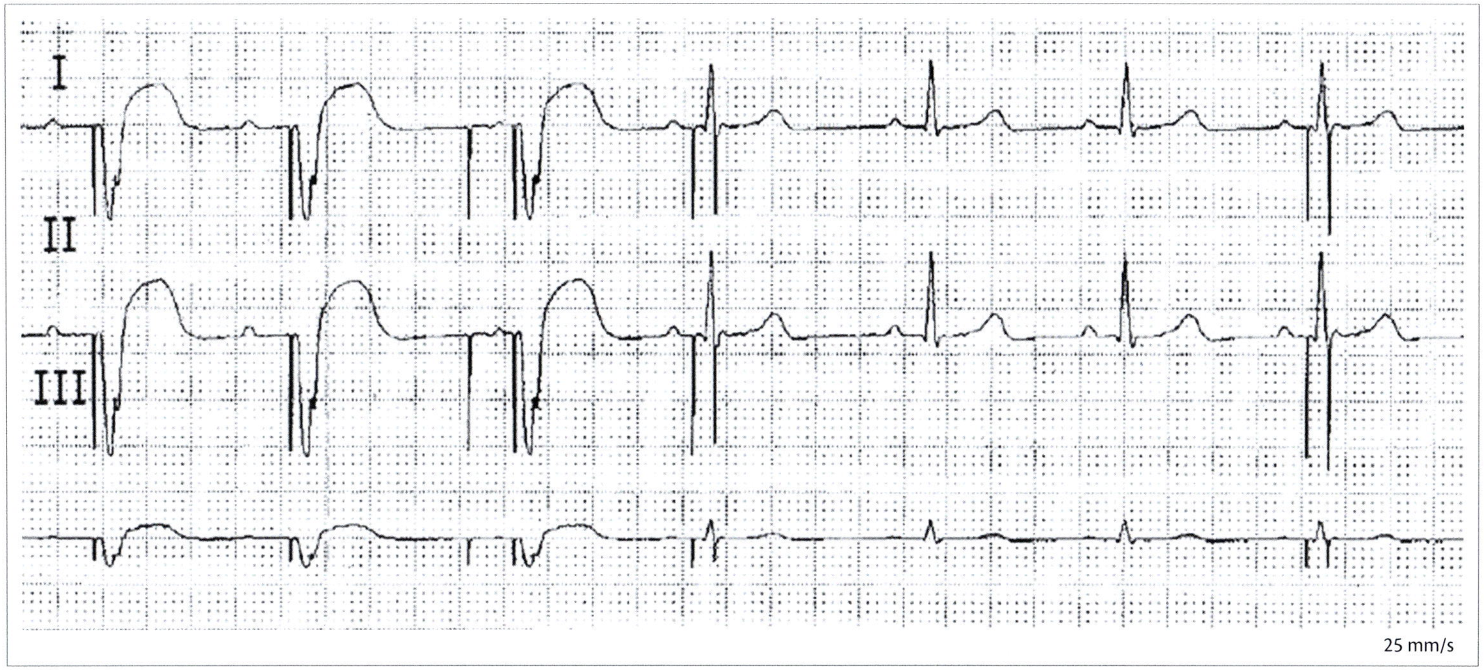

Courtesy of Mr T Bruggemann

Explain the variable AVIs.

A Sense compensation

B Rate-adaptive AVIs

C Crosstalk

D Ventricular safety pacing

Answer

D **Ventricular safety pacing**

Figure 17.2 Annotated ECG recorded at follow-up

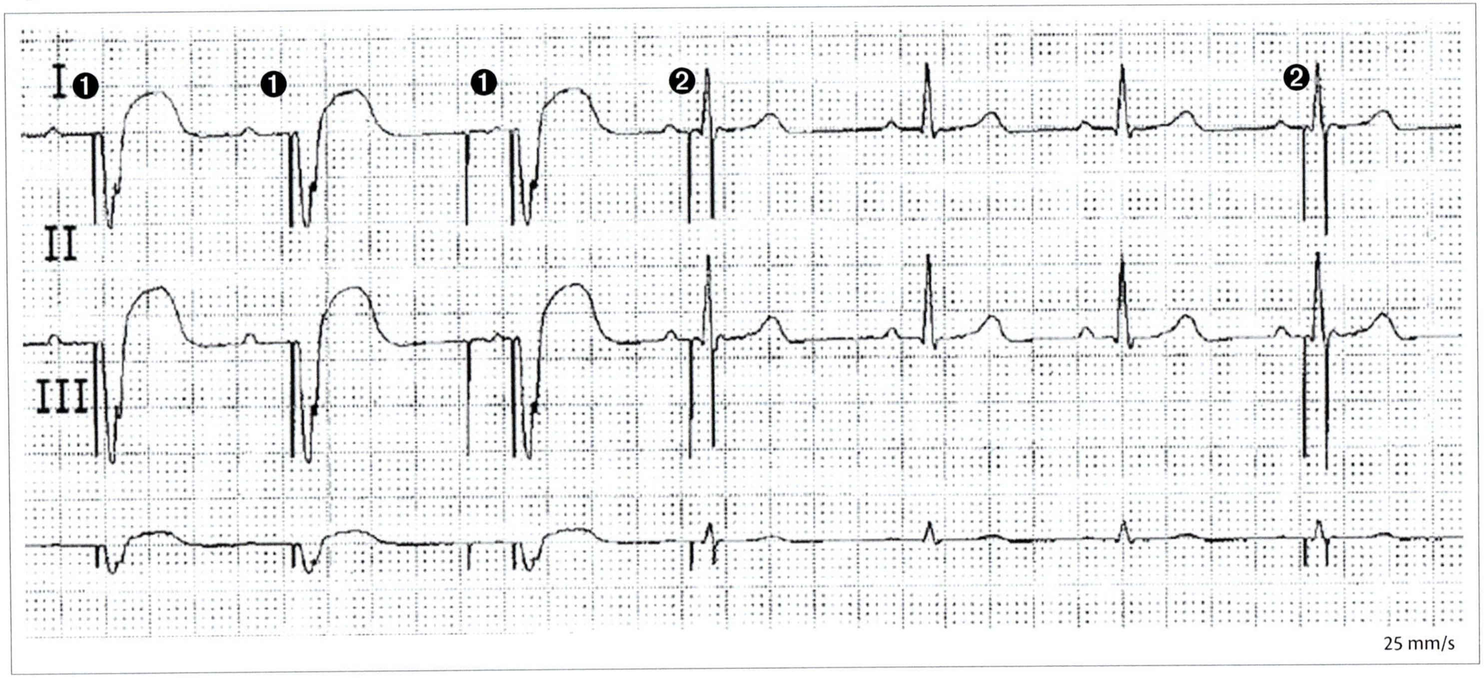

Courtesy of Mr T Bruggemann

❶ The 1st three cycles show usual pacemaker behaviour (Figure 17.2).

❷ The 4th and last cycle show atrial undersensing, with an atrial spike occurring after the P-wave. There is intrinsic AV conduction, with sensing of the conducted QRS shortly after the atrial spike in the ventricular safety pacing window. This leads to ventricular safety pacing at the end of the window of 100ms following AP.

Comments

Ventricular safety pacing

Ventricular safety pacing (Figure 17.3) is a feature designed to avoid the ill effect of AV crosstalk, which is a potentially lethal condition in pacemaker-dependent patients with complete heart block. After a paced atrial event (and not an AS event), if ventricular sensing occurs (after the PAVB) within a window of 90–120ms (depending on the manufacturer), the device delivers ventricular pacing at the end of the window. This will ensure the absence of asystole, if crosstalk had indeed occurred. In the event of the ventricular sensing being due to intrinsic AV conduction (which will not occur usually at such short intervals, unless there is another problem such as atrial undersensing, as in this example) or due to a VPB, the ventricular spike will fall during the myocardial refractory period, resulting in pseudofusion, which is harmless.

Figure 17.3 Schematic representation of ventricular safety pacing due to noise in the ventricular channel (VS)

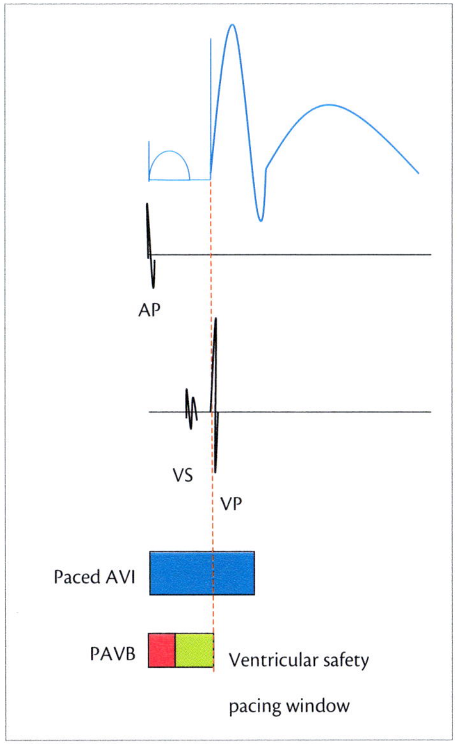

Introduction to the case

A patient with chronic AF and bradycardia was implanted with a single-chamber pacemaker. A ventricular high-rate episode was retrieved from the device memory and is shown in Figure 18.1. The device settings are shown in Table 18.1.

Table 18.1 Device settings

Pacing mode	VVIR
Lower rate	55bpm
Upper rate	130bpm
Ventricular output (bipolar)	2.5V@0.4ms
Ventricular sensitivity (bipolar)	2.8mV
VRP	330ms

Question

Figure 18.1 Ventricular high-rate episode EGM retrieved from the device memory

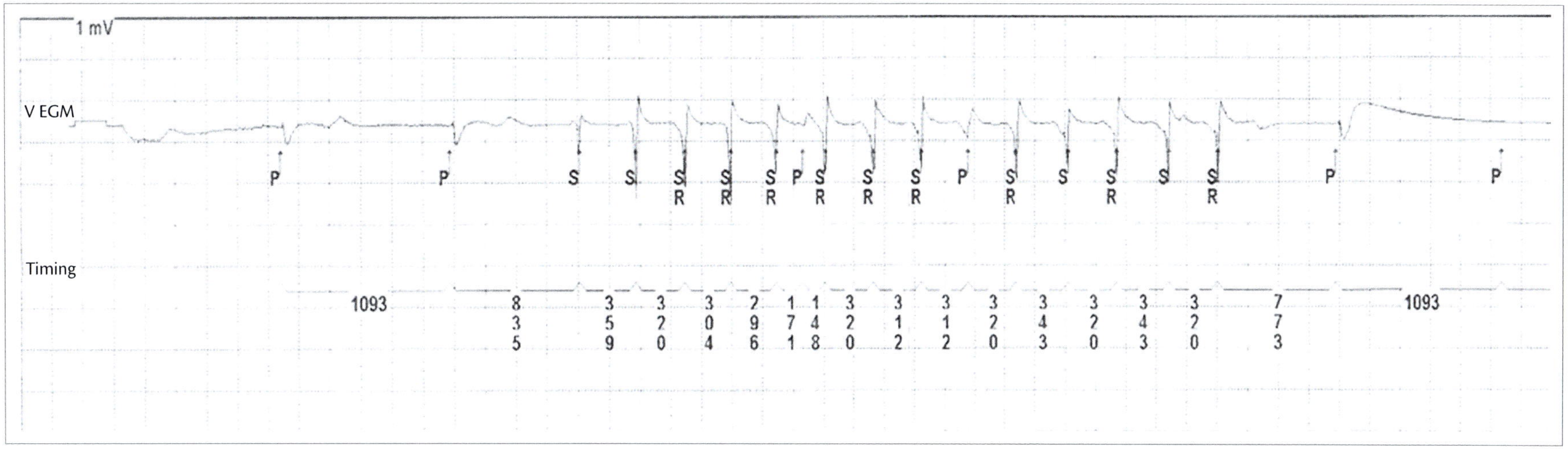

Courtesy of Dr A Menafoglio

Why does the pacemaker continue to pace during the ventricular high-rate episode?

A Noise reversion

B Ventricular rate smoothing

C Ventricular safety pacing

D Ventricular undersensing

Answer

A Noise reversion

Figure 18.2 Annotated ventricular high-rate episode EGM retrieved from the device memory

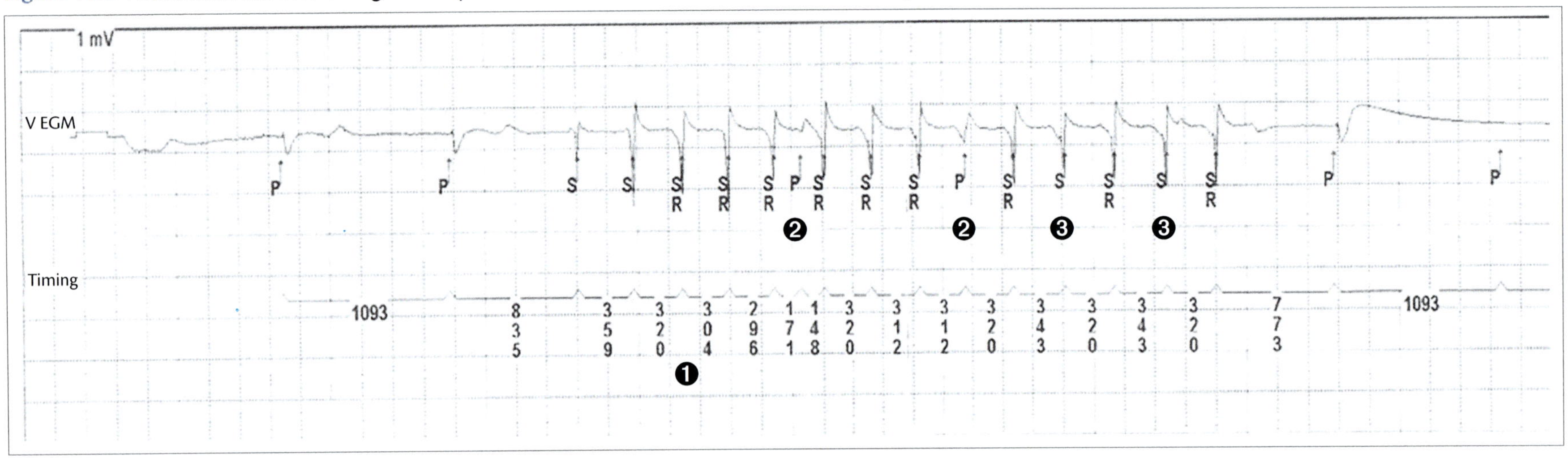

Courtesy of Dr A Menafoglio

The EGM in Figure 18.2 shows non-sustained VT with asynchronous ventricular pacing.

❶ All sensed ventricular events with a cycle length shorter than 330ms fall within the VRP and are classified as sensed refractory (SR) events.

❷ Repeated SR events trigger the noise reversion mode, resulting in asynchronous ventricular pacing at the baseline rate (55bpm).

❸ Cycles that are longer than 330ms are classified as sensed events (S) and interrupt the noise reversion mode.

Comments

Ventricular noise reversion

This is a safety feature that is activated in case of repeated detection of ventricular refractory events or very high-rate atrial events, which may be either tachyarrhythmia or noise (e.g. electromagnetic interference). In order to protect the patients from asystole, in the latter case resulting from inhibition of pacing, the device delivers asynchronous stimuli at the baseline rate. This may be interpreted erroneously as undersensing when visualizing spikes on the surface ECG. Asynchronous ventricular pacing on the T-wave may be proarrhythmic. However, noise is usually of short duration, limiting the risk to the patient.

Introduction to the case

A 72-year-old patient underwent implantation of a DDD pacemaker for paroxysmal complete AV block. The patient experienced syncope on the ward 30min after the intervention. The rhythm strip during the syncopal event is shown in Figure 19.1. The device settings are shown in Table 19.1.

Table 19.1 Device settings

Pacing mode	DDD
Lower rate	60bpm
Upper rate	120bpm
Atrial output (bipolar)	2.5V@0.4ms
Ventricular output (bipolar)	2.5V@0.4ms
Atrial sensitivity (bipolar)	0.4mV
Ventricular sensitivity (bipolar)	2.8mV
Paced AV delay	160ms
Sense compensation	40ms
PVARP	Auto

Question

Figure 19.1 Rhythm strip recorded on the ward during syncope

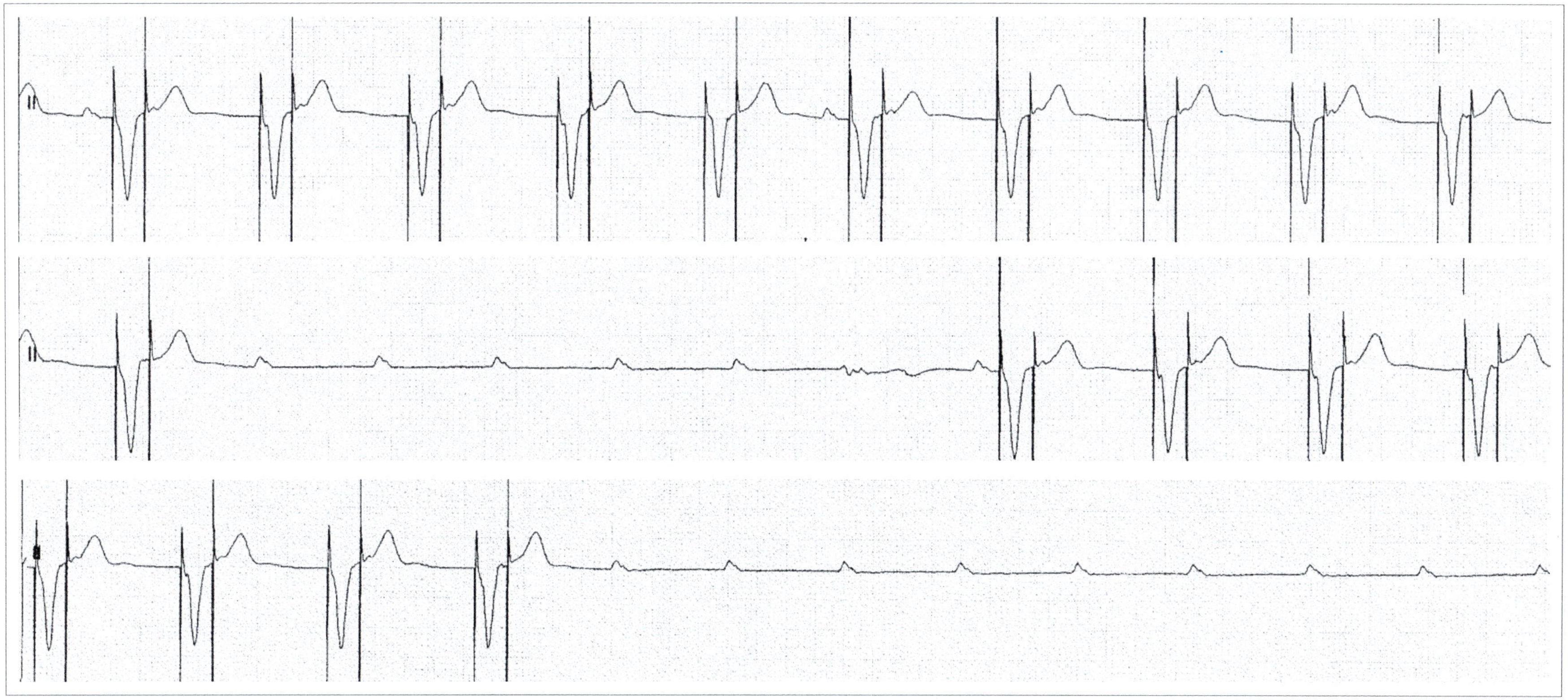

What is the problem?

A Atrial lead dislodged to the ventricle

B Ventricular lead dislodged to the atrium

C Atrial/ventricular lead switch on the header

D Ventricular oversensing

Answer

C Atrial/ventricular lead switch on the header

Figure 19.2 Annotated rhythm strip recorded on the ward during syncope

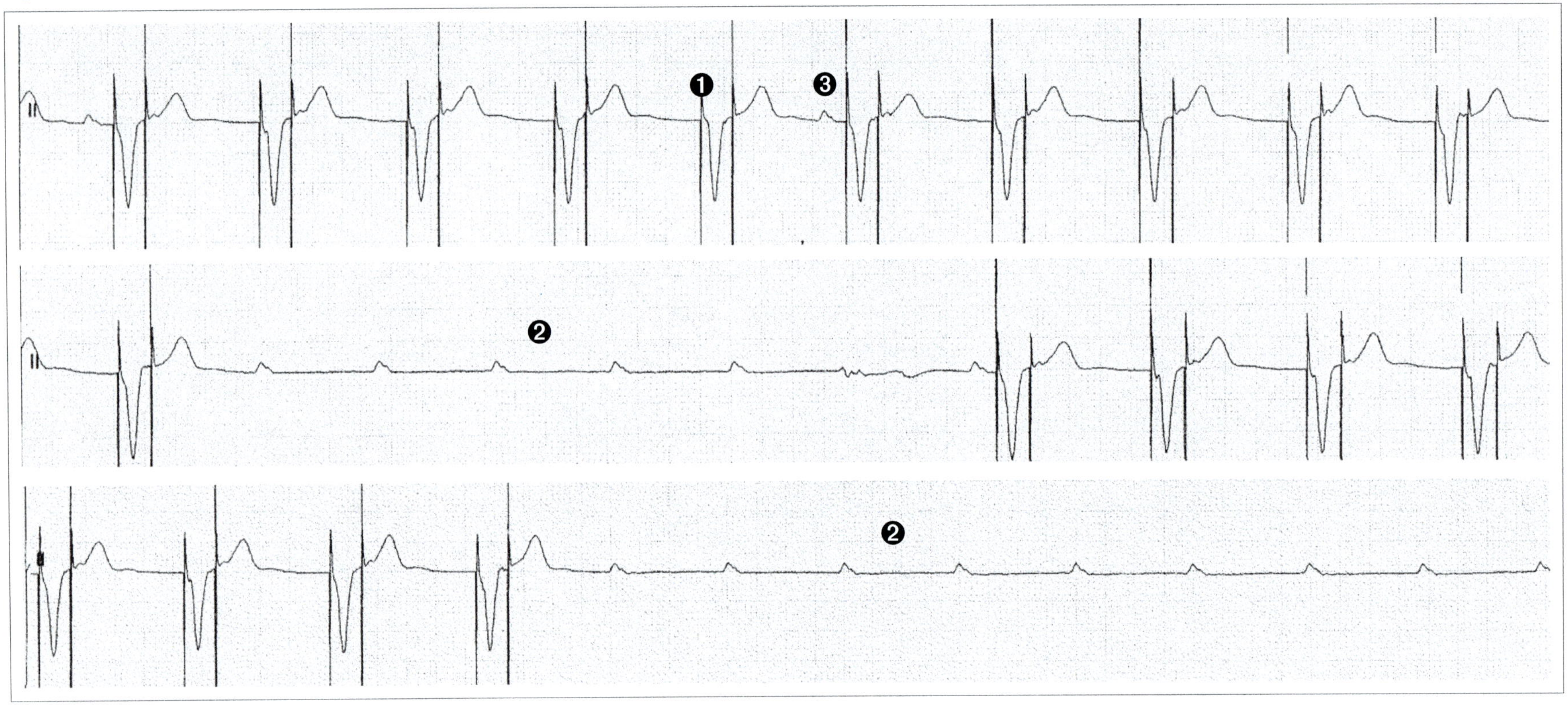

❶ The 1st spike, delivered by the atrial channel, entrains the ventricle (Figure 19.2). This may only result from A or C.

❷ Ventricular pacing is being inhibited by the P-waves, ruling out B (there needs to be a lead in the atrium). The P-waves are sensed in the ventricular channel at a rate that is faster than the pacing rate, thereby repeatedly inhibiting pacing in both channels (i.e. each P-wave sensed in the ventricular channel will trigger a VA interval, before the end of which a new ventricular sensed event will occur due to the next P-wave).

❸ Inhibition of ventricular pacing by the P-waves is intermittent (and absent here), as the sensitivity setting of the ventricular channel is similar to the amplitude of the P-waves.

Comments

Accidental atrial/ventricular lead switch

Atrial and ventricular switch on the header is a potentially lethal mistake that may occur, even to experienced implanters during a moment of distraction (as it did to the cardiac surgeon who performed this intervention). Operators often leave the atrial and ventricular crocodile clips fastened to the respective leads after testing and until insertion into the header, in order to avoid having to identify the leads by their serial numbers. A useful habit is to check always the rhythm monitor as soon as the leads are connected, in order to verify proper device function (this will, however, not be useful if the patient is in normal sinus rhythm). The advent of pacemakers and implantable cardioverter–defibrillators (ICDs) equipped with wireless telemetry also helps identify this issue per-operatively.

Introduction to the case

A patient implanted with a dual-chamber pacemaker complained of palpitations. During the atrial threshold test performed in the DDD mode, a tachycardia was triggered that reproduced the symptoms and is shown in Figure 20.1. The device settings are shown in Table 20.1.

Table 20.1 Device settings

Mode	DDDR
Lower rate	60bpm
UTR	140bpm
Atrial output (bipolar)	2.5V@0.4ms
Ventricular output (bipolar)	2.5V@0.4ms
Atrial sensitivity (bipolar)	0.3mV
Ventricular sensitivity (bipolar)	2.0mV
Sensed AVI	210ms
Paced AVI	250ms
PVAB	150ms
PVARP	150ms

Question

Figure 20.1 EGM recording during the atrial threshold test

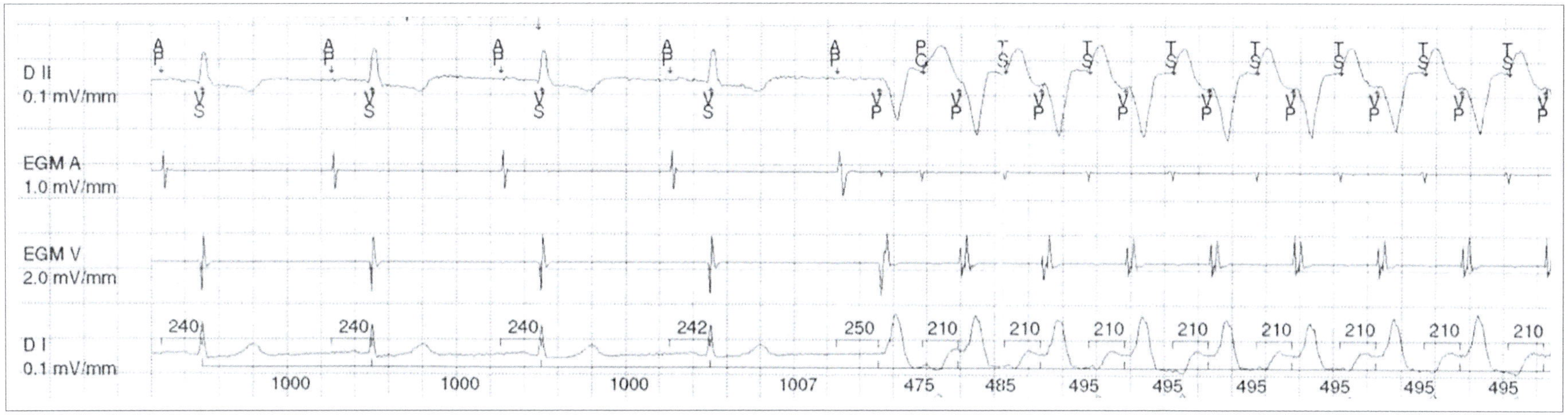

What is the mechanism of the tachycardia?

A AV node re-entrant tachycardia (AVNRT)

B Endless loop tachycardia

C AV re-entrant tachycardia (AVRT)

D Atrial tachycardia

Answer

B Endless loop tachycardia

Figure 20.2 Annotated EGM recording during the atrial threshold test

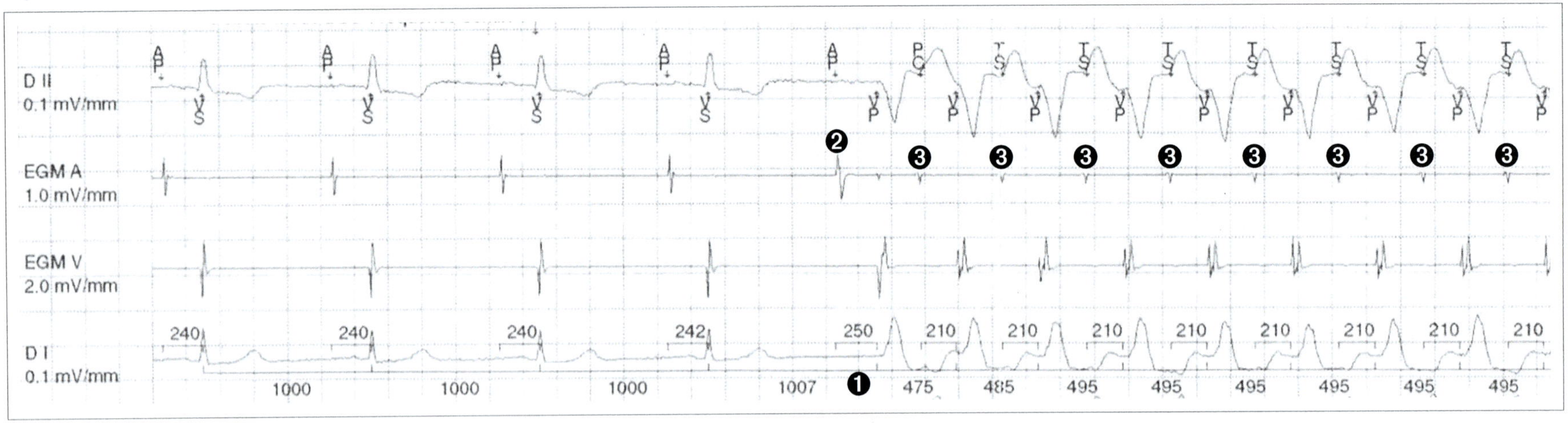

The 1st four atrial paced events (Figure 20.2) capture the atrium, with intrinsic AV conduction.

❶ This atrial paced event results in loss of capture, that is visible on lead I as absence of a P-wave (a low-amplitude P-wave is visible in the previous cycles). Ventricular pacing occurs at the end of the paced AVI of 250ms.

❷ The atrial EGM has a similar morphology, with or without atrial capture in this case, and is not very useful for determining the threshold here.

❸ Ventricular capture is followed by retrograde conduction, visible on the atrial channel and sensed by the device, as it falls outside the PVARP of 150ms. The 1st event is annotated on the marker channel as 'PC' (premature contraction), and the following events as 'TS' (tachycardia sense). These AS events trigger an AVI of 210ms (corresponding to the sensed AVI), at the end of which ventricular pacing occurs, resulting again in retrograde VA conduction and perpetuating endless loop tachycardia.

Comments

Endless loop tachycardia

Endless loop tachycardia is one form of pacemaker-mediated tachycardia. An easy way of testing whether this may be an issue with current settings in a device is to programme subthreshold atrial pacing output (or to perform an atrial threshold test, as in this example, although, in some devices, refractory periods are altered during threshold tests).

It requires:

1. a dual-chamber device set in a tracking mode (DDD or VDD) with ventricular capture and sensing of retrograde P-waves
2. the presence of VA conduction
3. a retrograde conduction interval greater than PVARP.

It is favoured by:

1. a short PVARP (more likely to have a retrograde P-wave falling outside the PVARP)
2. slow retrograde conduction (more likely to have a retrograde P-wave falling outside the PVARP)
3. high atrial sensitivity (more likely to sense retrograde P-waves)
4. low safety margin for atrial capture (leading to atrial non-capture)
5. long programmed AVIs in patients with AV block (this allows the conduction tissue to recover from the preceding event and be depolarized by retrograde conduction)
6. VDD programming with a sinus rate slower than the baseline rate.

It may be initiated by:

1. atrial non-capture (as in this example)
2. VPBs (the most frequent trigger)
3. atrial oversensing (initiating VP that is not preceded by a true atrial event, which, in essence, is similar to a VPB)
4. atrial undersensing (with AP and non-capture shortly after the intrinsic P-wave in a patient with AV block, which equates to a long AVI)
5. atrial premature beat falling outside the PVARP (with AVI extension due to the UTR, which also equates to a long AVI).

It may be terminated by:

1. magnet application (e.g. with initiation of device interrogation)
2. retrograde block: spontaneous, drugs (e.g. adenosine) or carotid sinus massage
3. undersensing of the retrograde P-wave
4. ventricular non-capture
5. atrial premature beat falling in the PVARP (which is therefore not tracked and results in a refractory atrium with retrograde block)
6. VPB (resulting in retrograde block or resetting of the timing cycles)
7. pacemaker algorithms: PVARP extension (Medtronic, Biotronik, Boston Scientific) or withholding ventricular pacing (St-Jude Medical).

It may be prevented by:

1. post-PVC PVARP extension algorithm
2. atrial pace on PVC algorithm (St-Jude Medical)
3. undersensing of retrograde P-waves (adjust sensitivity levels)
4. avoiding programming long AVIs in patients with AV block.

Introduction to the case

A dual-chamber pacemaker was implanted in a patient with sinus node dysfunction. The EGM recorded on the pre-discharge visit is shown in Figure 21.1. The device settings are shown in Table 21.1.

Table 21.1 Device settings

Pacing mode	DDDR
Lower rate	60bpm
Upper rate	120bpm
Atrial output (bipolar)	2.5V@0.4ms
Ventricular output (bipolar)	2.5V@0.4ms
Atrial sensitivity (bipolar)	0.4mV
Ventricular sensitivity (bipolar)	2.8mV
Paced AV delay	150ms
Sense compensation	−30ms

Question

Figure 21.1 Real-time EGM

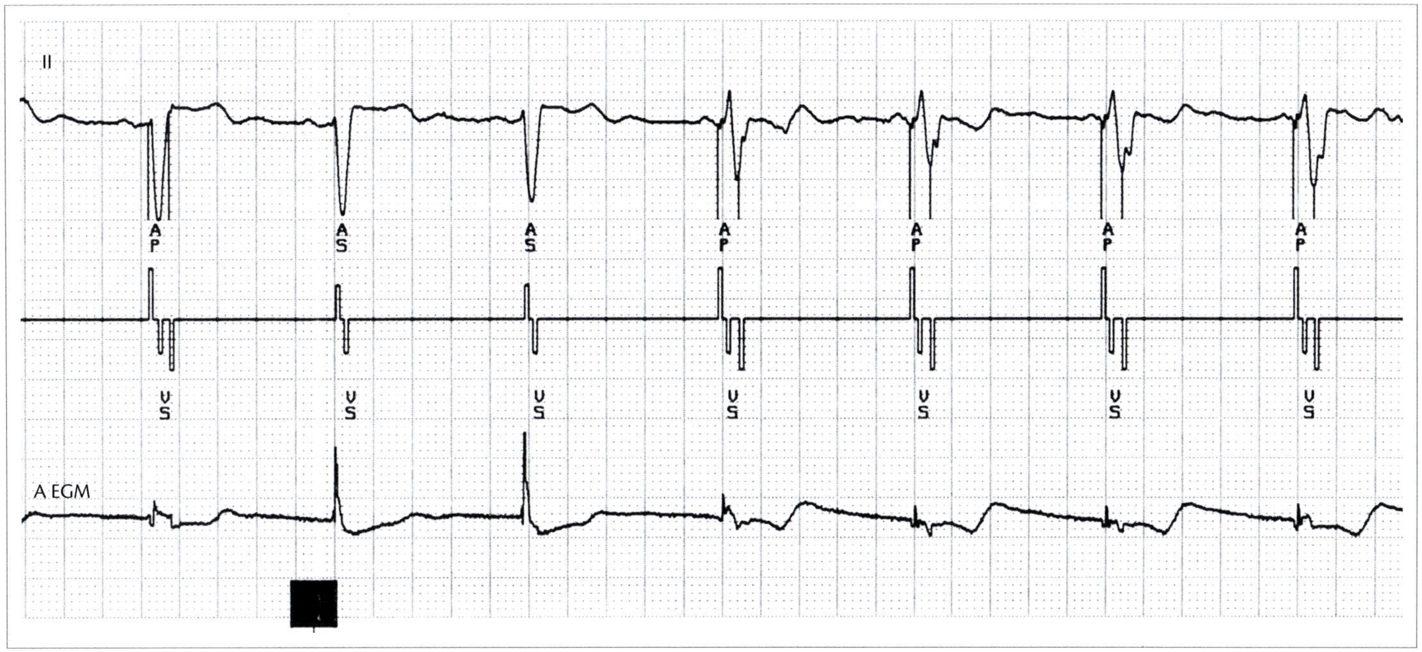

Courtesy of Dr M Anelli-Monti

What is your diagnosis?

A Normal device function

B A/V switch on the header

C Atrial lead dislodged to the ventricle

D Ventricular lead dislodgement

Answer

C **Atrial lead dislodged to the ventricle**

Figure 21.2 Annotated real-time EGM

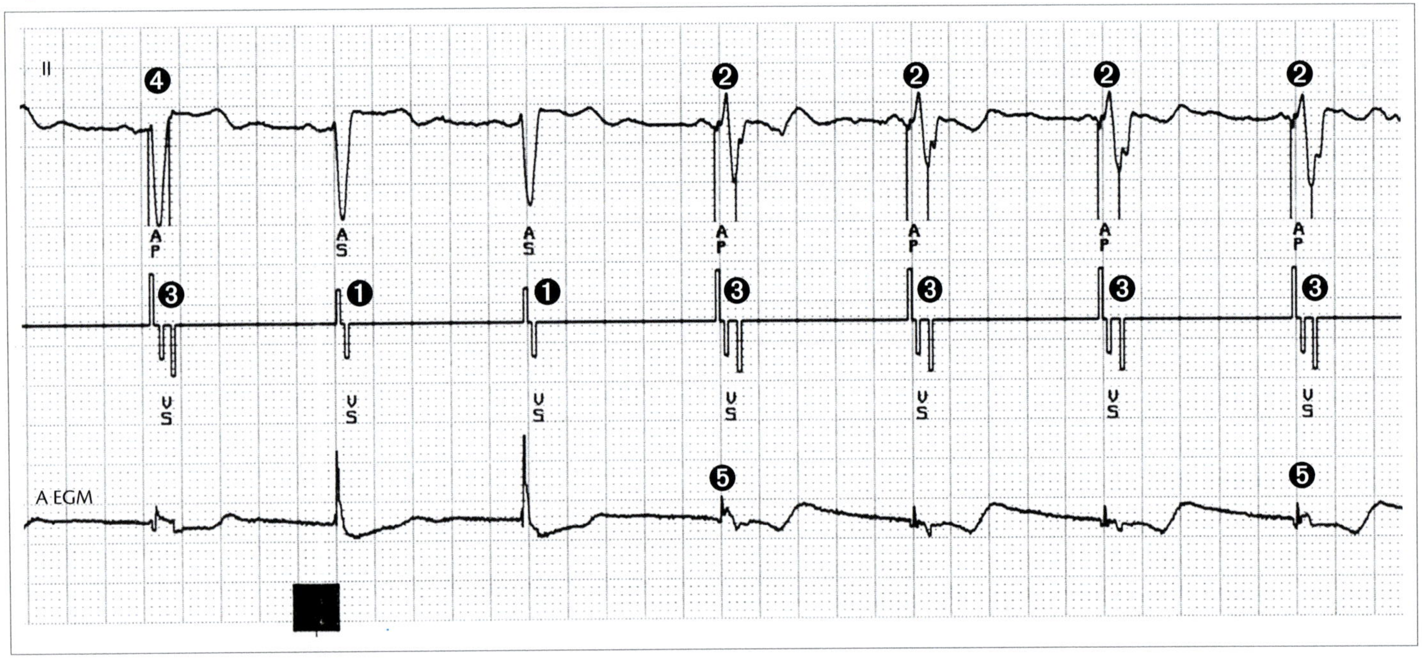

Courtesy of Dr M Anelli-Monti

A number of different elements can be observed in this example (Figure 21.2).

❶ Atrial sensing occurs simultaneously with the QRS complex, and none of the P-waves of the tracing are sensed. Note that ventricular sensing occurs just after 'atrial' sensing and is also simultaneous with the QRS complex. This rules out A/V lead switch.

❷ AP results in ventricular capture.

❸ The marker channel annotation indicates ventricular safety pacing. This occurs due to a VS event being detected in the safety pacing window of 110ms following atrial pacing. Note that no ventricular safety pacing occurs in ❶, due to the absence of this feature following AS events.

❹ This cycle shows ventricular pseudofusion due to intrinsic AV conduction. Note that the EGM morphology on the A channel (recording ventricular activity) is different, compared to the cycles with sensed event (even though the surface QRS is identical), due to differences in filter settings with sensed and paced events.

❺ Varying degrees of ventricular fusion occur during the paced cycles, as can be appreciated by the slightly different EGM morphology and deeper S-waves of the surface QRS of these two cycles (with more contribution of intrinsic conduction, compared to the two cycles in between).

Comments

Atrial lead dislodgement

A chest X-ray was performed and confirmed dislodgement of the atrial lead into the ventricle, as shown in Figure 21.3.

The main differential diagnosis in this case is A/V switch on the header (see Case 19) where atrial sensed and paced events occur simultaneously with the QRS complex. However, in this setting, ventricular safety pacing does not occur, as VA conduction takes longer than the duration of the ventricular safety pacing window, and VS events occur simultaneously with the P-wave (whereas P-waves are never detected in cases where the atrial lead has dislodged).

Figure 21.3 Chest X-ray showing atrial lead dislodgement into the ventricle

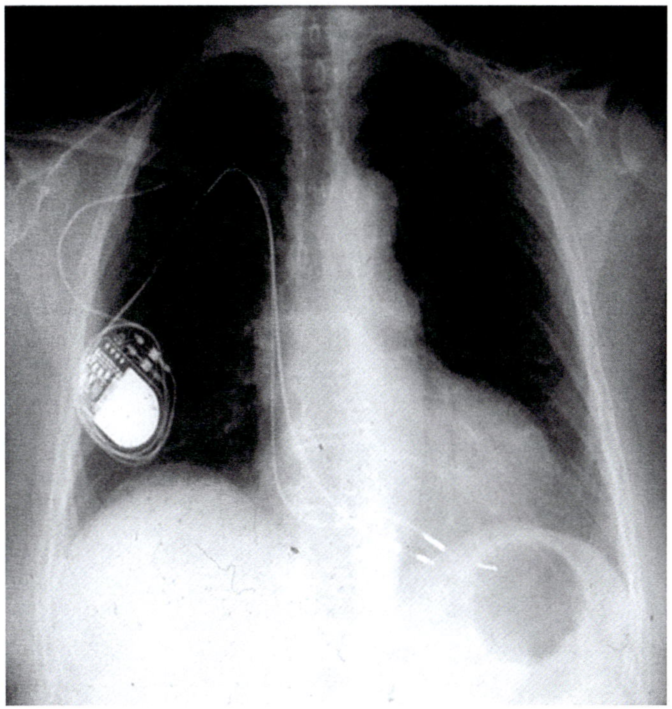

Courtesy of Dr M Anelli-Monti

Introduction to the case

A 45-year-old male had syncope while driving. Carotid sinus massage revealed a 7s sinus pause with malaise. Hypersensitive carotid sinus syndrome was diagnosed, and a dual-chamber pacemaker was implanted. After implantation, carotid sinus massage was repeated, and the patient remained asymptomatic. The EGM during the manoeuvre is shown in Figure 22.1.

Question

Figure 22.1 Real-time EGM recorded during a carotid sinus massage

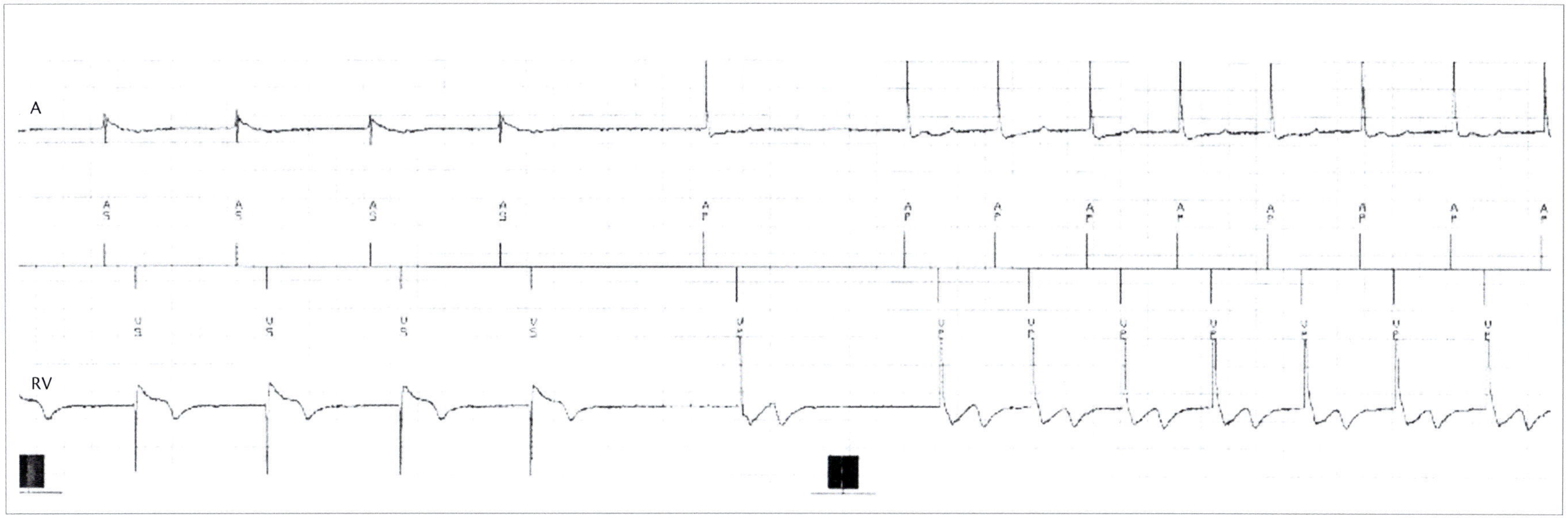

What do you observe?

A Rate drop response

B Atrial overdrive pacing

C Managed ventricular pacing

D Hysteresis

Answer

A **Rate drop response**

Figure 22.2 Annotated real-time EGM recorded during a carotid sinus massage

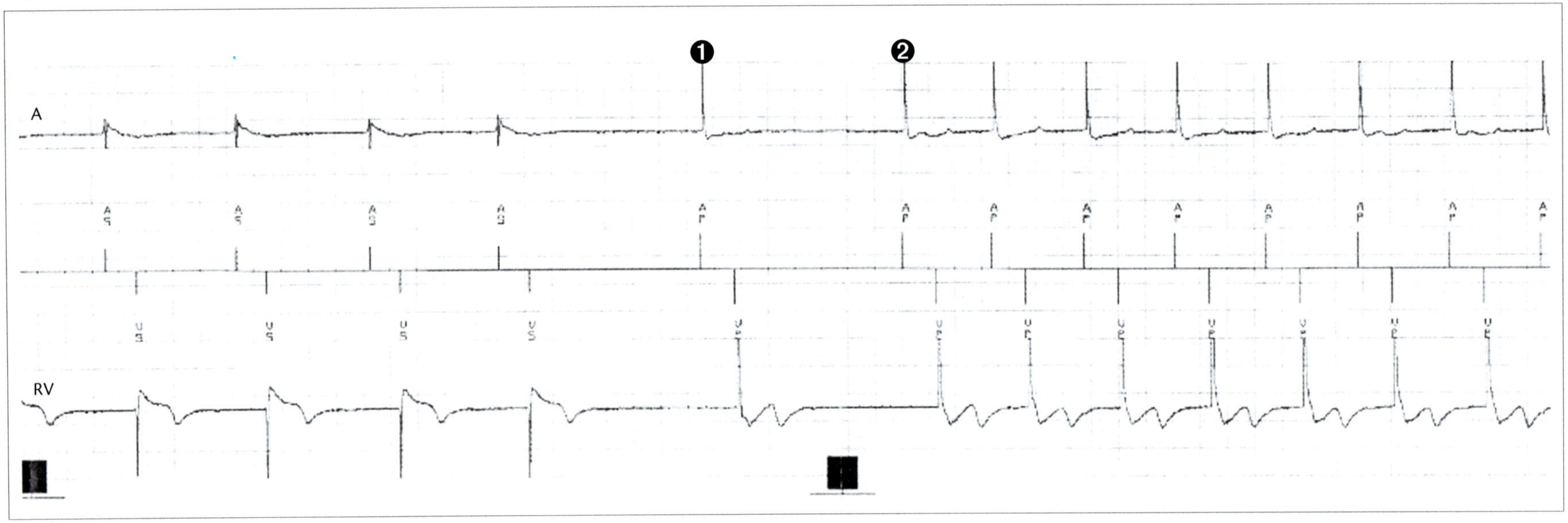

This is an illustration of the rate drop response algorithm (Figure 22.2).

❶ The device paces at the lower rate (40bpm) for two cycles.

❷ Following the drop in heart rate, the device paces at a predetermined rate (here 90bpm) for a programmable duration.

Comments

Rate drop response

Dual-chamber pacemakers are indicated for treatment of hypersensitive carotid sinus syndrome.[1] Specific algorithms detect a sudden fall in heart rate and respond by pacing at a higher rate (either at a set rate or at an average of previous P–P intervals, depending upon the model) for a predetermined duration. In the absence of such an algorithm and in case of persistence of symptoms with standard settings, the device can be programmed with a rapid baseline rate (e.g. 80bpm) and a hysteresis rate as low as possible (e.g. 30bpm). An inconvenience of these settings is possible rapid pacing during periods of increased vagal tone, e.g. during sleep, that may cause symptoms. In a small randomized study in patients with carotid sinus hypersensitivity, no difference in efficacy was found between pacing at VVI 40bpm or DDDR 60–120bpm, with or without a rate drop response algorithm.[2]

References

1. Brignole M, Auricchio A, Baron-Esquivias G, *et al.* 2013 ESC guidelines on cardiac pacing and cardiac resynchronization therapy: the task force on cardiac pacing and resynchronization therapy of the European Society of Cardiology (ESC). Developed in collaboration with the European Heart Rhythm Association (EHRA). *Europace* 2013; **15**: 1070–118.
2. McLeod CJ, Trusty JM, Jenkins SM, *et al.* Method of pacing does not affect the recurrence of syncope in carotid sinus syndrome. *Pacing Clin Electrophysiol* 2012; **35**: 827–33.

Introduction to the case

A 72-year-old man with symptomatic 2:1 AV block was implanted with a dual-chamber pacemaker. During follow-up, a real-time EGM was printed and is shown in Figure 23.1. The device settings are shown in Table 23.1.

Table 23.1 Device settings

Pacing mode	DDD
Lower rate	60bpm
Upper rate	120bpm
Atrial output (bipolar)	2.5V@0.4ms
Ventricular output (bipolar)	2.5V@0.4ms
Atrial sensitivity (bipolar)	0.75mV
Ventricular sensitivity (bipolar)	2.5mV
Paced AV delay (adaptive)	150–80ms
Sense compensation	30ms
PVAB after ventricular pace	120ms
PVARP	250ms
Post-PVC PVARP extension	400ms
Ventricular blanking after atrial pace	40ms
VRP	250ms

Question

Figure 23.1 Real-time EGM

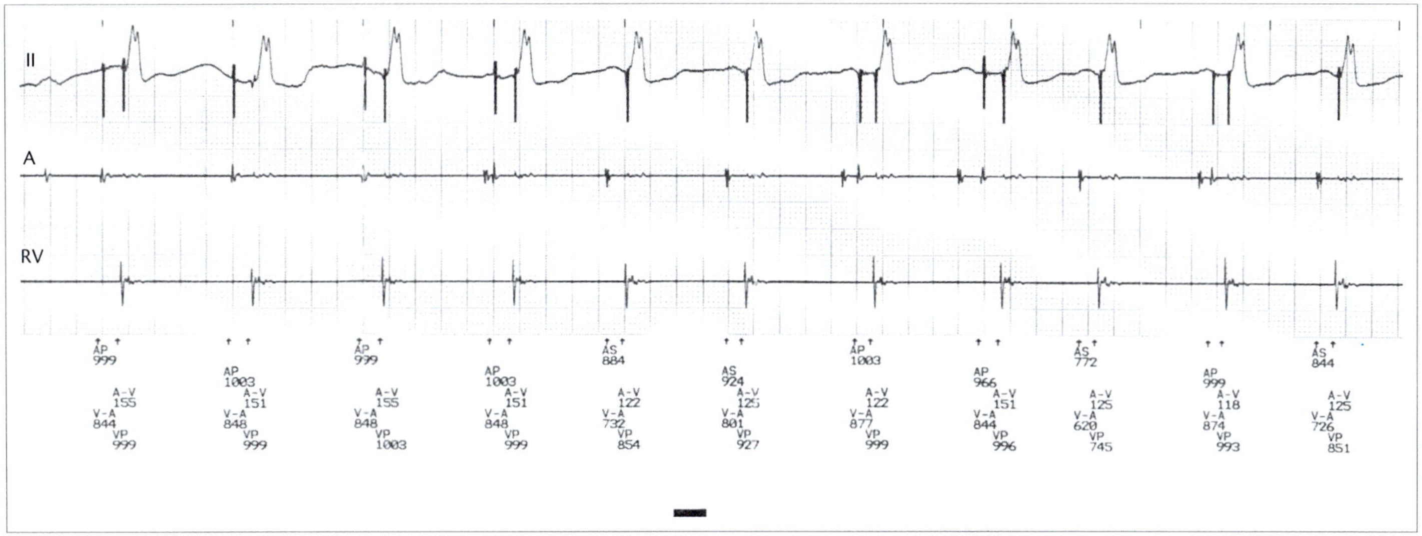

Which of the following is NOT observed?

A Atrial undersensing

B Adaptive AVIs

C Atrial-based timing

D Atrial non-capture

Answer

C **Atrial-based timing**

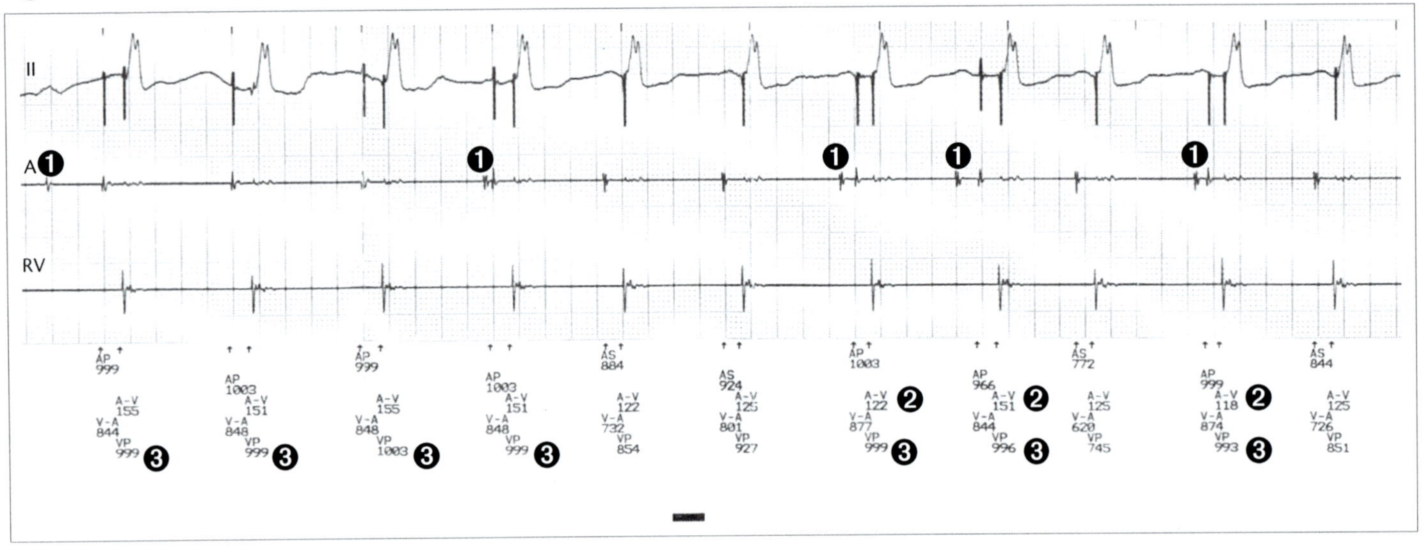

Figure 23.2 Annotated real-time EGM

A number of different observations can be made in Figure 23.2.

❶ Atrial undersensing, which is intermittent and observed for these cycles only (the other cycles have correctly identified AS events). Atrial sensitivity had been left at the nominal value of 0.75mV (and needs to be increased by programming to, e.g. 0.15mV). All the undersensed atrial events, except for the first cycle, lead to functional atrial non-capture (due to the atrium being refractory).

❷ The AVIs are adaptive (and shorter at higher heart rates). In this device, the AVI is based upon the A–A interval of the preceding cycle.

❸ The device is functioning with ventricular-based timing. The V–V intervals correspond to the lower rate of 60bpm (i.e. 1000ms), unless timing is reset by atrial sensing. The AP intervals may however vary. Note that for this cycle, the VA interval has reduced to 844ms in order to accommodate for the increase in AV interval (151ms) and maintain the VP interval close to 1000ms. The slight differences (993–1003ms) are due to the cycles of the device clock.

Comments

Atrial- and ventricular-based timing

Devices function with either atrial-based or ventricular-based timing in the DDD(R) mode, and knowledge of these timing cycles is important for advanced tracing interpretation. Many devices function with atrial-based timing, with a temporary switch to ventricular-based timing rules under certain circumstances (e.g. in the case of a suddenly shortened AVI, VPB, or mode switching). Basically, the Ax–AP intervals (AS–AP or AP–AP sequences) are constant with the former, and the Vx–VP intervals (VS–VP or VP–VP sequences) with the latter. Sensing of intrinsic atrial events and VPBs will reset the timers in both instances. For atrial-based timing, if intrinsic AV conduction occurs, the VA interval is only triggered at the end of the programmed AVI (versus directly after the VS event in case of ventricular-based timing). With ventricular-based timing, VA intervals are constant, as long as the AVIs are not adaptive and the rate is not sensor-driven. In the present case, the VA intervals are variable, due to the adaptive AVIs. Differences in these timing functions are illustrated in Figure 23.3. Note that, with atrial-based timing, the ventricular rate may be slightly below the programmed baseline rate (due to the difference between the sensed and paced AVI). For the same reason, with ventricular-based timing, the atrial rate may be slightly higher than the ventricular rate.

Figure 23.3 Atrial- and ventricular-based timing

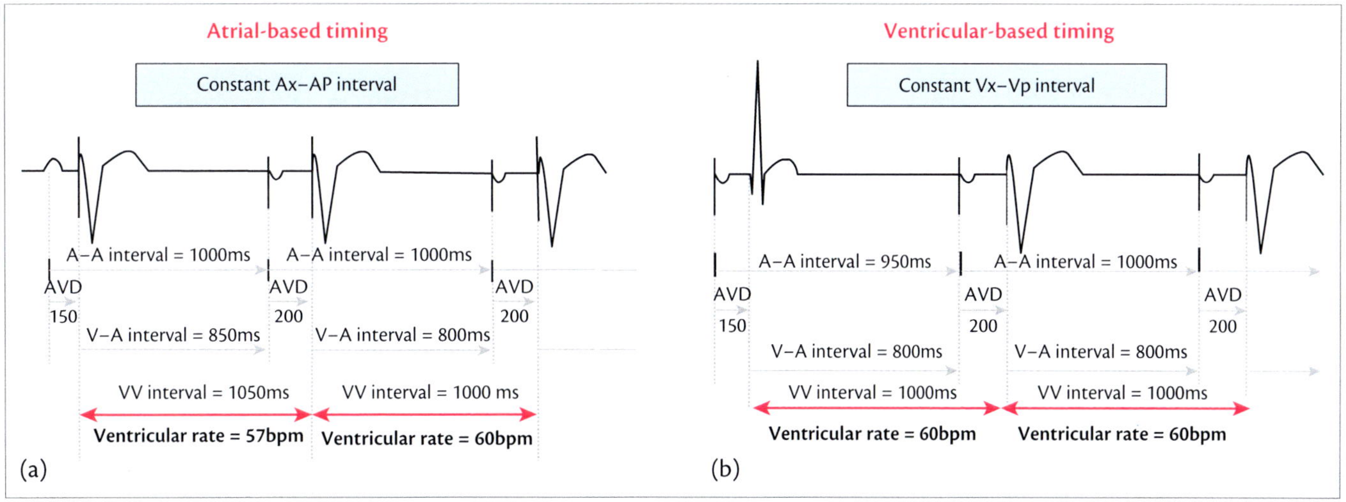

Introduction to the case

A patient with complete AV block and equipped with a dual-chamber pacemaker was seen at follow-up. The lower rate was programmed at 60bpm (see device settings in Table 24.1). The rate histograms are shown in Figure 24.1.

Table 24.1 Device settings

Pacing mode	DDDR
Lower rate	60bpm
Upper rate	120bpm
Atrial output (bipolar)	2.5V@0.4ms
Ventricular output (bipolar)	2.5V@0.4ms
Atrial sensitivity (bipolar)	0.4mV
Ventricular sensitivity (bipolar)	2.8mV
Paced AV delay	150ms
Sense compensation	−30ms

Question

Figure 24.1 Rate histograms

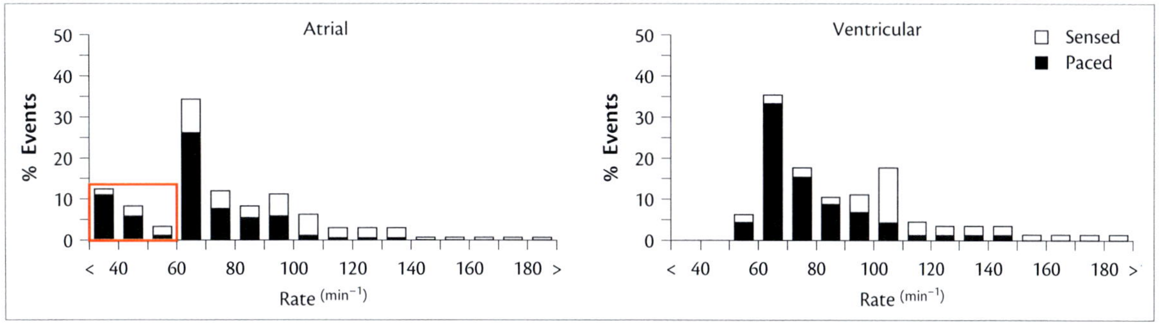

How do you explain AP at below the programmed lower rate (red square)?

A Atrial oversensing

B Atrial undersensing

C VPBs

D Hysteresis

Answer

C **VPBs**

Figure 24.2 Annotated real-time EGM

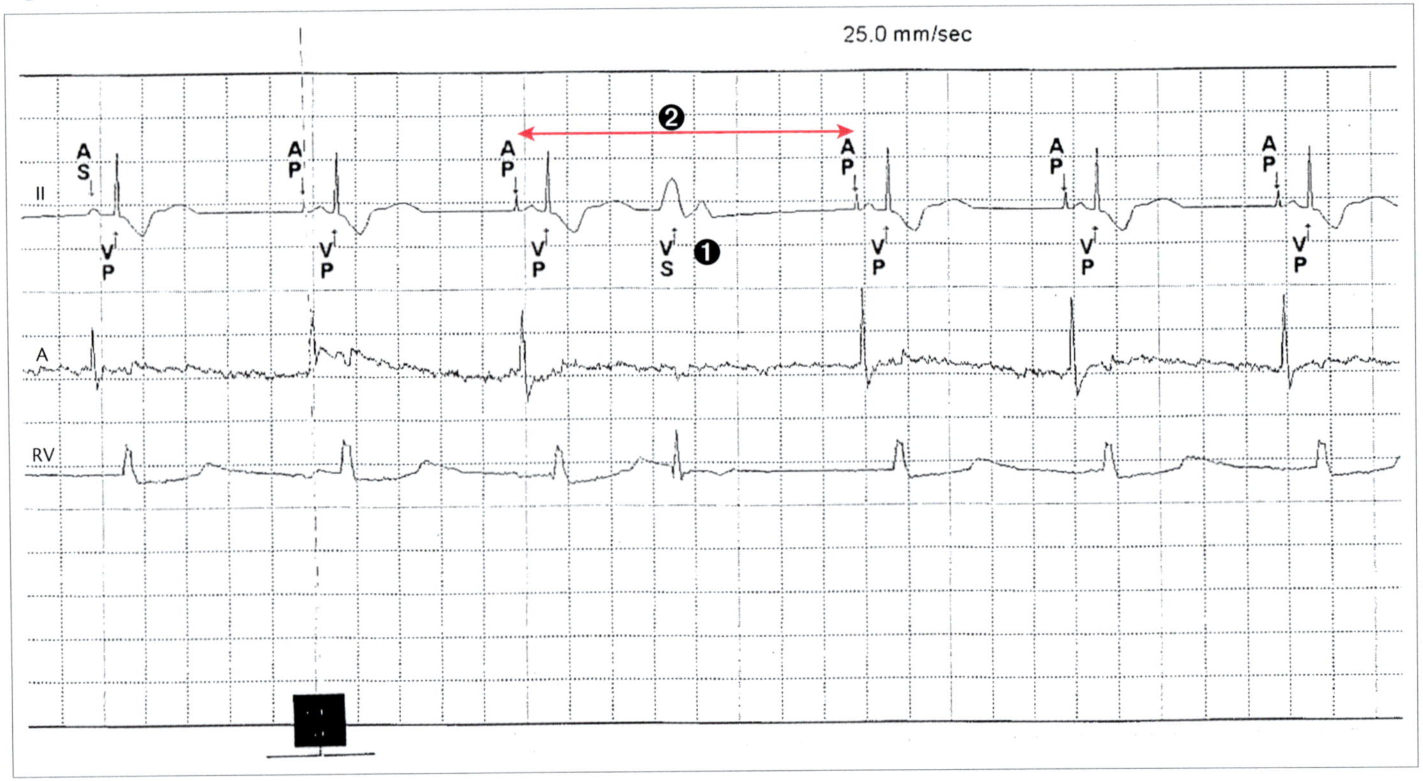

Pacing occurs at a sensor-driven rate of 968ms. This patient had VPBs, shown by the VS events at 100bpm on the rate histogram (Figure 24.1), which resulted in low atrial rates on the histogram.

❶ A VPB occurs (Figure 24.2), resetting the timers and triggering a VA interval of 968 – 148 = 820ms.

❷ This results in an AP–AP interval of 148 + 593 + (968–148) = 1561ms (which corresponds to a rate of 38bpm).

The paced events at 50–60bpm on the ventricular histogram in Figure 24.1 may be explained by atrial-based timing of the device, resulting in ventricular pacing at slightly below the baseline rate (Figure 23.3).

Comments

Premature ventricular contractions

PVCs may result in a number of observations of pacemaker behaviour. These include:

1 atrial pacing at below the lower rate limit (as in this example)
2 non-tracking of P-waves (due to post-PVC PVARP extension)
3 ventricular safety pacing (when the PVC closely follows an atrial paced event)
4 endless loop tachycardia
5 VVT response (in some biventricular devices).

A potential risk of PVCs is FFRW oversensing in the atrial channel, with tracking of the event and ventricular pacing on the T-wave, which may be arrhythmogenic (Figure 24.3).

Figure 24.3 Consequence of programming the PVARP < VRP in the case of a VPB falling in the VRP (without resetting the timers) and tracking of FFRW oversensing, resulting in ventricular pacing on the T-wave (a). This is why the PVARP should always be programmed at least as long as the VRP (b).

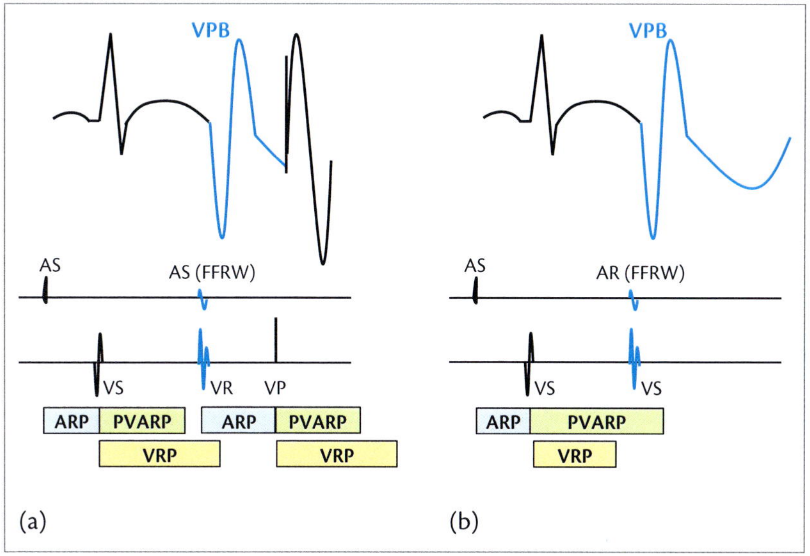

Introduction to the case

An 82-year-old patient with a history of brady–tachy syndrome and implanted with a DDD pacemaker presented with palpitations. The presenting ECG (Figure 25.1) showed AF with an irregular paced ventricular rhythm. The device memory revealed a high burden of atrial arrhythmia (Figure 25.2). The device settings are shown in Table 25.1, and a real-time EGM is shown in Figure 25.3.

Figure 25.1 Presenting ECG showing irregular paced ventricular rhythm

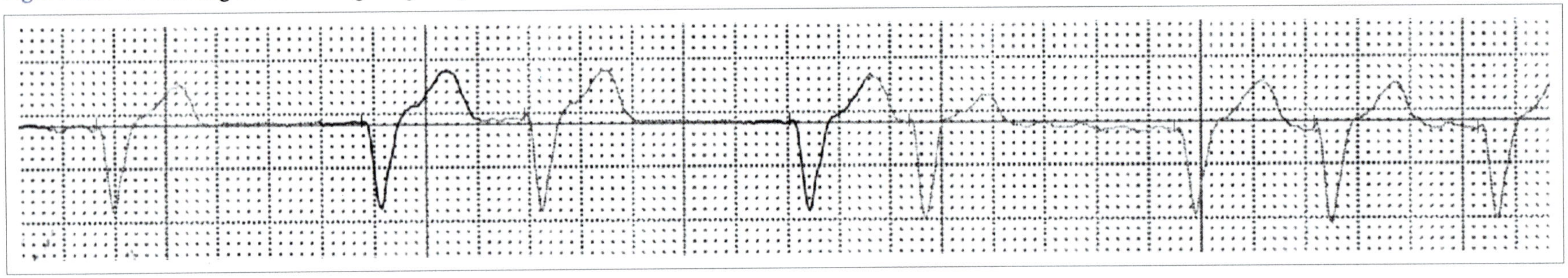

Figure 25.2 History of atrial arrhythmia retrieved from the device memory

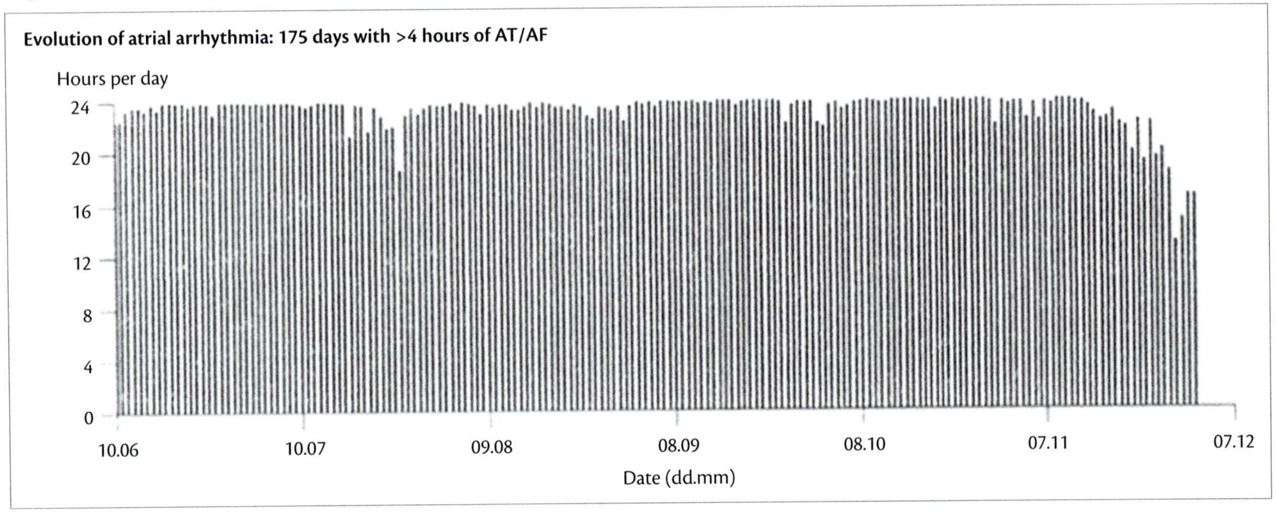

Courtesy of Dr C Vuille

Table 25.1 Device settings

Pacing mode	DDDR
Lower rate	60bpm
Upper rate	130bpm
Atrial output (bipolar)	2.5V@0.4ms
Ventricular output (bipolar)	2.5V@0.4ms
Atrial sensitivity (bipolar)	0.18mV
Ventricular sensitivity (bipolar)	2.8mV
Paced AV delay	150ms
Sense compensation	−30ms
Atrial rate for mode switch	175bpm
Pacing mode during mode switch	DDIR
PVARP	310ms

Question

Figure 25.3 Real-time EGM

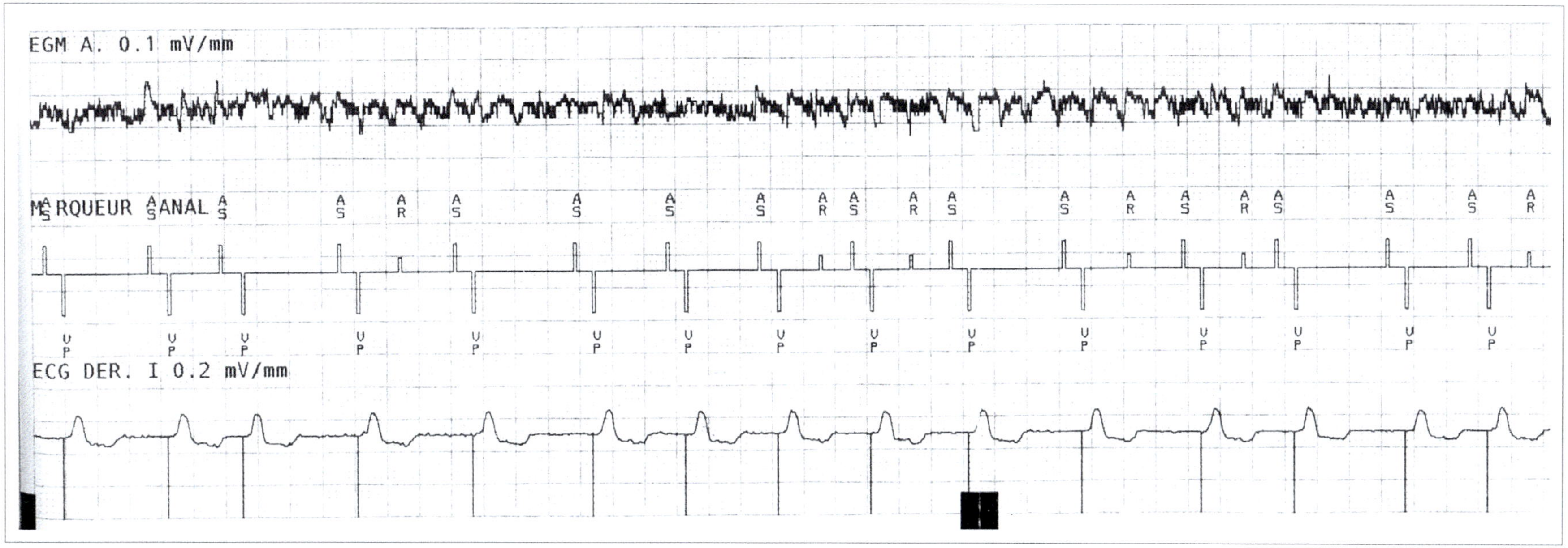

Courtesy of Dr C Vuille

Why is the ventricular rhythm irregular?

A Atrial undersensing

B Mode switch programmed off

C Rate response

D Ventricular safety pacing

Answer

A Atrial undersensing

Figure 25.4 Annotated real-time EGM

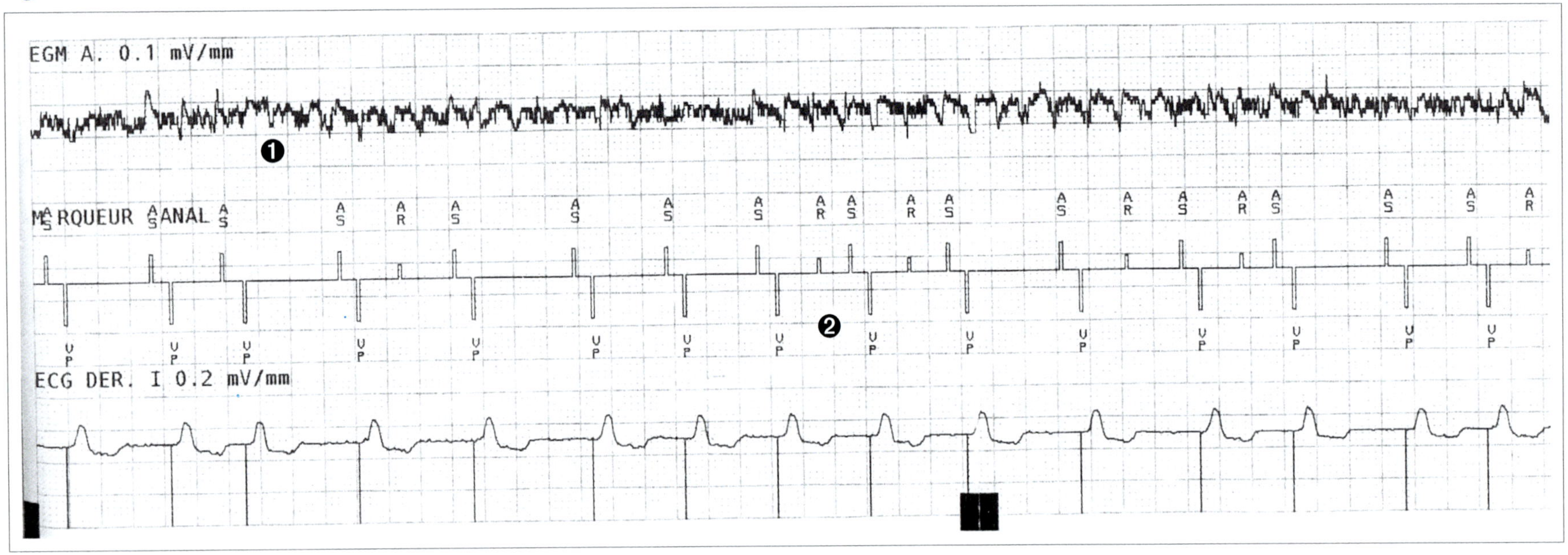

The pacemaker is functioning in a tracking mode (DDD), as AS events are followed by VP at the programmed sensed AV delay of 120ms. Mode switch had been programmed on but was not activated in this instance, due to atrial undersensing (Figure 25.4).

❶ The atrial EGM shows AF with low-amplitude signals (scale of 0.1mV/mm), resulting in atrial undersensing.

❷ The high-rate AS events are too few and far in between to fulfil the criteria for triggering mode switch. Intermittent atrial sensing results in variable ventricular pacing rate.

Comments

Pacemaker-mediated tachycardia due to undersensing of atrial fibrillation

Figure 25.5 Decrease in detected AF burden due to atrial undersensing ❶

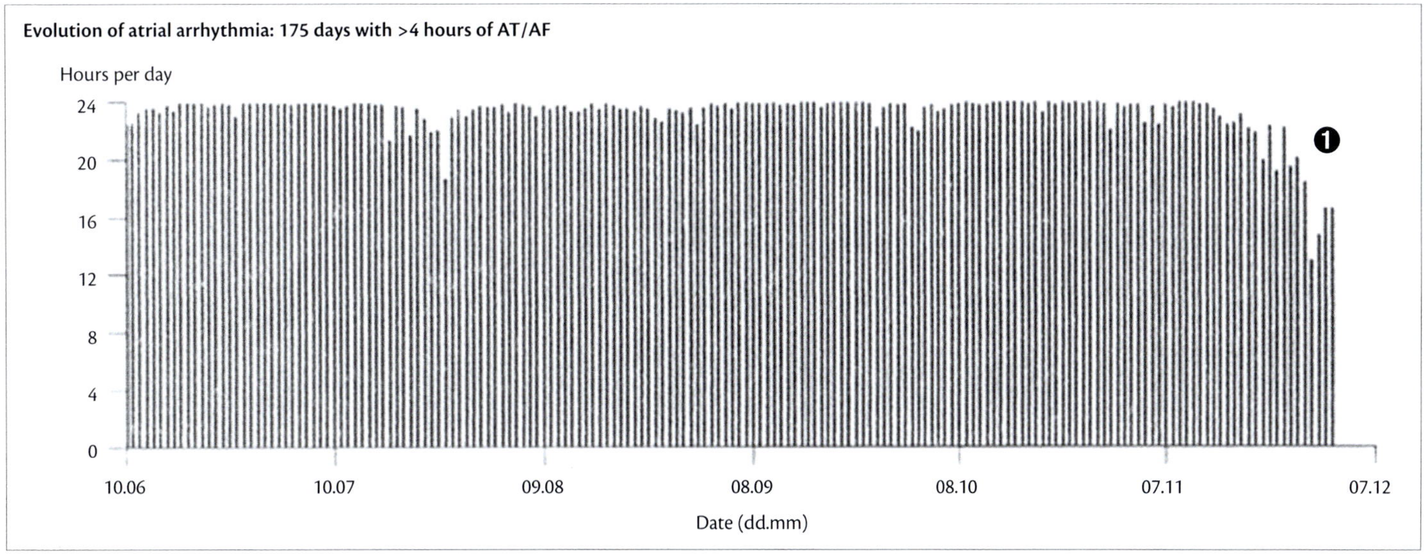

Courtesy of Dr C Vuille

This example shows how intermittent undersensing of AF can lead to irregular ventricular pacing. In addition to lack of mode switch, these events will not be stored in the device memory as atrial high-rate episodes. Atrial EGM amplitude tends to decrease, as AF becomes chronic. In the present case, atrial undersensing resulted in a decrease in the daily AF burden since a few days before device interrogation (Figure 25.5).

Atrial sensing had already been programmed to its most sensitive value, so continued undersensing was unavoidable. Due to the unlikely event of the patient reverting to sinus rhythm, the device was programmed to the VVIR mode.

Introduction to the case

A 74-year-old patient implanted with a dual-chamber pacemaker for complete AV block was admitted to the intensive care unit for sepsis. The baseline rate was increased to 80bpm, but an irregular paced rhythm was observed. The real-time EGM strip is shown in Figure 26.1. Device settings are shown in Table 26.1.

Table 26.1 Device settings

Pacing mode	DDD
Lower rate	80bpm
Upper rate	130bpm
Atrial output (bipolar)	2.5V@0.4ms
Ventricular output (bipolar)	2.5V@0.4ms
Atrial sensitivity (bipolar)	0.1mV
Ventricular sensitivity (bipolar)	2.0mV
Paced AV delay	180–140ms
Sense compensation	−45ms
Atrial high rate for mode switch	180bpm
Pacing mode for mode switch	DDIR
Baseline rate during mode switch	90bpm
PVARP	Auto

Question

Figure 26.1 Real-time EGM

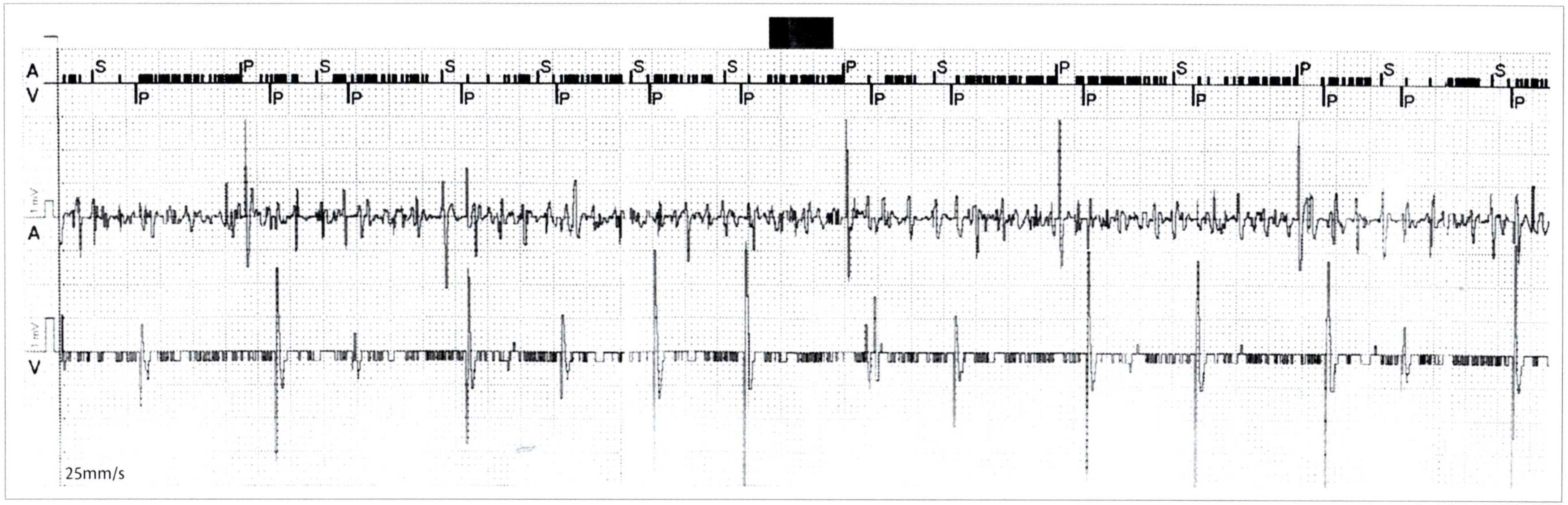

How do you explain the irregular ventricular pacing rate?

A Atrial undersensing

B Atrial noise reversion

C Mode switch was not programmed on

D Rate stabilization algorithm

Answer

B Atrial noise reversion

Figure 26.2 Annotated real-time EGM

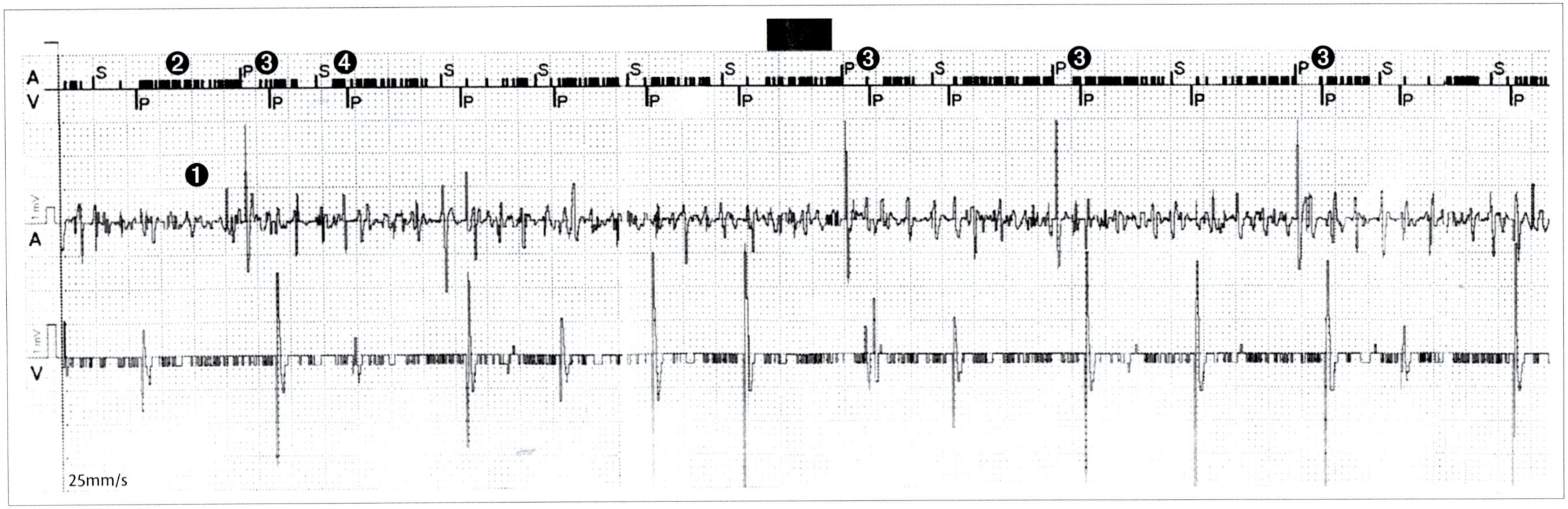

The atrial EGM (Figure 26.2) shows AF, but the device is functioning in a tracking (DDD) mode, due to atrial noise reversion, which is inhibiting mode switch.

❶ The atrial EGM shows low-amplitude signals with a very high frequency that are sensed due to the high sensitivity setting (0.1mV).

❷ Repeated high-rate sensing in the atrial channel is interpreted by the device as noise.

❸ Due to the noise (occurring repeatedly in windows of 50ms for this device), asynchronous pacing occurs at the baseline rate. Note that all cycles with atrial pacing have VP–VP intervals that are slightly below the baseline rate (at approximately 800ms/75bpm). This is due to atrial-based timing sequences (Figure 23.3).

❹ When noise ends, the sensed atrial events (that are outside the PVARP) are tracked to the ventricles, resulting in an irregular ventricular rhythm. The sensed AVIs may be longer than the programmed value (this is apparent for this cycle and the 1st one), due to limitation of the UTR at 130bpm, with Wenckebach response.

Comments

Atrial noise reversion due to oversensing of atrial fibrillation

This example shows how an atrial sensitivity level that is set too high can lead to atrial oversensing, noise reversion, and absence of mode switch, with tracking of atrial events that fall outside the noise reversion window. A compromise should be made with sufficient sensitivity to avoid undersensing of AF, but not too high to result in oversensing (e.g. FFRW oversensing or sensing of fractionated potentials, as in this case). The problem was corrected by reducing the sensitivity level from 0.1mV to 0.4mV.

Paradoxical atrial undersensing of AF has been shown to occur in 13% of patients programmed at the maximum atrial sensitivity level[1] and may occur due to either noise reversion or 'ringing'. The latter entity corresponds to saturation of the sense amplifier (usually due to atrial arrhythmias with high-amplitude signals) and can be distinguished from noise reversion by the absence of sense markers.[2]

References

1. Kolb C, Halbfass P, Zrenner B, Schmitt C. Paradoxical atrial undersensing due to inappropriate atrial noise reversion of atrial fibrillation in dual-chamber pacemakers. *J Cardiovasc Electrophysiol* 2005; **16**: 696–700.
2. Van Gelder BM, Van Den Broek W, Bracke FA, Meijer A. Paradoxical atrial undersensing: noise rate reversion or amplifier ringing? *J Cardiovasc Electrophysiol* 2006; **17**: 1371–4.

Introduction to the case

A 75-year-old woman in chronic AF had been implanted with a single-chamber pacemaker 2 years ago. The pacemaker was programmed to VVI 60bpm (see settings in Table 27.1). Device counters revealed 72% VP, and the rate histogram is shown in Figure 27.1. A real-time EGM recorded at follow-up is shown on in Figure 27.2.

Table 27.1 Device settings

Pacing mode	VVI
Lower rate	60bpm
Ventricular output (bipolar)	2.5V@0.4ms
Ventricular sensitivity (bipolar)	2.5mV
VRP	250ms

Figure 27.1 Ventricular rate histogram

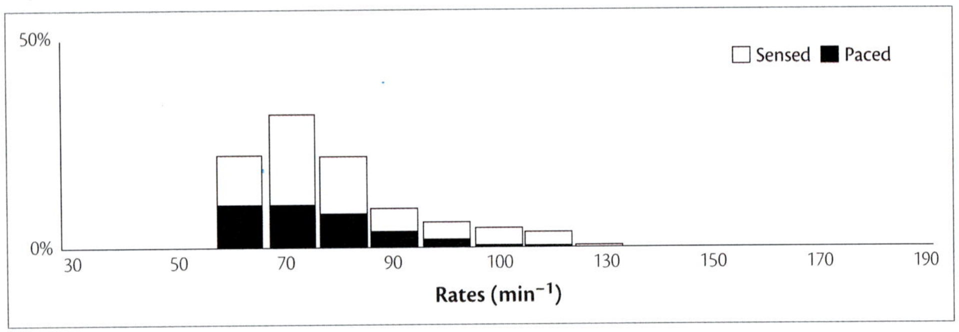

Question

Figure 27.2 Real-time EGM

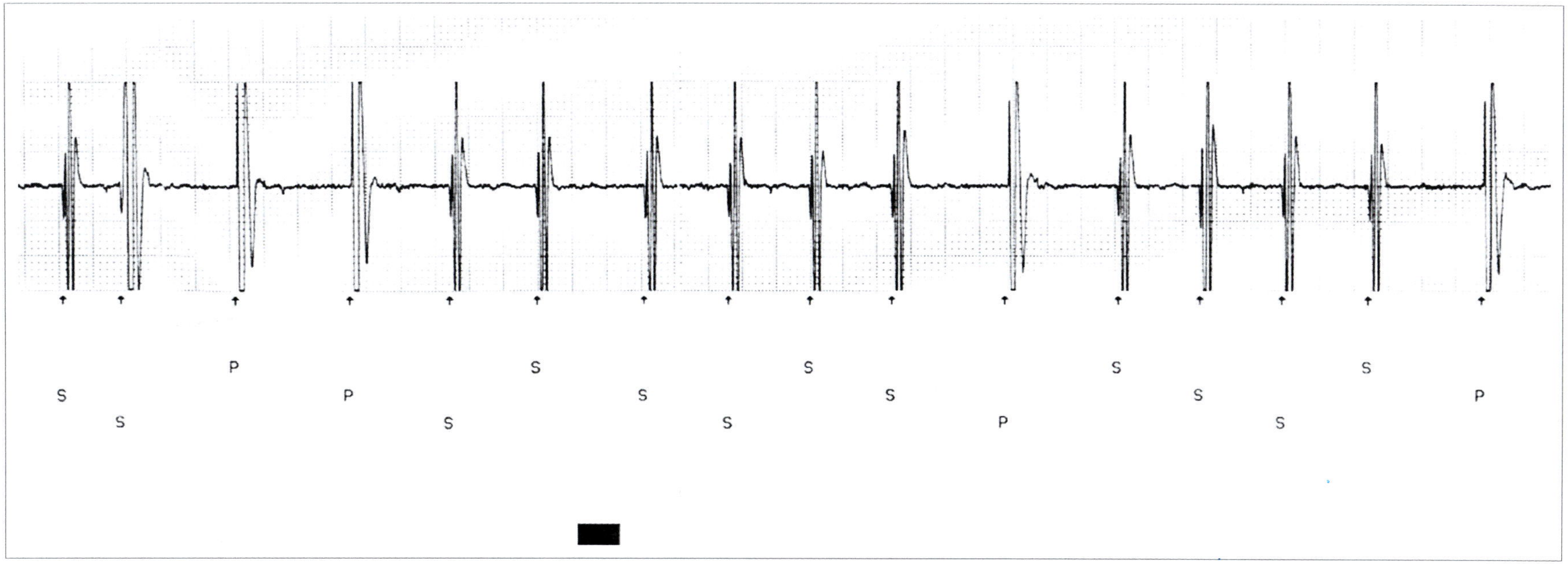

How do you explain pacing at above the lower rate?

A Rate regularization algorithm

B Sensor-driven rate

C Runaway pacemaker

D Magnet response

Answer

A **Rate regularization algorithm**

Figure 27.3 Annotated real-time EGM

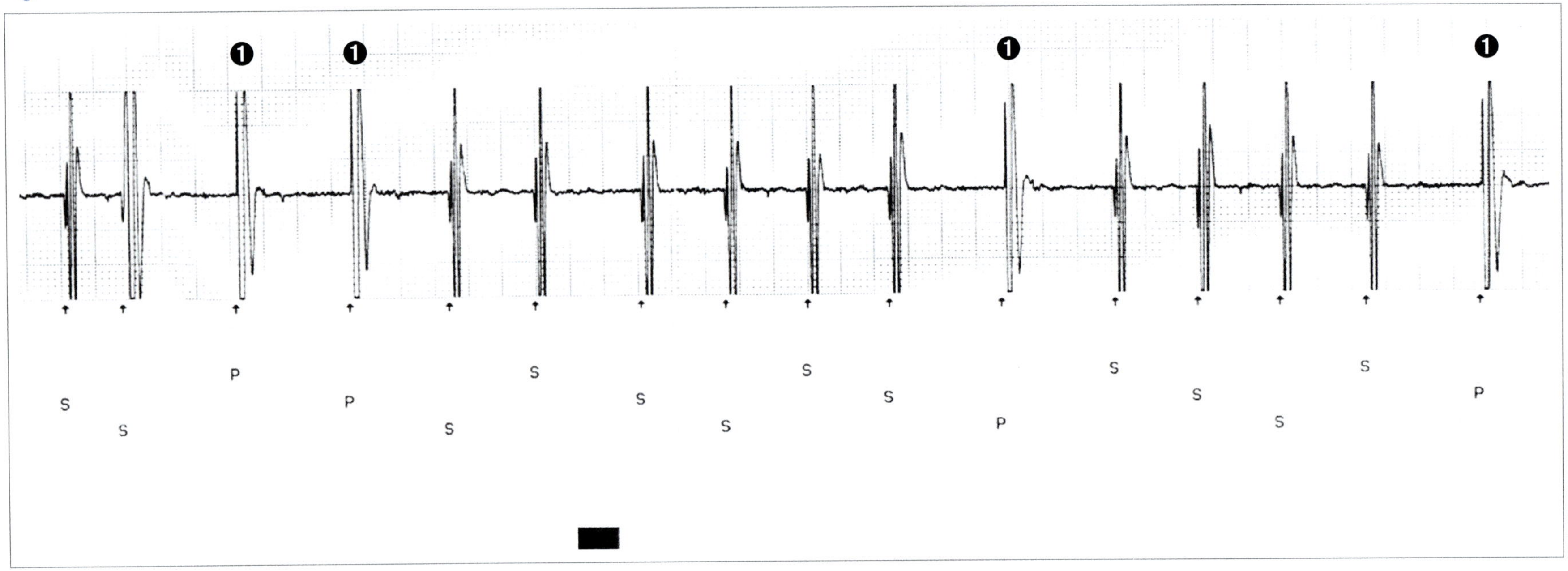

The EGM (Figure 27.3) shows relatively rapidly conducted AF with irregular heart rates.

❶ Ventricular pacing occurs above the baseline rate of 60bpm (here at about 90bpm), due to the rate regularization (smoothing) algorithm that aims to reduce irregularities in the heart rate, and thereby improve the patient's symptoms.

Comments

Pacing at an unexpectedly fast rate

Rate regularization/rate-smoothing algorithms are designed to avoid sudden changes in the heart rate, especially in the setting of AF, in order to reduce symptoms of arrhythmias in patients with single- and dual-chamber devices. The upper rates at which these algorithms can pace may be programmable but never exceed the UTR or sensor-driven rate. Symptoms may be improved, but at the expense of an increased percentage of pacing. Causes for pacing at a faster than expected rate are:

1 rate-smoothing/rate regularization algorithms
2 rate drop response
3 AP preference algorithms (designed to override the intrinsic atrial activity, in order to prevent AF, and seldom used nowadays due to lack of efficacy).[1] Repetitive non-re-entrant ventriculoatrial synchrony (RNRVAS)[1,2] may also be observed with these algorithms
4 automatic threshold measurements
5 inadequately programmed sensor (threshold too low or slope too steep)
6 AF/atrial flutter/atrial tachycardia with inactivated mode switch or intermittent atrial undersensing (see Cases 11 and 25)
7 endless loop tachycardia
8 exposure to magnetic fields (pacing at magnet rate)
9 runaway pacemaker (device dysfunction).

References

1. Healey JS, Connolly SJ, Gold MR, *et al*. Subclinical atrial fibrillation and the risk of stroke. *N Engl J Med* 2012; **366**: 120–9.

2. Barold SS, Stroobandt RX, Van Heuverswyn F. Pacemaker repetitive nonreentrant ventriculoatrial synchrony. Why did automatic mode switching occur? *J Electrocardiol* 2012; **45**: 420–5.

Introduction to the case

An 82-year-old patient with symptomatic sinus node dysfunction and second-degree AV block was implanted with a biventricular pacemaker. A Holter was performed, due to dizziness occurring at the same time every afternoon, with the rhythm during symptoms shown in Figure 28.1. Device follow-up was normal. The device settings are shown in Table 28.1.

Table 28.1 Device settings

Pacing mode	DDDRV
Lower rate	60bpm
Upper rate	120bpm
Atrial output (bipolar)	2.5V@0.4ms
RV output (bipolar)	2.5V@0.4ms
LV output (bipolar)	2.5V@0.4ms
Atrial sensitivity (bipolar)	0.3mV
RV sensitivity (bipolar)	2.5mV
LV sensitivity (bipolar)	2.5mV
Paced AV delay (fixed)	120ms
Sense compensation	30ms
PVAB after ventricular pace	150ms
PVARP	280ms
Post-PVC PVARP extension	400ms
Ventricular blanking after atrial pace	40ms
VRP	250ms

The 'V' of DDDRV corresponds to multisite ventricular pacing, according to the NBG code.

Question

Figure 28.1 Holter recording

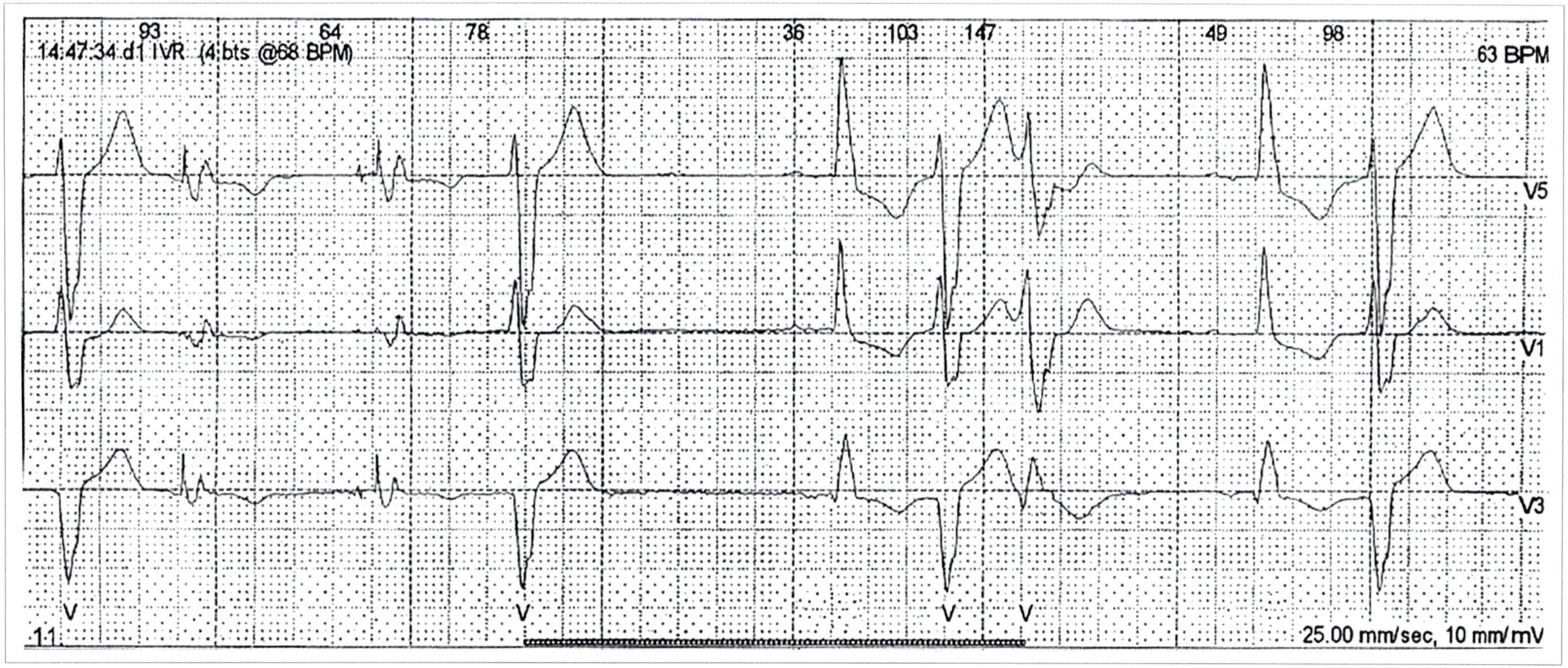

What is the most likely reason for the bradycardia?

A T-wave oversensing

B Atrial undersensing

C ADI/DDD mode

D Autosensing algorithm

Answer

D Autosensing algorithm

Figure 28.2 Annotated Holter recording

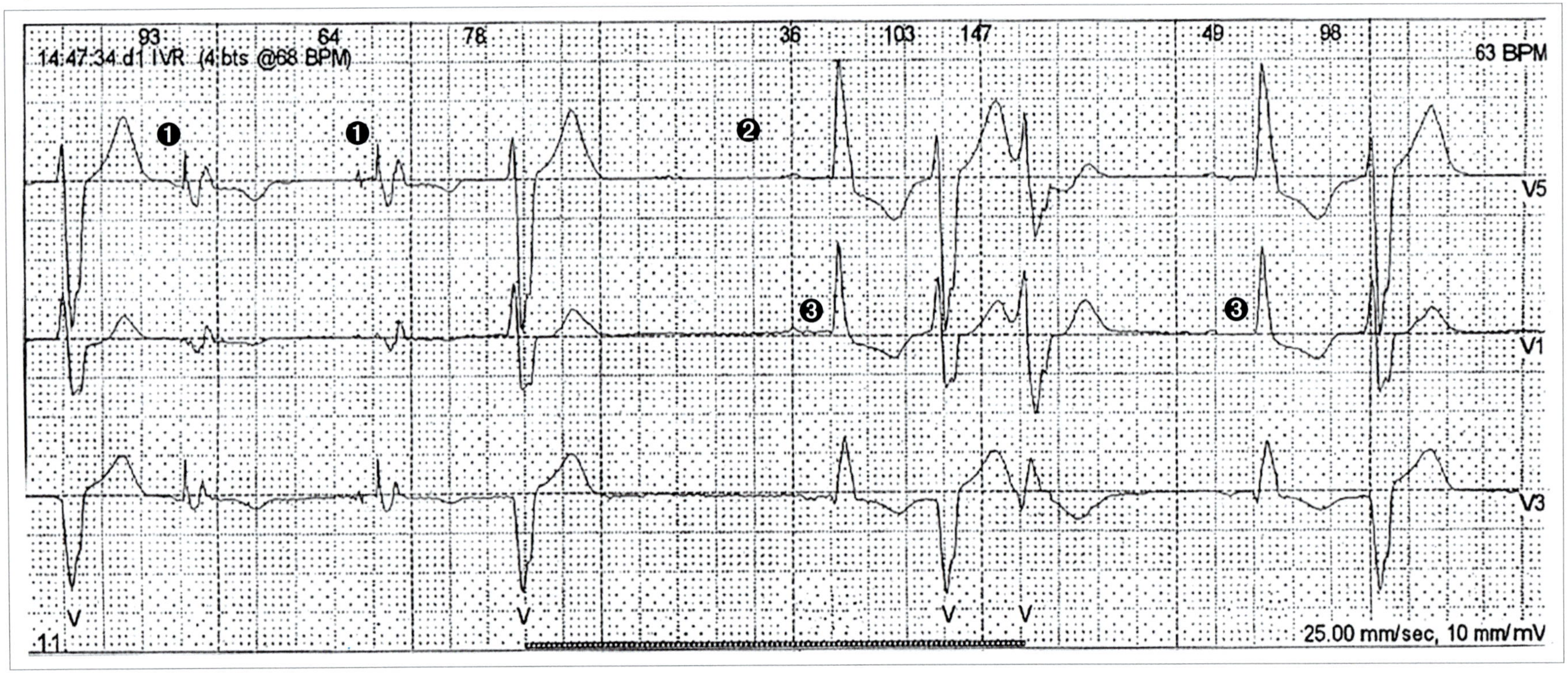

The Holter (Figure 28.2) shows an intrinsic rhythm occurring below the programmed lower pacing rate, due to an algorithm sensing intrinsic atrial and ventricular signal amplitude.

❶ The first complex is an AS–VP, followed by an AP–VP event, with a pacing rate of 60bpm.

❷ If the reason for the low pacing rate had been T-wave oversensing, one would expect to have a VP event at approximately this timepoint, based upon the intervals between the preceding paced ventricular events. There is no evidence of atrial pacing during the pause, which should have occurred with a device programmed with an ADI/DDD algorithm.

❸ These two cycles are sinus beats with intrinsic AV conduction. The other QRS complexes (other than those indicated in ❶) are VPBs.

Comments

Unexpectedly slow pacing rates

Symptoms that occur repeatedly at the same time of the day are suggestive of a device algorithm. In this case, the bradycardia was caused by the pacemaker functioning temporarily in a DDI mode at a rate of 30bpm, in order to measure daily intrinsic atrial and ventricular amplitudes. For this model, this takes place on a daily basis at the time the device was implanted. Timing of this feature varies between models. Other automatic algorithms that may cause symptoms are automatic threshold tests or lead impedance tests (with delivery of unipolar pulses that may cause pectoral twitching).

Heart rates that are lower than the programmed lower rate may occur with:

1. ventricular oversensing (T-wave, myopotentials, lead fracture artefacts, electromagnetic interference, etc.)*
2. rate hysteresis
3. programmed night heart rate
4. specific device algorithms (ADI/DDD mode, autosensing algorithm, automatic threshold algorithms, non-competitive atrial pacing algorithm, etc.)
5. non-capture (threshold rise, lead or generator dysfunction, programming error, etc.).

* Atrial oversensing will result in mode switch and pacing in VDI(R)/DDI(R) or in triggering of an AV delay with ventricular pacing (and thus there is no bradycardia).

Introduction to the case

A patient with a dual-chamber pacemaker had a atrial high-rate episode retrieved from the device memory. The retrieved EGM is shown in Figure 29.1. The device parameters are listed in Table 29.1.

Table 29.1 Device settings

Pacing mode	DDDR
Lower rate	70bpm
Upper rate	120bpm
Atrial output	2.5V@0.4ms (bipolar)
Ventricular output	Auto@0.4ms (unipolar)
Atrial sensitivity	0.3mV (bipolar)
Ventricular sensitivity	2.0mV (bipolar)
Paced AV delay	300ms
Sense compensation	−50ms

Question

Figure 29.1 EGM of atrial high-rate episode

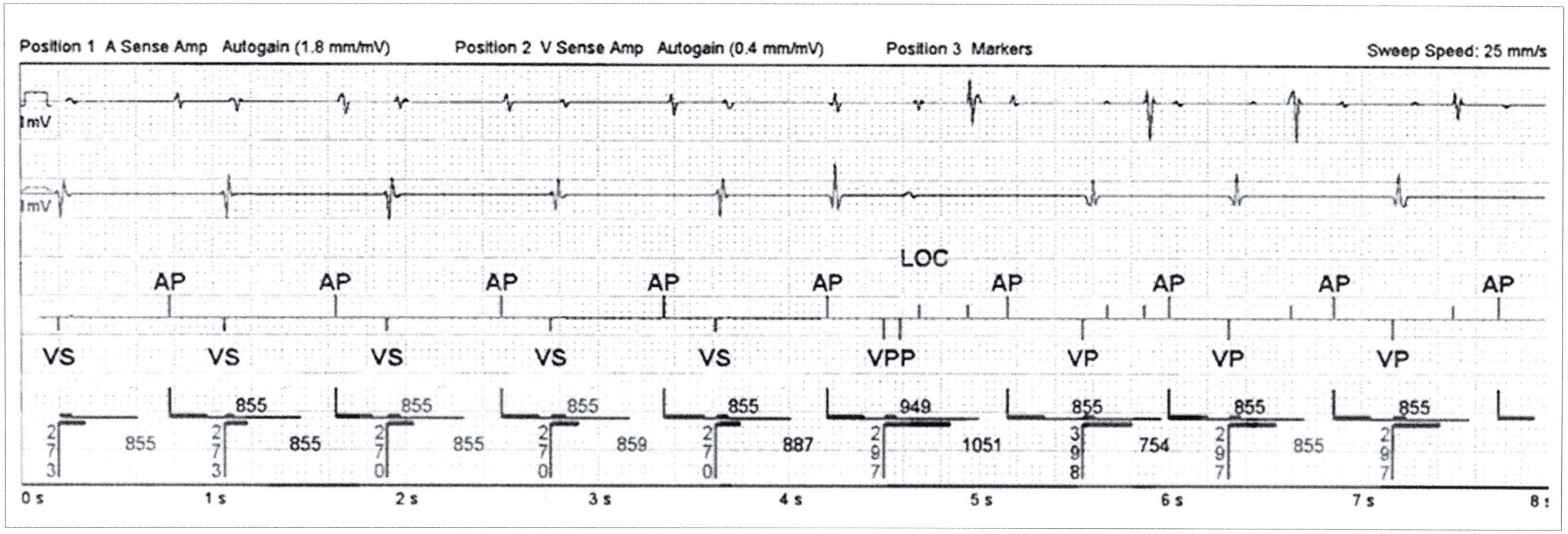

Courtesy of Mr H Leersen

What is happening at 'LOC' on the upper tracing?

A Loss of ventricular capture due to a premature beat

B Loss of ventricular capture due to fluctuating threshold

C Loss of atrial capture due to a premature beat

D Loss of atrial capture due to fluctuating threshold

Answer

A **Loss of ventricular capture due to a premature beat**

Figure 29.2 Annotated EGM of atrial high-rate episode

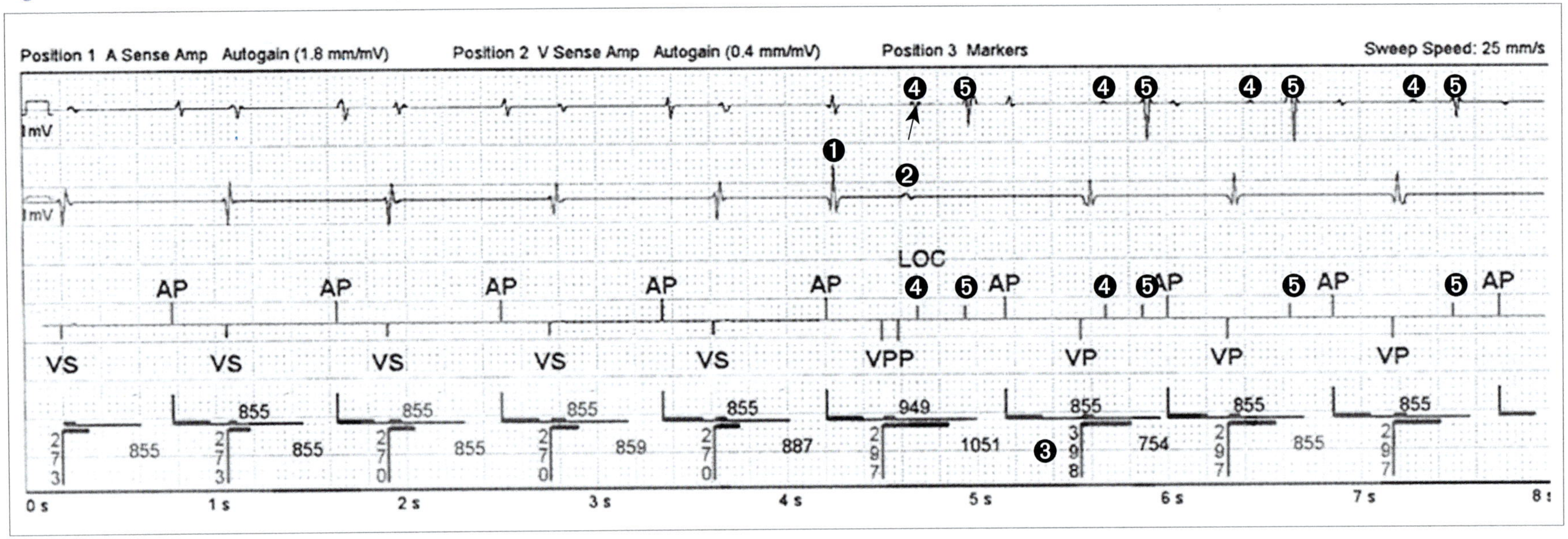

Courtesy of Mr H Leersen

This example (Figure 29.2) illustrates the function of an automatic capture algorithm (of St-Jude Medical) which detects loss of capture on a beat-to-beat basis.

❶ A VPB occurs by chance simultaneously with atrial pacing and is not sensed, as it falls in the PAVB (functional undersensing). ventricular pacing occurs at the end of the 300ms paced AVI, with absence of capture, as the ventricle is refractory after the premature beat. Loss of capture (LOC) is detected by the device, which then delivers a backup pace at 5V (VPP).

❷ Ventricular capture of the backup pace is not evident on the EGM but does occur, as there is a FFRW visible on the atrial EGM (arrow).

❸ The AVI is extended by 100ms for a single cycle, in order to avoid pseudofusion (without an evoked potential) that may have led to erroneous diagnosis of loss of capture of the previous cycle. Capture of this cycle is confirmed (no VPP sequence), with resumption thereafter of the programmed paced AVI.

❹ FFRWs of the paced QRS complexes are visible on the atrial EGM but are sensed as atrial refractory events for the 1st two VP cycles only, as the signals of the two following VP cycles are too small to be sensed.

❺ Retrograde P-waves are visible. All these events fall in the PVARP and therefore do not reset the timers for AP. There is no capture of the AP events, as the atrial myocardium is still refractory, following the retrograde P-waves. Notice that the morphology of the EGM during AP is different here, compared to before the LOC event (when atrial capture occurred).

Comments

Automatic ventricular capture algorithms

The automatic capture algorithm evaluates the presence of an evoked response (ER) potential resulting from myocardial capture and has to differentiate it from the after-potential resulting from the polarization of the tissue–electrode interface (which may be present also without ventricular capture (Figure 29.3).

It performs beat-to-beat confirmation of ventricular capture, thus allowing the delivery of pacing at an amplitude slightly above the capture threshold (e.g. 0.25–0.5V). It is particularly useful to save battery drain in case of a high capture threshold (thus avoiding having to double the programmed amplitude) and also to maintain capture in case of a rise in threshold.

This feature is currently available on St-Jude Medical, Boston Scientific, and Biotronik devices. It should be distinguished from automatic threshold tests, which perform thresholds on a daily basis (and may use this information to adjust the pacing output) but do not verify beat-to-beat capture.

Figure 29.3 Evoked response and polarization

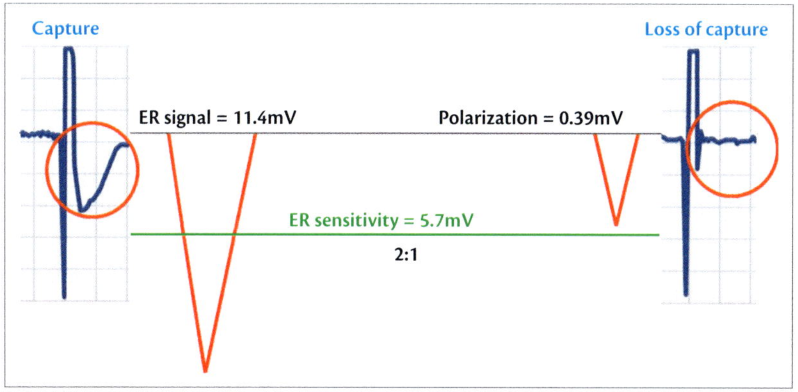

Reproduced with permission from St-Jude Medical (St Paul, MN, USA)

Introduction to the case

A patient implanted with a CRT-P had the incidental finding of spikes on T-waves during a Holter recording, shown by the asterisks in Figure 30.1. During device follow-up, the same phenomenon was observed, with the EGM tracing shown in Figure 30.2. Additionally, the device settings are mentioned in Table 30.1.

Figure 30.1 Holter recording

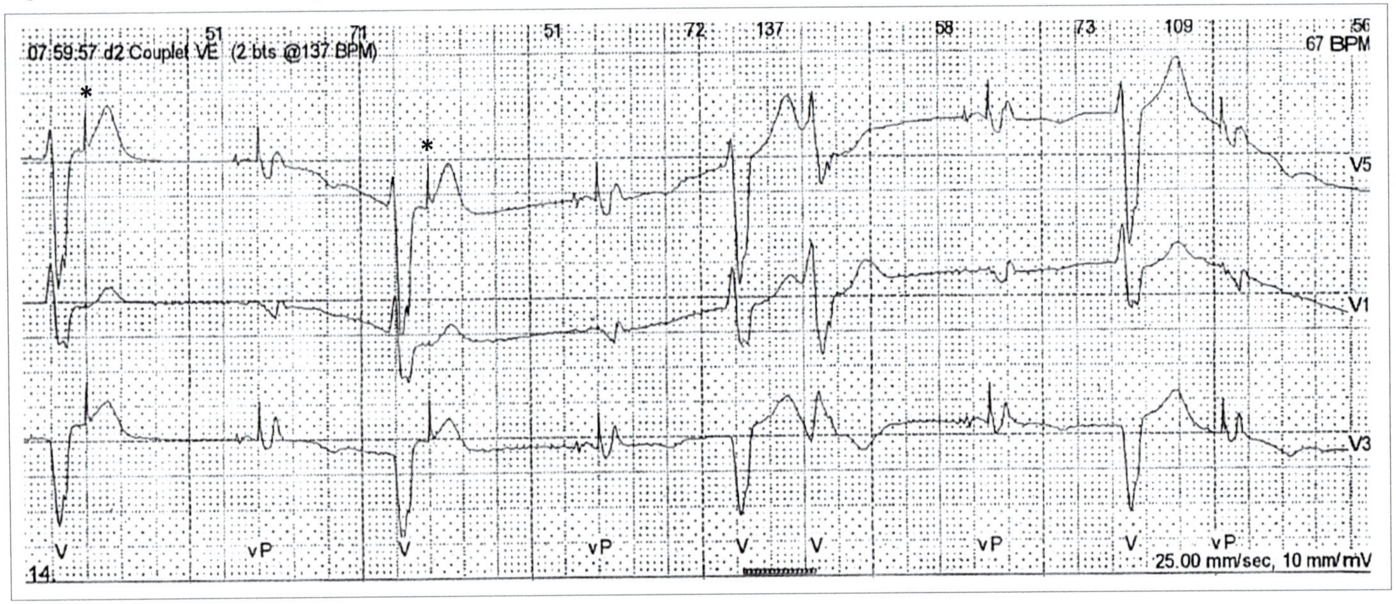

Table 30.1 Device settings

Pacing mode	DDDRV
Lower rate	60bpm
Upper rate	120bpm
Atrial output	2.5V@0.4ms
RV output	2.5V@0.4ms
LV output	2.5V@0.4ms
Atrial sensitivity (bipolar)	0.3mV
RV sensitivity (bipolar)	2.5mV
LV sensitivity (bipolar)	2.5mV
Paced AV delay (fixed)	120ms
Sense compensation	30ms
Interventricular delay (LV first)	20ms
PVAB after ventricular pace	150ms
PVARP	280ms
Post-PVC PVARP extension	400ms
Ventricular blanking after atrial pace	40ms
VRP	250ms

Question

Figure 30.2 Real-time EGM

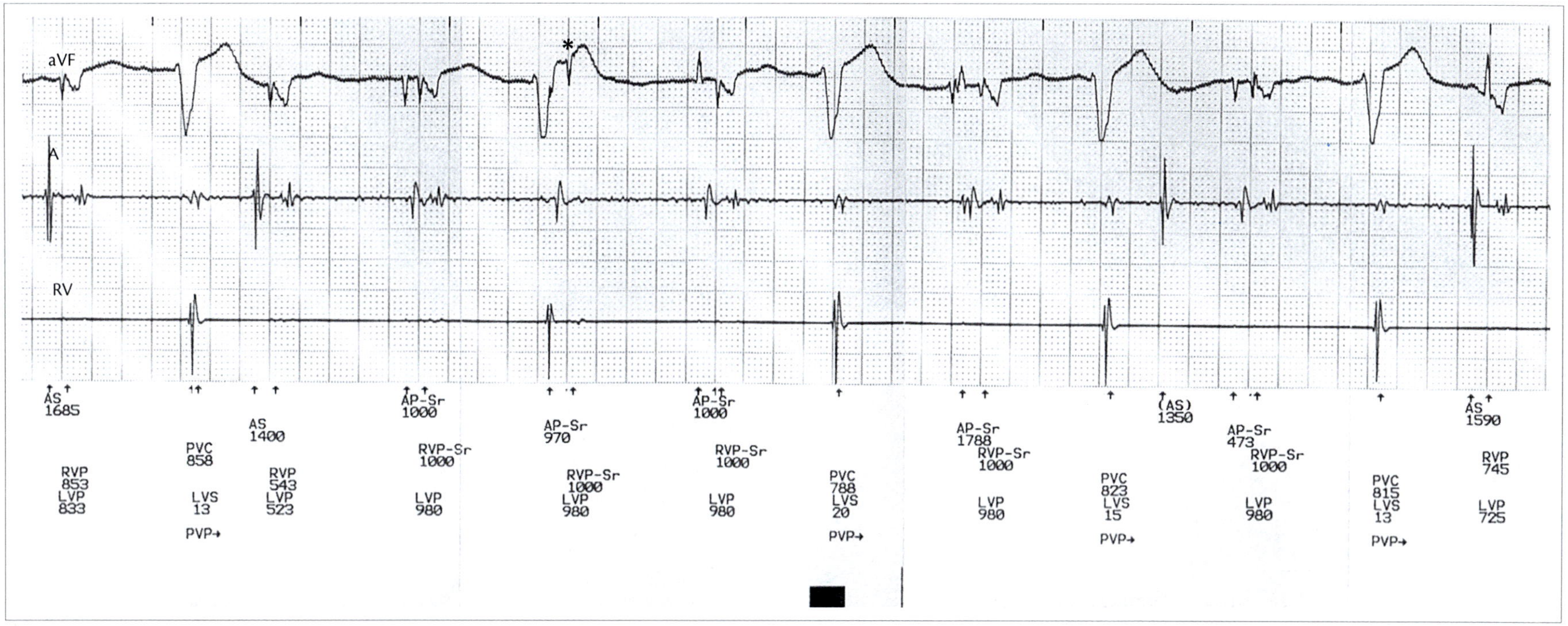

How do you explain the spike on the T-wave (*)?

A Ventricular safety pacing

B Atrial pacing

C Atrial oversensing

D Functional ventricular undersensing

Answer

D Functional ventricular undersensing

Figure 30.3 Annotated real-time EGM

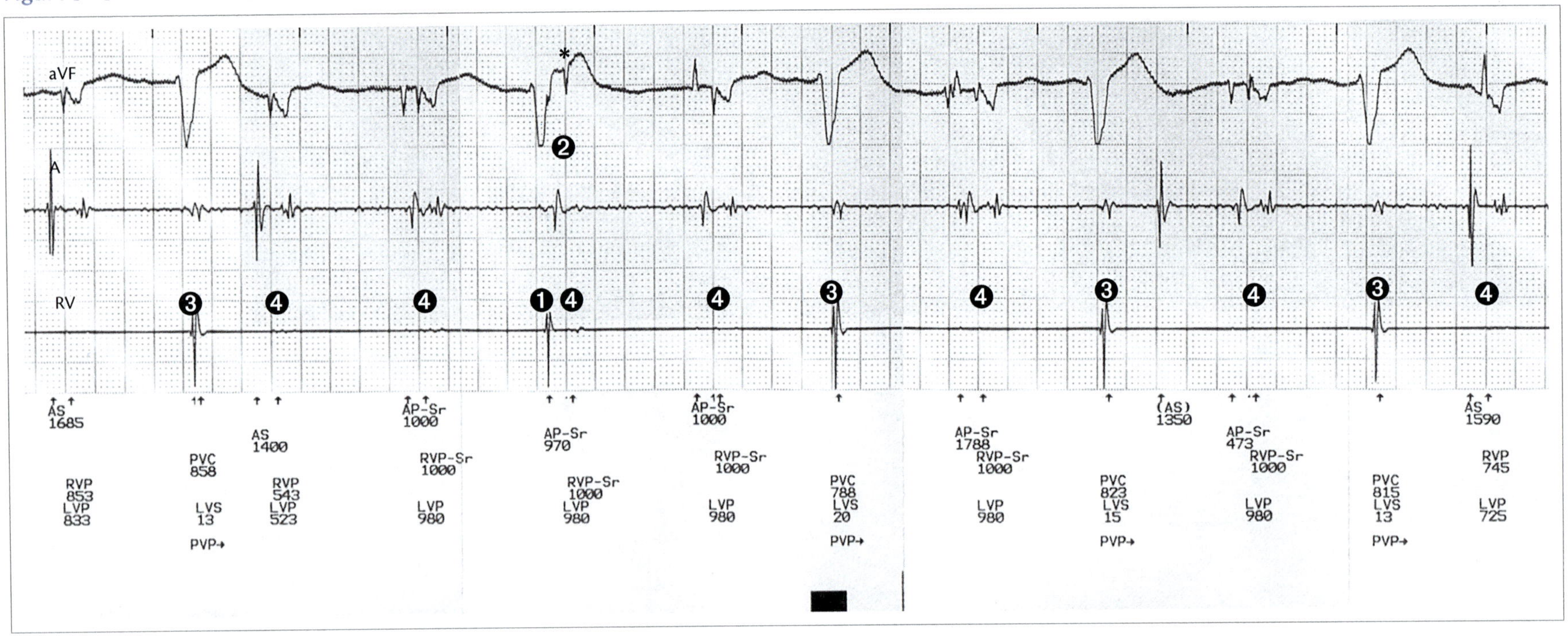

This example (Figure 30.3) shows functional undersensing of a VPB.

❶ A VPB falls coincidentally with an atrial paced event. Due to the PAVB, the premature beat is not sensed.

❷ A ventricular spike follows after the atrial paced event and falls on the T-wave.

❸ These VPBs are properly sensed.

❹ The automatic gain on the RV channel decreases the scale during ventricular pacing explaining why the EGM is flat during these events.

❺ As this device has RV-based timing, the Vx–VP cycles are at the baseline/sensor-driven rate (1000ms for this cycle). The AP timing at 970ms can be explained by the AVI which is longer by 30ms for this cycle, compared to the previous one (due to the specific behaviour of this device, the details of which are not relevant for the purposes of this book).

Comments

Hazards of programming long atrioventricular intervals

In the case of functional undersensing of a ventricular event in patients with a long programmed AVI (or AV hysteresis), pacing on the T-wave may result, which may be proarrhythmic. In patients with a shorter AVI, pacing will occur shortly after the QRS complex, i.e. during the myocardial refractory period, which is not a problem.

Other potential drawbacks with programming long AVIs may be haemodynamic compromise due to the 'P on T' phenomenon (see Case 14), endless loop tachycardia (see Case 20), and limitation of the maximum 1:1 tracking rate (which is limited by the TARP, see Case 7).

Introduction to the case

A patient implanted 6 months ago with a dual-chamber pacemaker for intermittent AV block presented to his cardiologist for follow-up. The ECGs recorded at presentation and with magnet application are shown in Figure 31.1. The cardiologist faxed the tracings, but the device settings are unknown.

Question

Figure 31.1 ECG

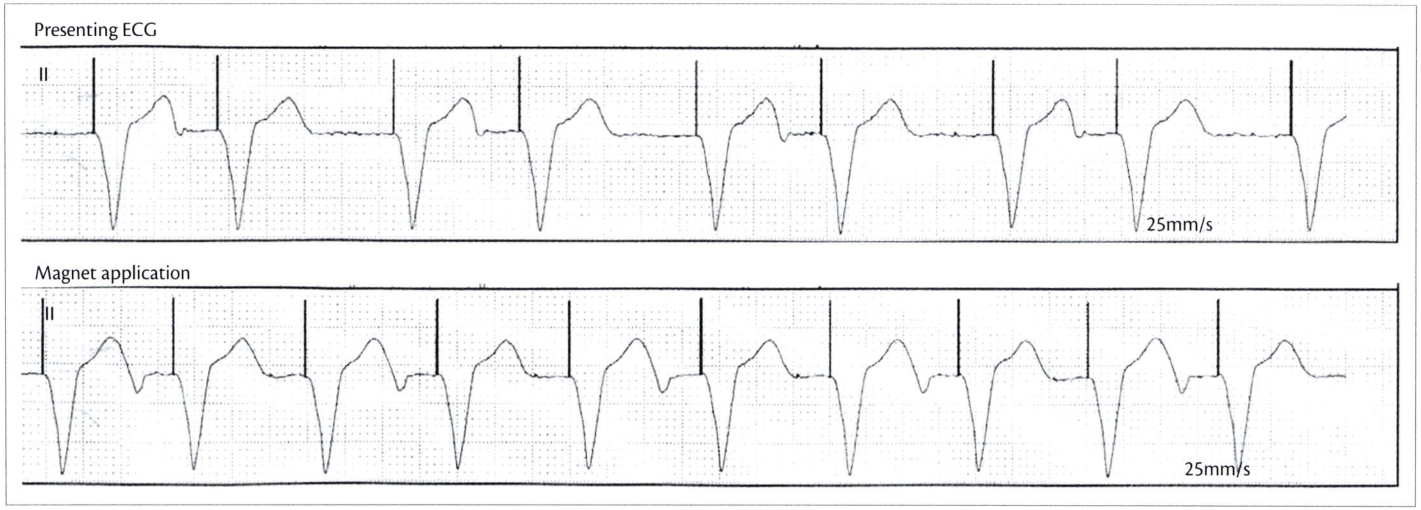

Courtesy of Dr C Vuille

What is the cause for the irregular heart rate on the presenting ECG?

A Atrial non-capture

B Upper rate behaviour

C Atrial bigeminy

D Hysteresis

Answer

A Atrial non-capture

Figure 31.2 Annotated ECG

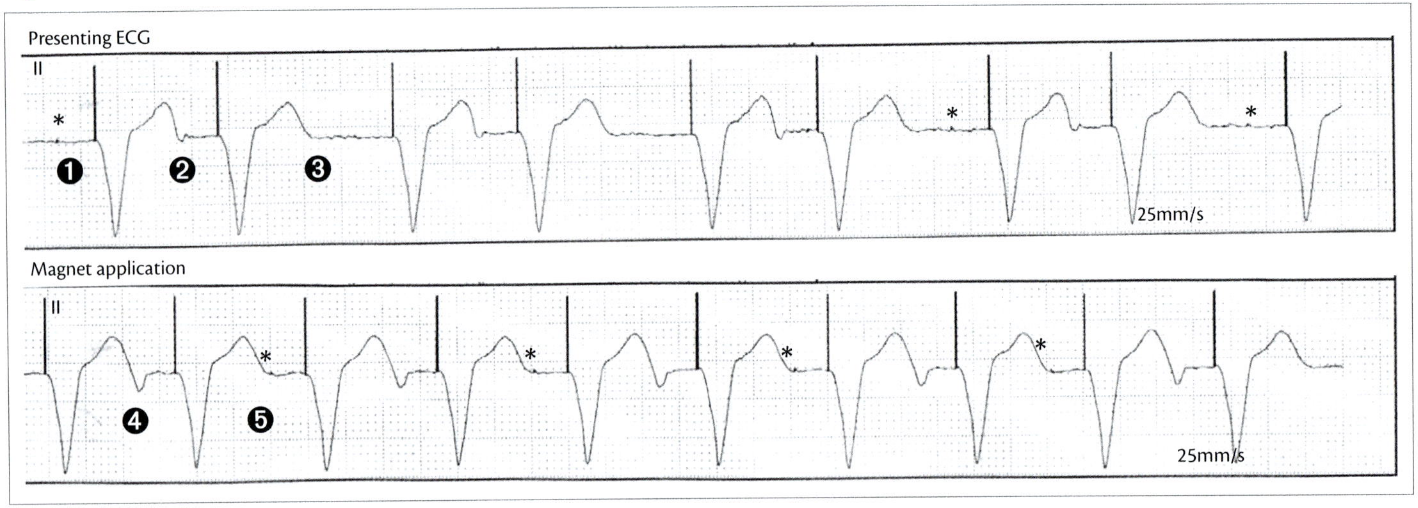

Courtesy of Dr C Vuille

❶ A P-wave following the pacing artefact (*) is not visible, indicating atrial non-capture (Figure 31.2). The atrial pacing artefact is of low amplitude (bipolar pacing) and is not always visible (i.e. before the 3rd and 5th cycles of the presenting ECG).

❷ A P-wave is visible at the end of each 2nd T-wave, corresponding to retrograde conduction, following the ventricular paced event. This P-wave is tracked and initiates an AVI, at the end of which ventricular pacing occurs.

❸ There is no retrograde P-wave visible at the end of this cycle, indicating a 2:1 retrograde VA block. The cycles then repeat.

❹ During magnet application, the pacing mode is DOO 85bpm. The RP interval is longer than during the presenting rhythm, due to the faster pacing rate with decremental VA conduction, detaching the P-wave from the T-wave and making it more visible (and speaks against atrial bigeminy). An atrial pacing artefact is not visible but must be occurring simultaneously with the retrograde P-wave (and is hidden by it).

❺ Again, a 2:1 VA block occurs during magnet application.

Comments

Utility of magnet application

The magnet application was used as an indication of the battery status (by measuring the magnet pacing rate) and as a rough indication of capture threshold (by decremental pacing output of consecutive beats). Magnet application is seldom used nowadays since the advent of modern devices. It nevertheless still has its uses. These include:

1. indication of the battery status and capture thresholds in case a programmer is not available
2. identification of the device manufacturer (company-specific magnet rates)
3. temporary programming in the DOO or VOO mode during surgery to avoid interference with electrocautery
4. temporary programming in the DOO or VOO mode to elucidate device malfunction (as in this case)
5. interruption of pacemaker-mediated tachycardia
6. bailout solution in case of A/V switch on the header (see Case 19).

A detailed review of the magnet function of pacemakers and ICDs has been published.[1]

Reference

1. Jacob S, Panaich SS, Maheshwari R, Haddad JW, Padanilam BJ, John SK. Clinical applications of magnets on cardiac rhythm management devices. *Europace* 2011; **13**: 1222–30.

Introduction to the case

A patient implanted with a dual-chamber pacemaker for syncopal complete heart block presented for routine device follow-up. The tracing in Figure 32.1 was observed during the ventricular threshold test performed in the DDD mode at 75bpm. The pacemaker settings are shown in Table 32.1.

Table 32.1 Device settings

Pacing mode	DDD
Lower rate	50bpm
Upper rate	130bpm
Atrial output (unipolar)	2.5V@0.4ms
Ventricular output (unipolar)	2.5V@0.4ms
Atrial sensitivity (bipolar)	0.5mV
Ventricular sensitivity (bipolar)	2.0mV
Paced AV delay	170ms
Sense compensation	−20ms
PVAB	100ms
PVARP	275ms
Ventricular blanking	12ms
VRP	250ms

Question

Figure 32.1 EGM during a ventricular threshold test

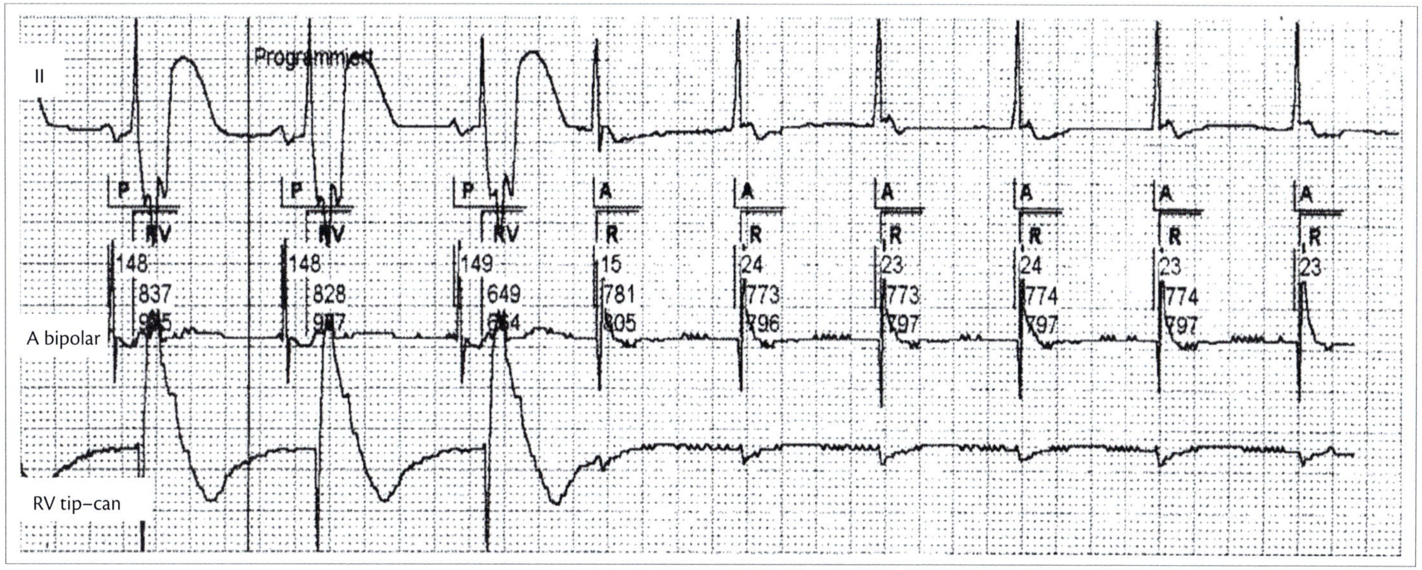

Courtesy of Dr C Israel

What do you observe?

A AV crosstalk

B FFRW oversensing

C Far-field P-wave oversensing

D Ventricular non-capture

Answer

A **AV crosstalk**

Figure 32.2 Annotated EGM during the ventricular threshold test

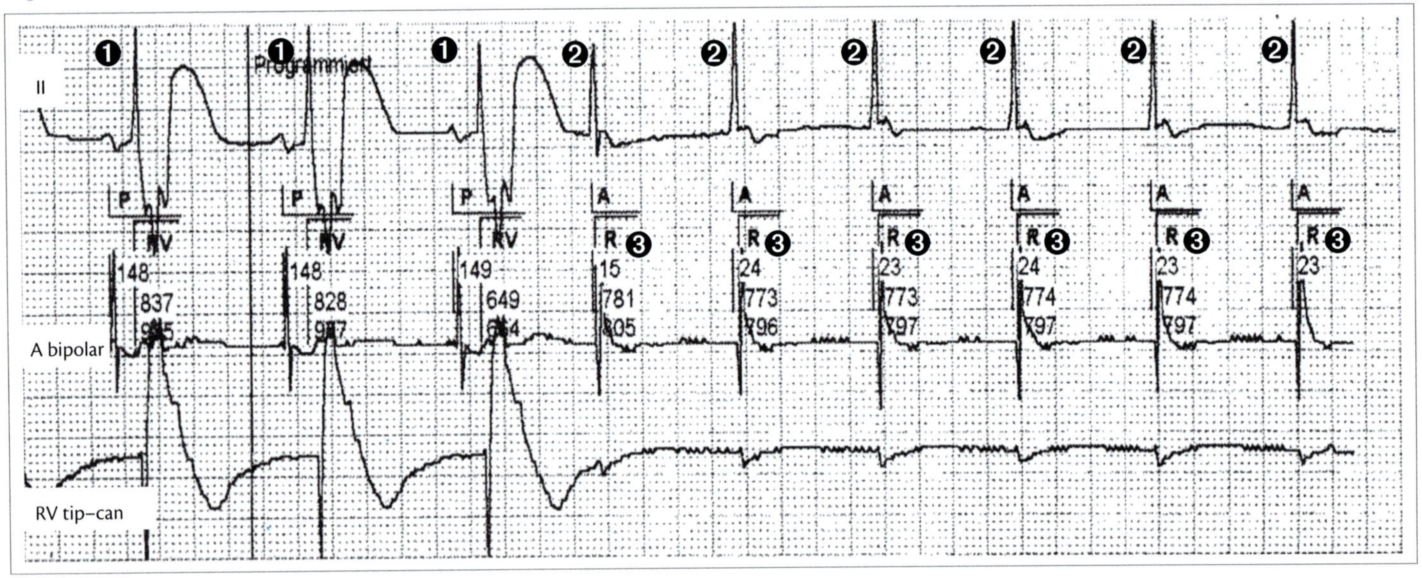

Courtesy of Dr C Israel

This is an illustration (Figure 32.2) of the potentially lethal condition known as crosstalk.

❶ The 1st three cycles before the onset of the ventricular threshold test are in sinus rhythm with ventricular pacing and ventricular capture.

❷ The ventricular threshold test is being performed in DDD 75bpm with delivery of atrial pacing and atrial capture.

❸ A VS event occurs 15–24ms after atrial pacing, inhibiting ventricular pacing, corresponding to AV crosstalk with ventricular asystole.

Comments

Atrioventricular crosstalk

Crosstalk is a potentially lethal condition in patients with complete heart block. It results from sensing of the pacing spike in one chamber by a lead implanted in another chamber. It should be distinguished from far-field oversensing (of the R-wave by the atrial lead and, more rarely, the P-wave by the ventricular lead), although there is some confusion of these terms in the medical literature.

Crosstalk is favoured by high pacing amplitude/duration, high sensitivity settings, and short blanking periods. It is, however, seldom observed in modern devices, due to protection of the phenomenon by blanking periods (PVAB and PAVB), as well as porous leads which reduce polarization and generators which discharge polarization currents. Blanking periods are significantly longer in duration (e.g. 40ms) than the pacing spike duration (e.g. 0.4ms). This is to avoid oversensing of the after-potential (resulting from polarization at the electrode–tissue interface after delivery of the pacing spike).

During threshold tests, blanking and refractory periods may be temporarily modified in some devices, exceptionally resulting in crosstalk. In this case, the ventricular threshold test was successfully performed in the VVI mode.

Introduction to the case

A patient with sick sinus syndrome was implanted with a dual-chamber pacemaker. A Holter was performed about a year after implantation, due to chest pain while walking. A strip from the Holter is shown in Figure 33.1. The device parameters are shown in Table 33.1. Pacemaker follow-up was normal.

Table 33.1 Device settings

Pacing mode	ADIR/DDDR
Lower rate	60bpm
Upper rate	130bpm
Atrial output (bipolar)	Auto@0.4ms
Ventricular output (bipolar)	Auto@0.4ms
Atrial sensitivity (bipolar)	Auto mV
Ventricular sensitivity (bipolar)	Auto mV
Paced AV delay (fixed)	150ms
Sense compensation	−30ms
Non-competitive AP	On
PVAB	180ms
PVARP	Auto
Ventricular blanking after atrial pace	28ms
VRP	230ms

Question

Figure 33.1 Holter recording

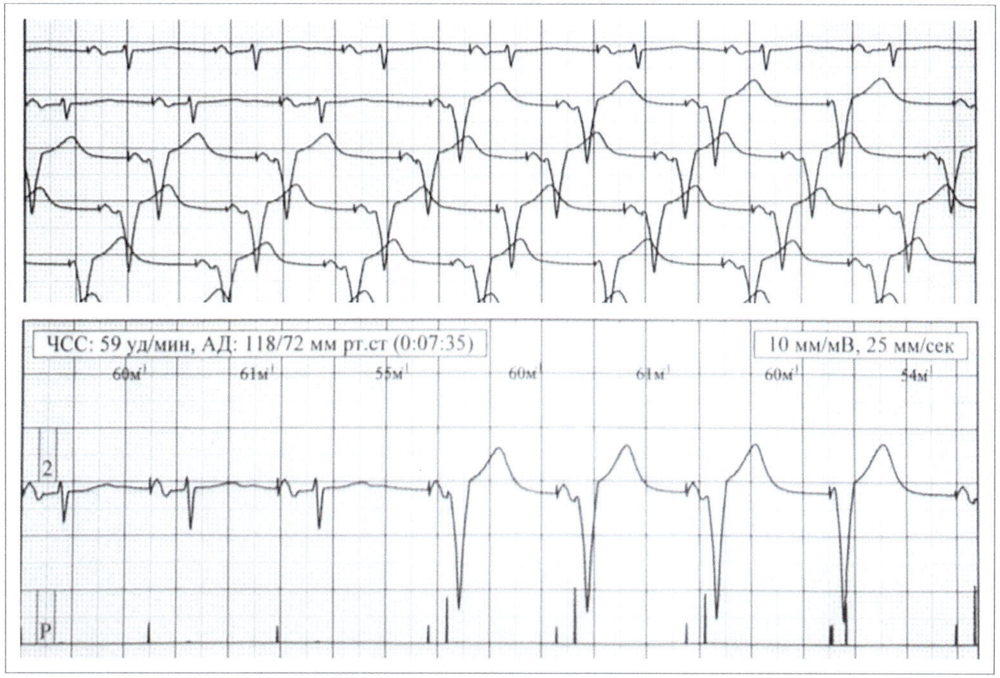

Courtesy of Dr S Moiseenko

What do you observe?

A Non-competitive atrial pacing

B Ventricular safety pacing

C Accelerated ventricular rhythm

D Automatic RV threshold test

Answer

D Automatic RV threshold test

Figure 33.2 Annotated Holter recording

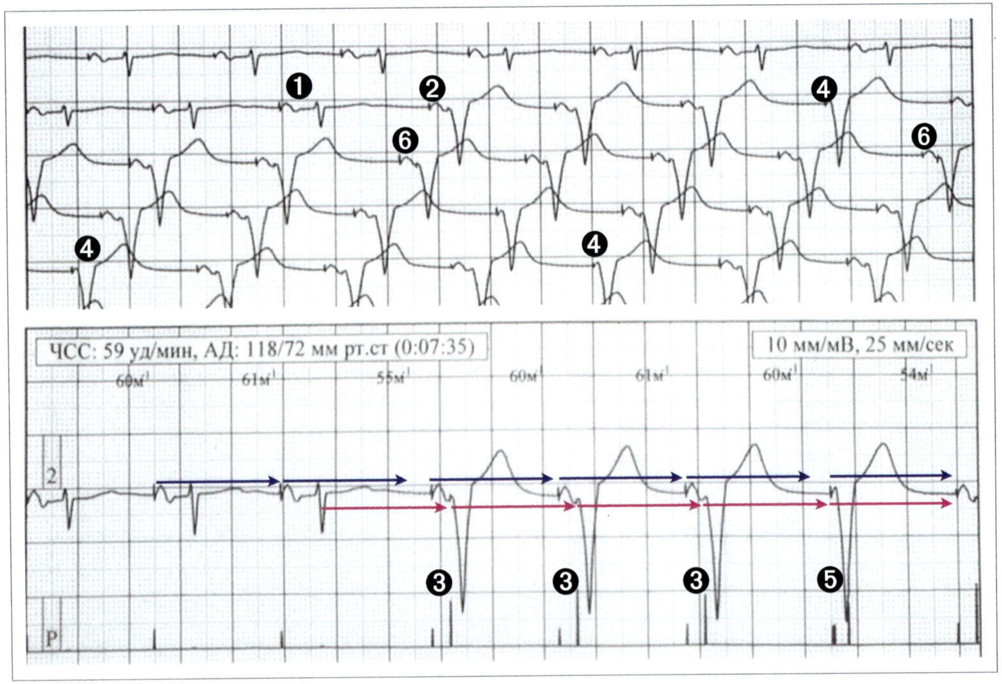

Courtesy of Dr S Moiseenko

The observed sequence (Figure 33.2) of ventricular pacing is due to the Medtronic automatic RV threshold test.

❶ Pacing is in the ADI mode at the baseline (rest) rate of 60bpm up to this cycle (the PR interval is much longer than the programmed paced AVI of 150ms).

❷ The automatic threshold test is initiated by DDD pacing. A prolonged A–A interval, resulting from the non-competitive atrial pacing algorithm (e.g. because of atrial oversensing), would not result in a switch to DDD pacing.

❸ The Holter displays reconstructed pacing artefact signals, showing AV pacing at the programmed AVI of 150ms for three cycles (ventricular safety pacing would result in an interval of 110ms).

❹ The 4th beat does not have a clearly visible P-wave (although the slightly larger R-wave corresponds, in fact, to summation with the onset of the P-wave).

❺ The reconstructed pacing artefacts show closely spaced lines, corresponding to atrial pacing, followed immediately by ventricular pacing at the test amplitude, which captures the ventricle. This sequence is followed by a backup spike at 110ms (at the programmed amplitude and pulse width of 1ms).

❻ These two cycles show the same sequence of three support cycles, followed by a test cycle with a longer AP interval. This time, the test spike (invisible) results in loss of capture, with the backup spike (visible due to the 1ms duration) capturing the ventricle.

All the arrows are of the same length. The blue arrows serve to illustrate prolongation of the A–A interval when there is sudden shortening of the AVI (due to onset of DDD pacing after the 2nd arrow and due to very short AVI with the test cycle after the 5th arrow). The red arrows show that the V–V intervals are constant, except for the last arrow which shows sudden prolongation of the V–V interval. This device functions with atrial-based timing and switches to what is, in essence, ventricular-based timing for the cycles with suddenly shortened AVIs, and it then reverts to atrial-based timing for cycles with lengthening of the AVI (see Comments in Case 23, p. 93).

Comments

Recognizing patterns to deduce device algorithms

Many modern pacemakers have a number of automatic tests that verify lead impedance, sensing and pacing thresholds. The details of all these tests (which differ between manufacturers) are almost impossible to memorize. Nevertheless, intriguing device behaviour that is observed to be repetitive most often results from one of these automatic algorithms. The clinician can then refer to the device technical manual or online resources (e.g. <http://www.medtronicfeatures.com> for this case), in order to identify the algorithm.

This case also illustrates that devices may temporarily function with different timing rules under certain circumstances. A full understanding of atrial- and ventricular-based timing explains why A–A or V–V intervals may suddenly change.

Introduction to the case

A patient with a dual-chamber pacemaker (and an atrial lead in the right atrial appendage) presented with atrial flutter 2 months after radiofrequency pulmonary vein isolation for paroxysmal AF. The ECG is shown in Figure 34.1. The atrial cycle length was measured at 280ms, and a non-invasive electrophysiological study (NIPS), with right atrial pacing via the pacemaker at a cycle length of 260ms, was performed. The real-time EGM at the end of the atrial burst is shown in Figure 34.2.

Figure 34.1 The 12-lead ECG at presentation

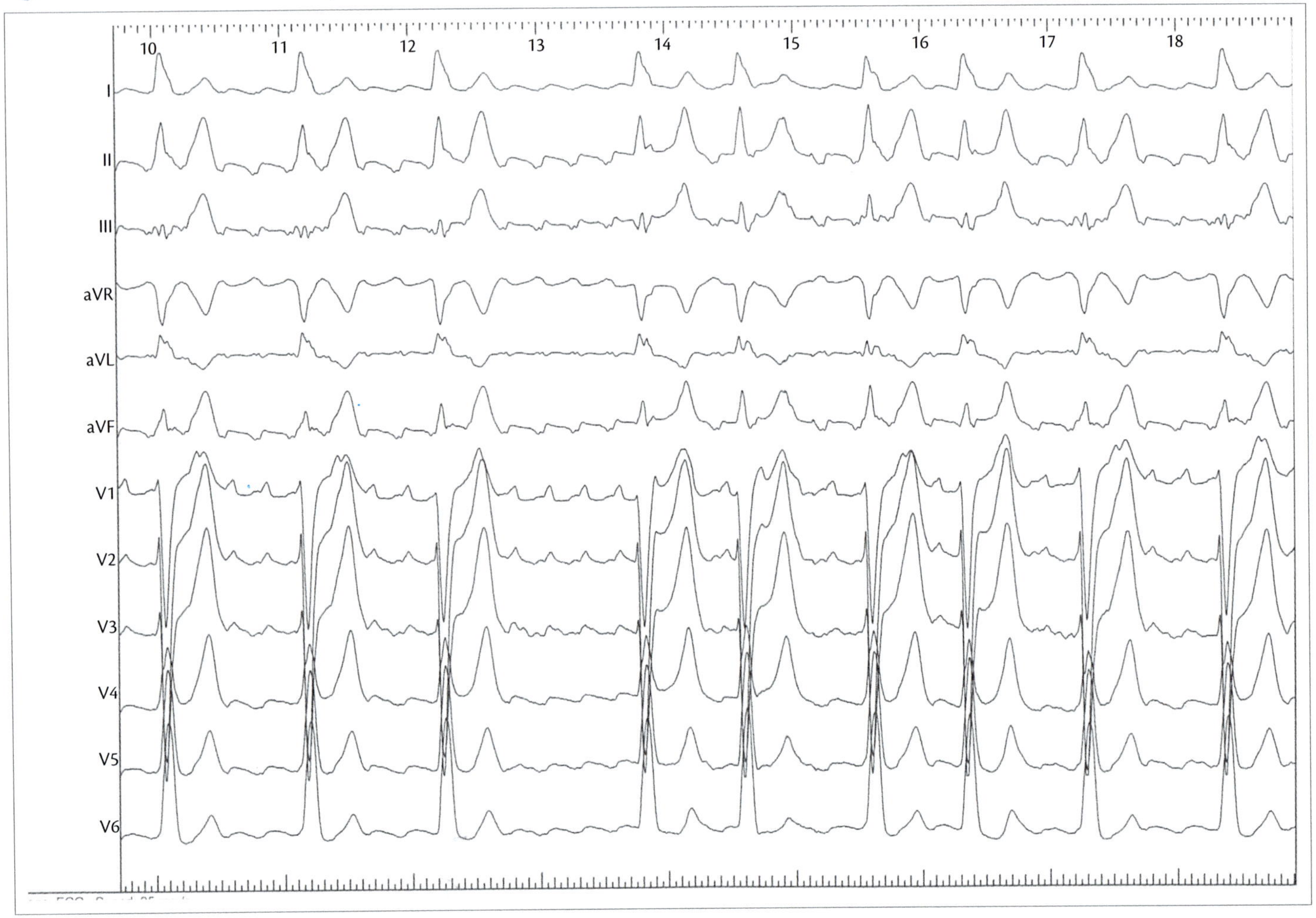

Question

Figure 34.2 Real-time EGM during the non-invasive electrophysiological study with overdrive atrial pacing

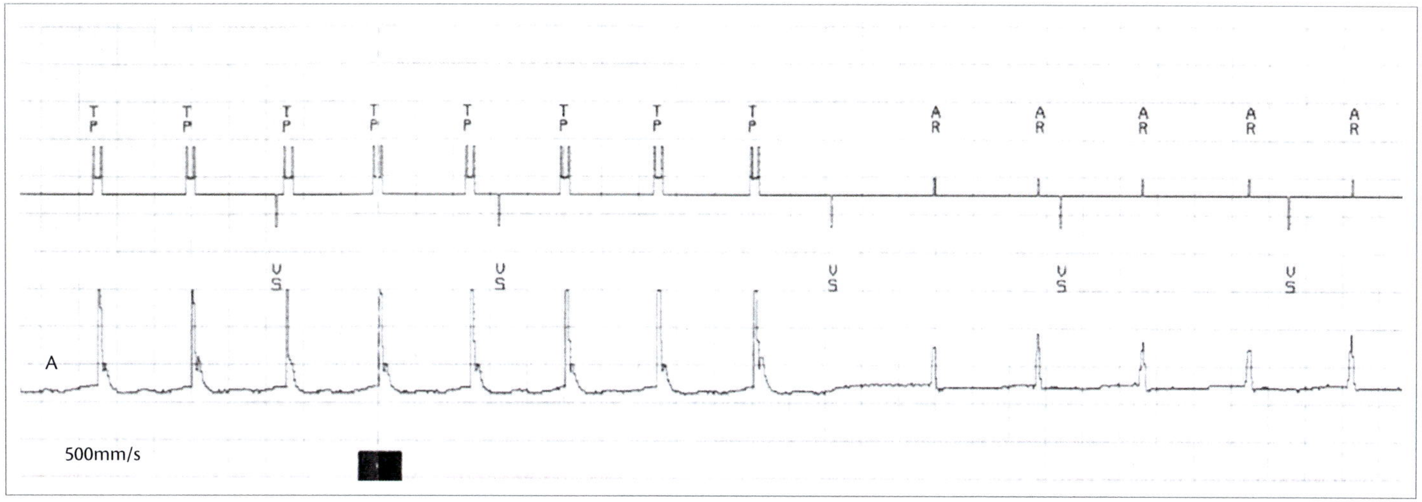

Which of the following is most likely to be true regarding the flutter circuit?

A Counterclockwise typical flutter

B Clockwise typical flutter

C Left atrial flutter

D Impossible to say

Answer

C **Left atrial flutter**

Figure 34.3 Annotated real-time EGM during the non-invasive electrophysiological study with overdrive atrial pacing

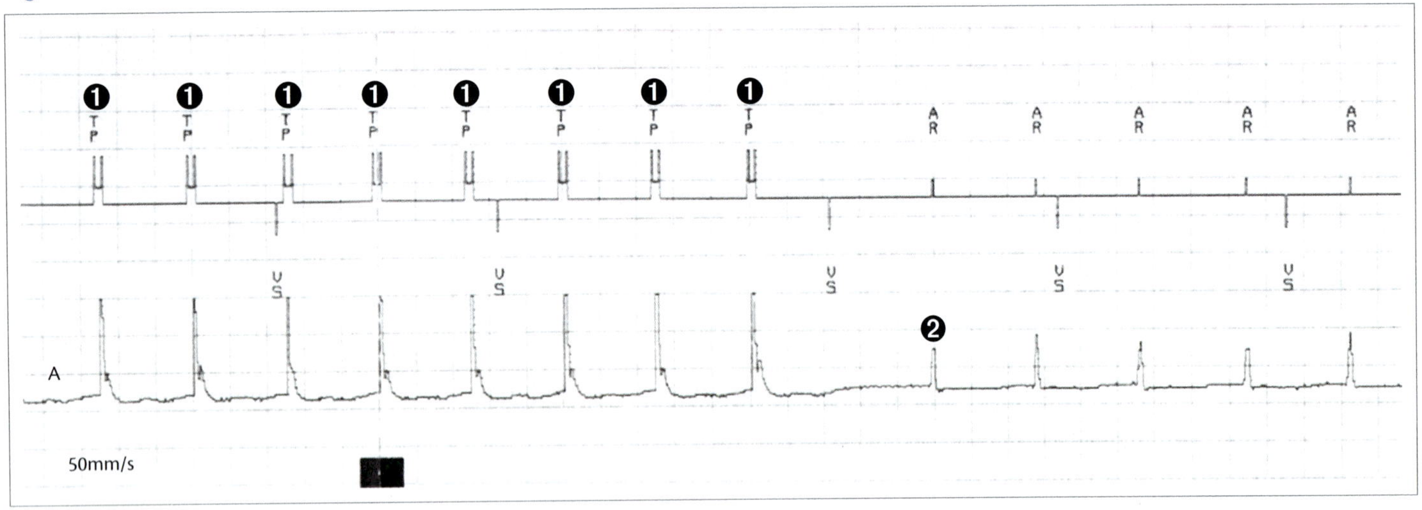

The surface ECG may suggest typical counterclockwise atrial flutter. However, the post-pacing interval performed by overdrive pacing from the right atrial appendage is very long, suggesting a left atrial circuit (Figure 34.3).

❶ Atrial tachycardia pacing (TP) captures the right atrium, as is apparent from the atrial EGM.

❷ The post-pacing interval is long (500ms), and significantly longer than the tachycardia cycle length (260ms).

Comments

Non-invasive pacing studies with pacemakers (1)

The patient underwent a redo radiofrequency ablation procedure, with localization of the flutter circuit in the left atrium near the ostium of the left inferior pulmonary vein, which was successfully ablated. It has been shown that entrainment mapping via pacemakers and ICDs, with a post-pacing interval that is <100ms longer than the tachycardia cycle length, allows to distinguish right atrial from left atrial circuits.[1] Atrial overdrive pacing may also be used to reduce atrial flutters by applying bursts, and some devices have algorithms that do this automatically.

Reference

1. Burri H, Zimmermann M, Sunthorn H, *et al.* Non-invasive pacing study via pacemakers and implantable cardioverter defibrillators for differentiating right from left atrial flutter. *Heart Rhythm* 2015 (in press).

Introduction to the case

A 78-year-old patient with a history of symptomatic sinus node dysfunction was implanted with a dual-chamber pacemaker. Upon return to the ward, the patient felt palpitations (which he had previously experienced), and the nurse noted a regular tachycardia at 110bpm, with a left bundle branch block QRS pattern (that was also present at baseline). Device interrogation was performed, and the real-time EGM is shown in Figure 35.1. A non-invasive pacing study (NIPS) was performed via the pacemaker, with ventricular pacing at a cycle length of 500ms (the tachycardia cycle length was measured at 540ms). The EGM at the end of the pacing sequence is shown in Figure 35.2.

Figure 35.1 Real-time EGM

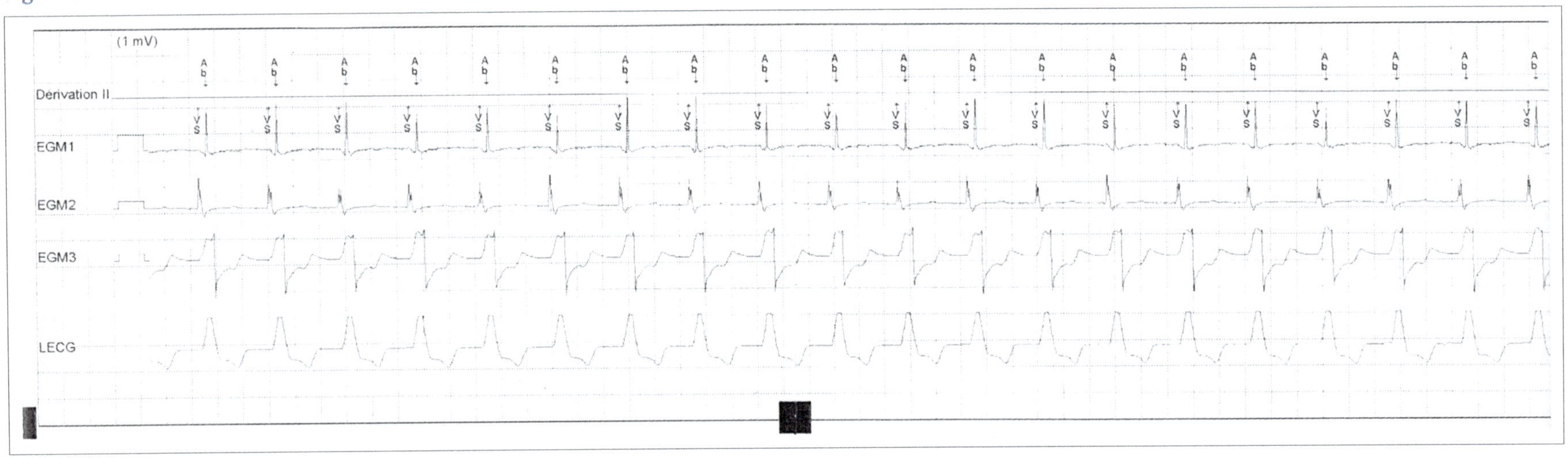

Question

Figure 35.2 Real-time EGM of the non-invasive pacing study (NIPS)

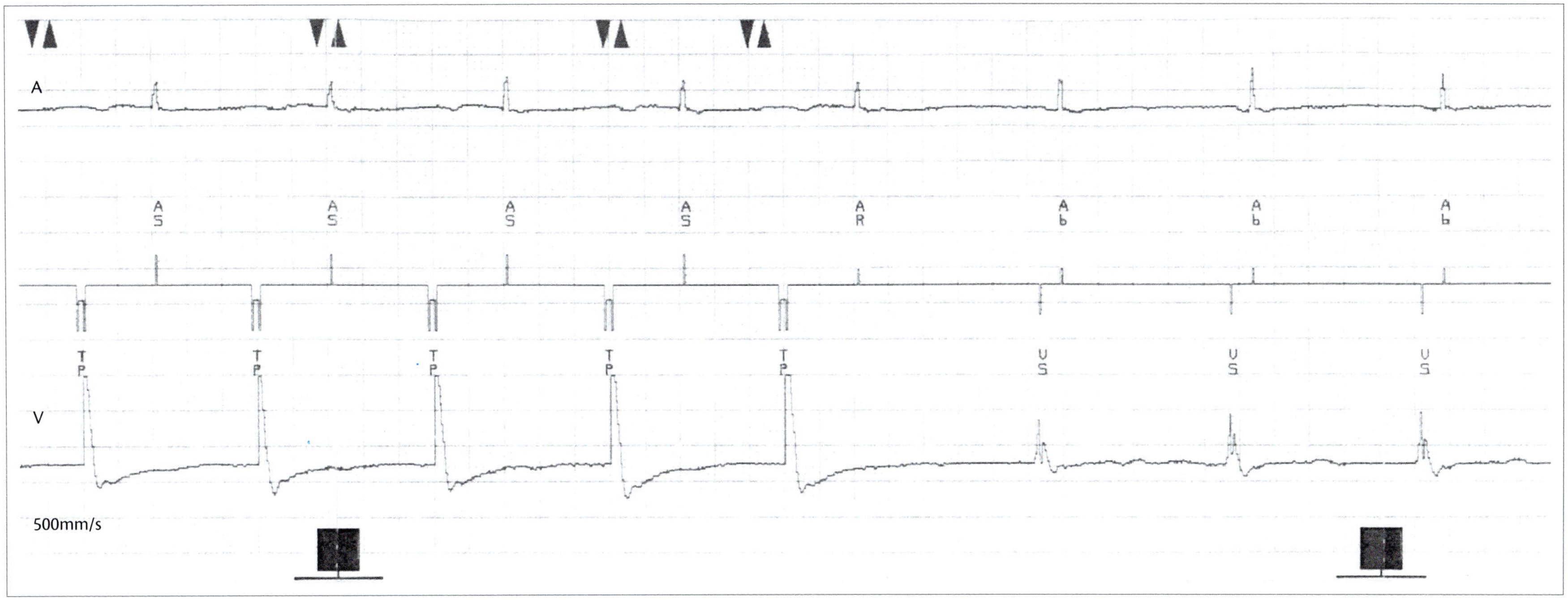

What is your diagnosis?

A Pacemaker-mediated tachycardia

B Atrial tachycardia

C VT

D AVNRT

Answer

D AVNRT

Figure 35.3 Annotated real-time EGM of the NIPS

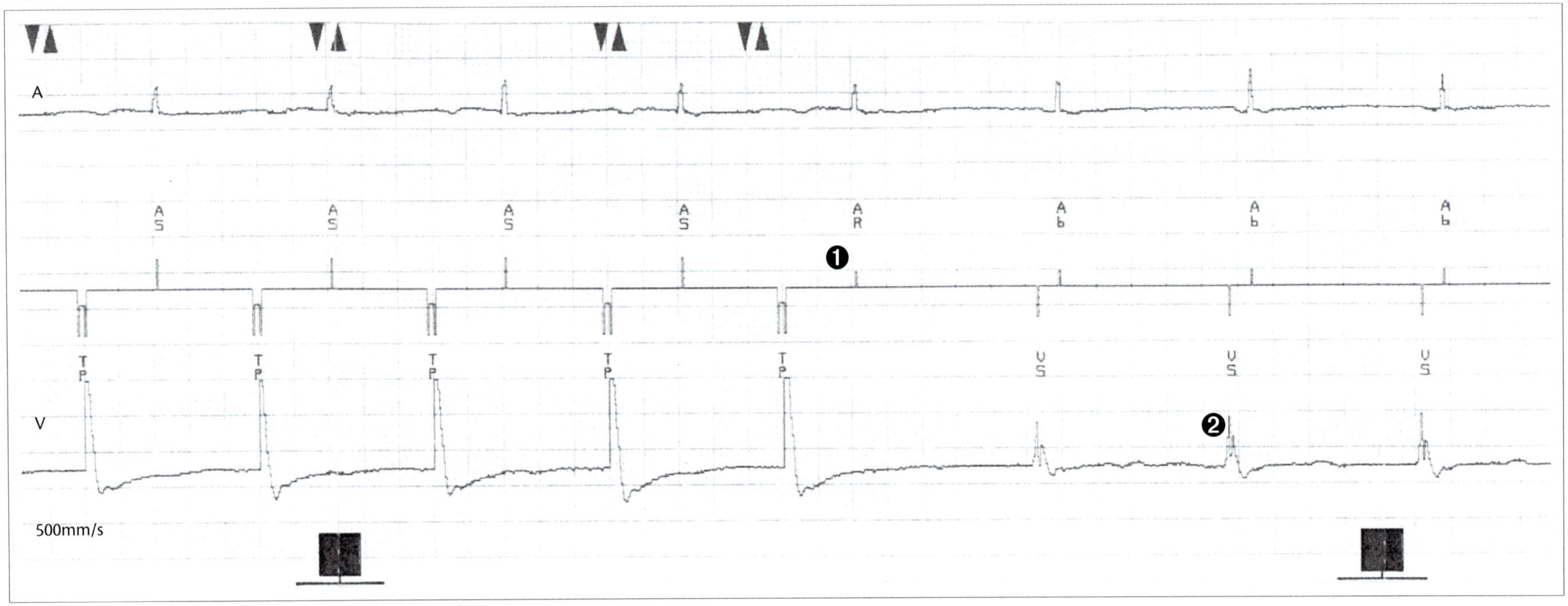

Pacemaker-mediated tachycardia is excluded by the fact that there is no pacing during the tachycardia. The pacing manoeuvres led to the diagnosis of AVNRT (Figure 35.3).

❶ Ventricular overdrive pacing results in retrograde conduction to the atrium (with constant VA intervals).

❷ Tachycardia resumes after interruption of ventricular overdrive pacing.

The following can be observed which confirm the diagnosis of AVNRT:

- a 'VAV' sequence
- a (stimulation-A)–(VA) interval of 120ms
- a post-pacing interval—tachycardia cycle length of 160ms.

Comments

Non-invasive pacing studies with pacemakers (2)

AVNRT was confirmed by an electrophysiological study, and radiofrequency modification of the slow pathway was performed.

NIPS can be useful in case of tachycardias with a 1:1 AV ratio where the differential diagnosis is atrial tachycardia, AVNRT, and AVRT. Almost all devices allow performing NIPS, which can use the same criteria for diagnosis as for standard electrophysiological studies.

Section 2

ICD

Cases 36–53

Introduction to the case

A 73-year-old patient with ischaemic heart disease and a history of sustained VT and a single-chamber ICD presented for follow-up. The patient did not report any complaints. A stored event was retrieved from the device memory. The tachogram is shown in Figure 36.1, and the EGM of the event in Figure 36.2.

Figure 36.1 Tachogram of the stored event

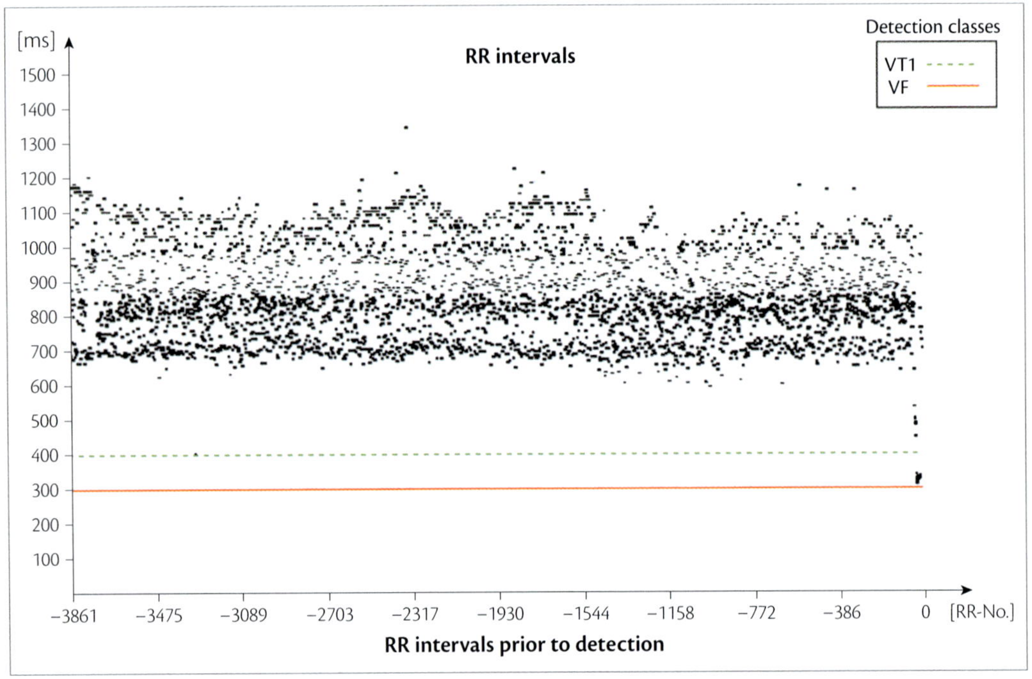

Question

Figure 36.2 EGM of stored event

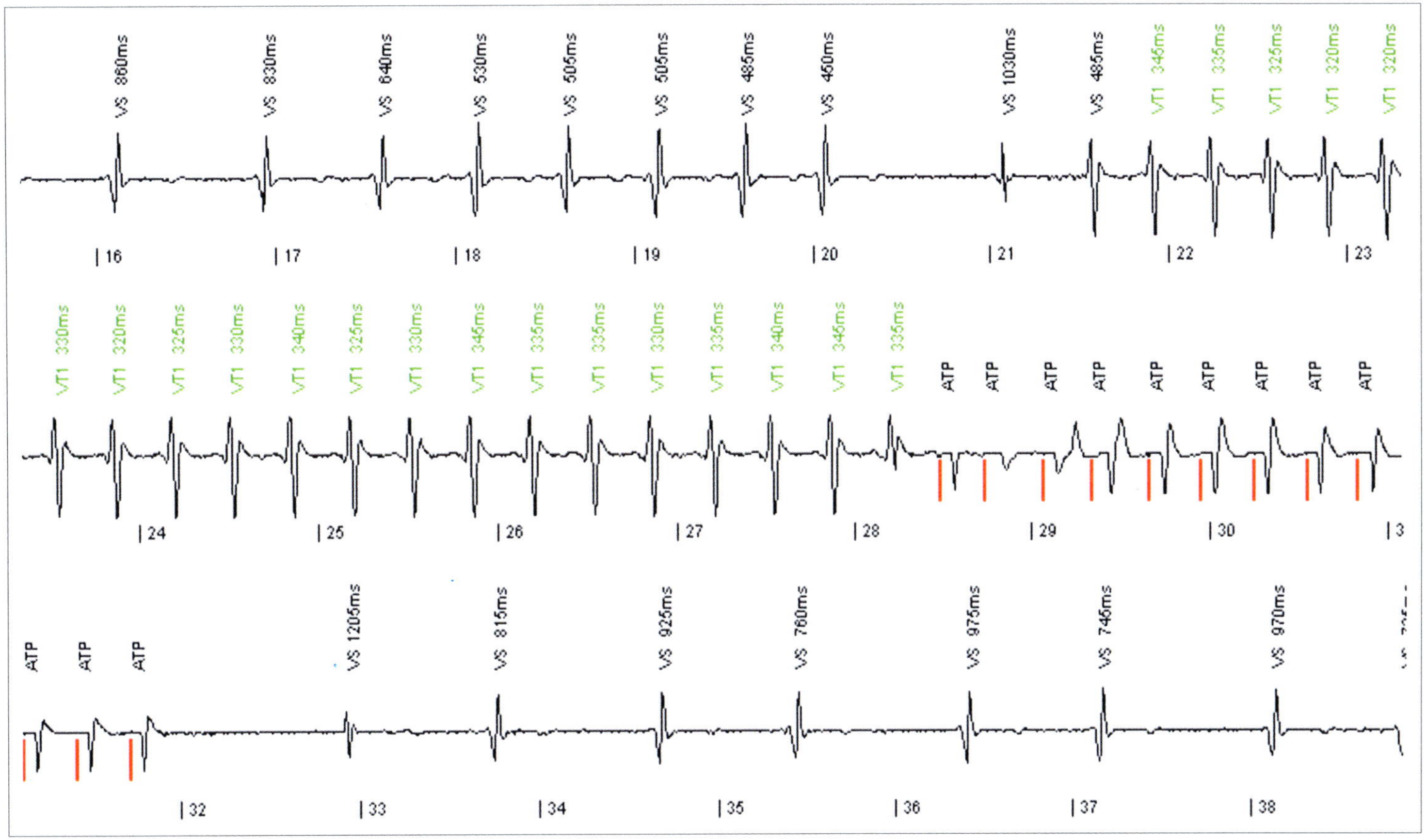

What is your diagnosis?

A Sinus rhythm with appropriate therapy for VT

B AF with appropriate therapy for VT

C Sinus rhythm with inappropriate therapy for SVT

D AF with inappropriate therapy for SVT

Answer

B AF with appropriate therapy for VT

Figure 36.3 Annotated EGM of stored event

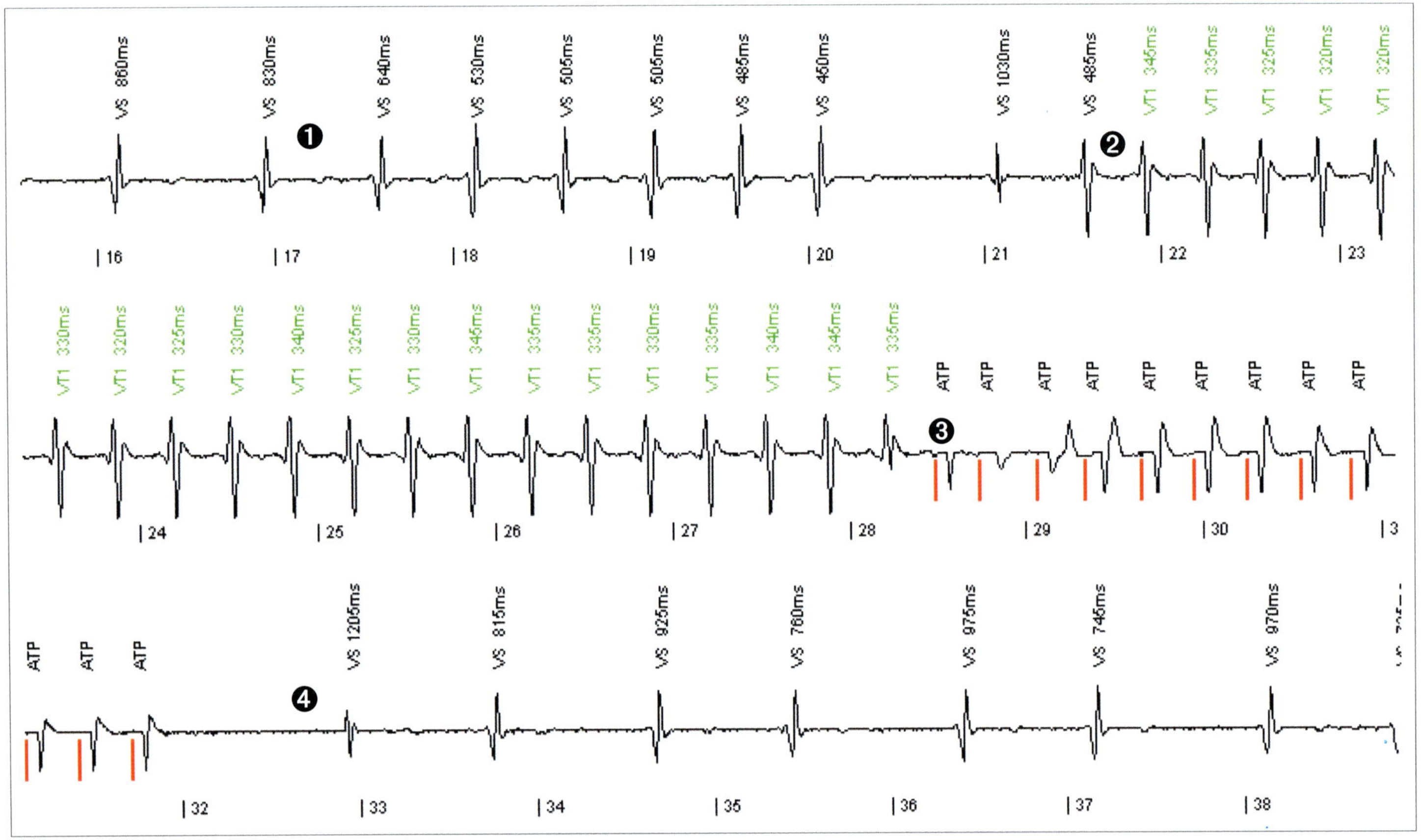

The patient is in AF, with the onset of monomorphic VT that is successfully treated by a burst of antitachycardia pacing (ATP) (Figure 36.3).

❶ The RR intervals are very irregular, indicating AF.

❷ A relatively regular tachycardia (cycle length of 320–345ms) of sudden onset with a different EGM morphology is indicative of VT.

❸ After 20 rapid cycles (the programmed number of intervals to detect VT), an ATP sequence is delivered which successfully interrupts the VT.

❹ Baseline rhythm resumes (the 1st beat is probably ventricular, due to the different morphology).

Comments

Ventricular tachycardia/supraventricular tachycardia discrimination in single-chamber implantable cardioverter–defibrillators

In this example, the three discriminatory criteria were fulfilled to distinguish VT from SVT:

- sudden onset, which distinguishes sinus tachycardia from VT but will not distinguish VT from atrial or junctional tachycardia (AVNRT, AVRT)
- regularity, which distinguishes VT from AF but will not be useful to discriminate VT from regular SVT (e.g. atrial tachycardia, atrial flutter, or AVNRT)
- morphology, which will distinguish VT from SVT, unless aberrant intraventricular conduction is present (e.g. due to rate dependence).

The examples shown in the 1st three cases of this book are taken from older devices, dating from around 2000, and do not reflect modern-day technology and programming. However, the principles for interpreting tracings remain the same.

Introduction to the case

A patient with a single-chamber ICD was seen for routine follow-up. He had no complaints. An episode classified as VT was retrieved from the device memory. The tachogram of the episode is shown in Figure 37.1, and the EGM of the episode is shown in Figure 37.2.

Figure 37.1 Tachogram of the stored event

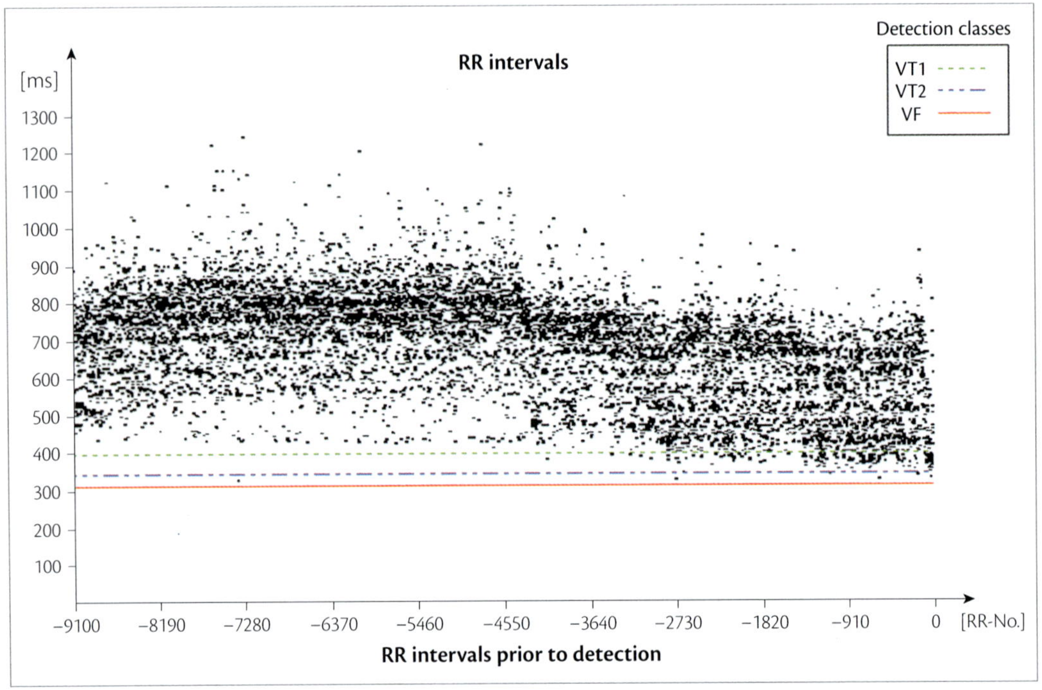

Question

Figure 37.2 EGM of the stored event

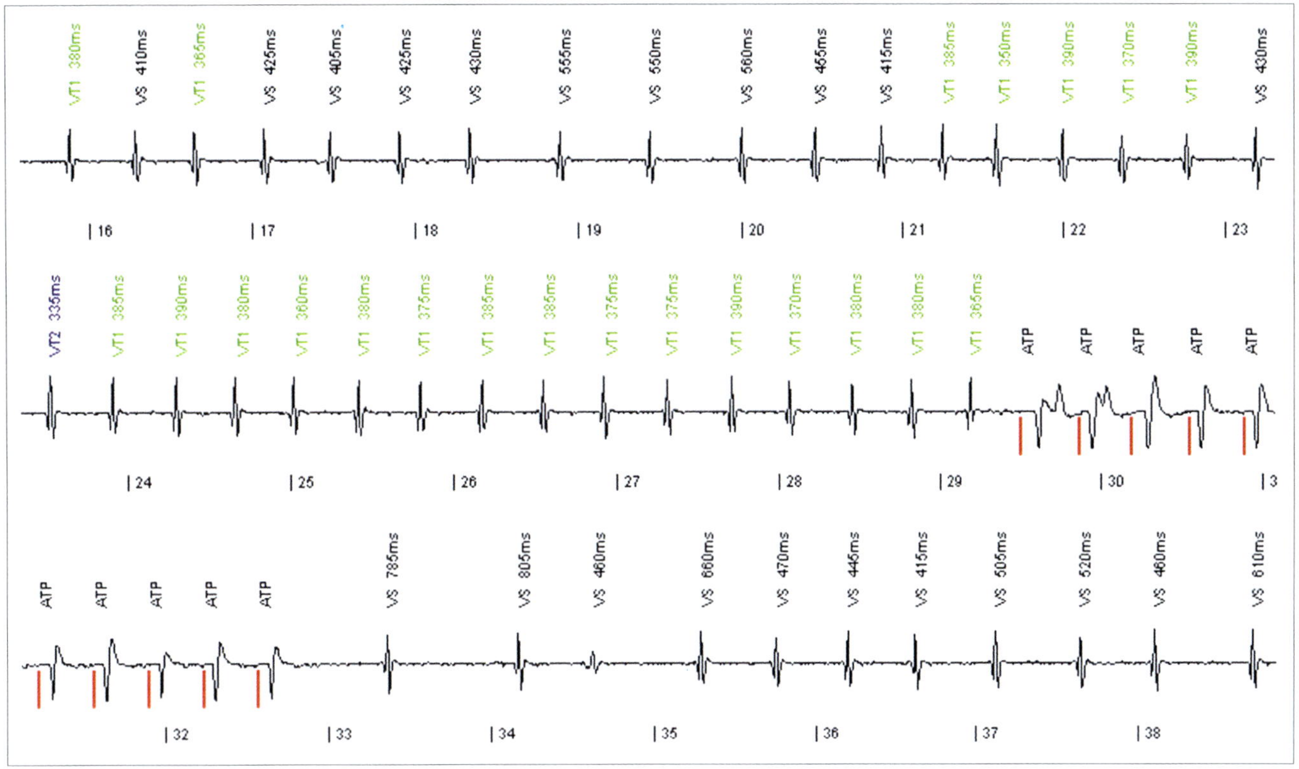

What is your diagnosis?

A Sinus rhythm with appropriate therapy for VT

B AF with appropriate therapy for VT

C Sinus rhythm with inappropriate therapy for SVT

D AF with inappropriate therapy for SVT

Answer

D **AF with inappropriate therapy for SVT**

Figure 37.3 Annotated EGM of the stored event

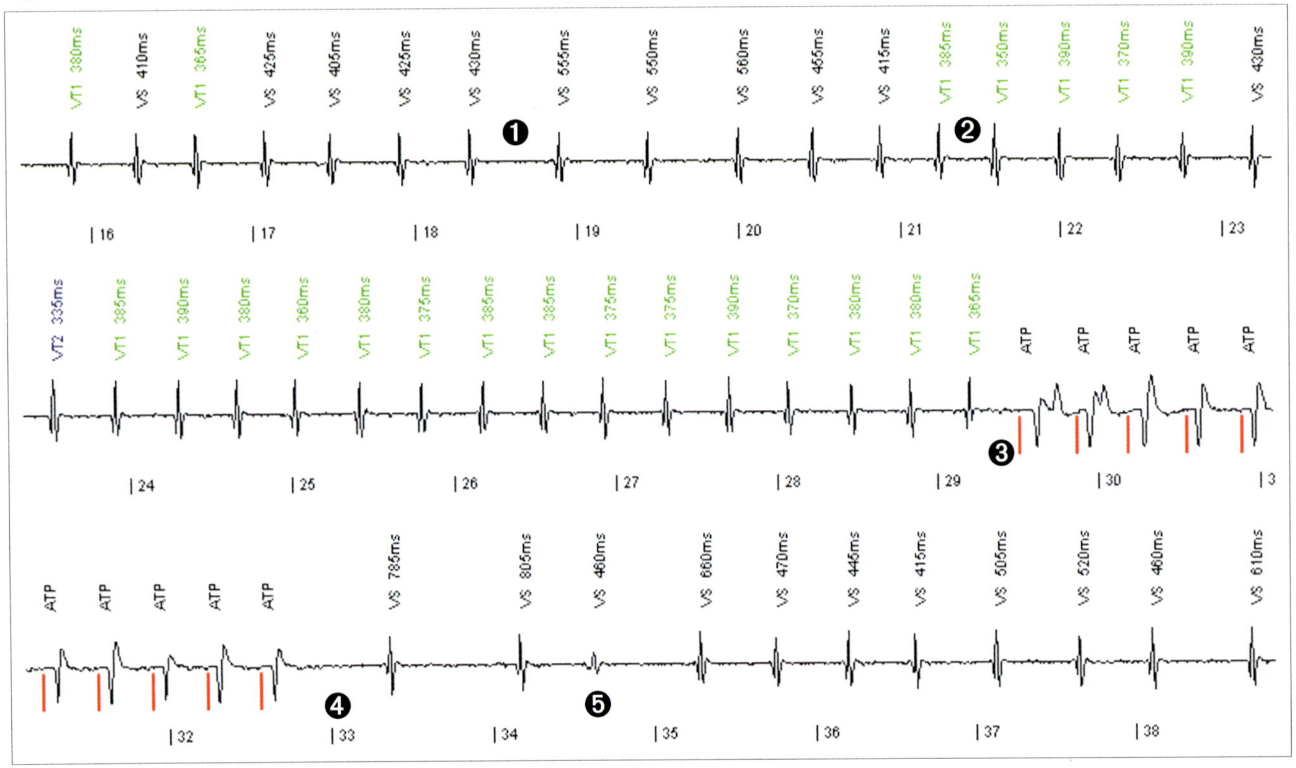

The patient had AF, with increasing heart rates which gradually entered the VT zone, resulting in ATP therapy (Figure 37.3).

❶ The RR intervals are very irregular (this can be appreciated by the tachogram on the preceding page), strongly suggesting underlying AF.

❷ The RR intervals enter the VT zone (400ms), without any change in EGM morphology. Note that the intervals before delivery of ATP are relatively regular (between 360ms and 390ms), despite AF.

❸ An ATP burst is delivered, because the number of intervals to detect VT was reached (which was 16 consecutive intervals in this case) and because therapy was not inhibited by a VT/SVT discriminatory algorithm.

❹ There is a pause after ATP delivery, which is probably due to concealed retrograde conduction into the AV node, delaying the consecutive anterograde conduction of AF. This should not be mistaken as being an effective therapy of VT.

❺ This beat with a different EGM morphology could be intraventricular aberration or a VPB.

Comments

Ventricular tachycardia and ventricular fibrillation counters

Inappropriate therapy would probably have been avoided in this case by programming a morphology discrimination algorithm (unavailable on this device) or by the sudden onset criterion.As can be appreciated by the tachogram, cycles had already been entering the VT zone since >2700 RR intervals. However, VT was not detected, due to resetting of the counters by events slower than the tachy zone. Manufacturers use different criteria for detecting VT and ventricular fibrillation (VF):

- Biotronik and Medtronic devices require a prespecified number of consecutive intervals to fall within the VT zone. VF detection, on the other hand, is based upon a sliding window probabilistic counter (e.g. 24/30 intervals falling in the window)
- Boston Scientific ICDs require that three consecutive fast intervals be detected, in order to initiate analysis, with a sliding window probabilistic counter that functions during a predefined duration of time for tachycardia detection
- Sorin devices also use a sliding window probabilistic counter for the VT and VF zones. Once this is satisfied, a 'duration' counter of intervals is incremented. The probabilistic and duration counters are programmable. The counters are reset, if slow intervals or SVT is classified by the discriminatory criteria
- St-Jude devices use a binning system, in which an interval will be binned (as sinus, VT, VF, or not binned at all), depending on the average of the current and last three intervals. VT and VF counters keep on incrementing up to the programmable duration of numbers of intervals, as long as five sinus intervals are not detected.

Details of these criteria have been published previously in a comprehensive article.[1]

Reference

1. Mansour F, Khairy P. ICD monitoring zones: intricacies, pitfalls, and programming tips. *J Cardiovasc Electrophysiol* 2008; **19**: 568–74.

Introduction to the case

A patient with a single-chamber ICD and implanted for the primary prevention of sudden death, was followed up at the device clinic. He complained of palpitations without any malaise. An episode of arrhythmia was retrieved from the device memory. The tachogram is shown in Figure 38.1, and the EGM in Figure 38.2.

Figure 38.1 Tachogram of the stored episode

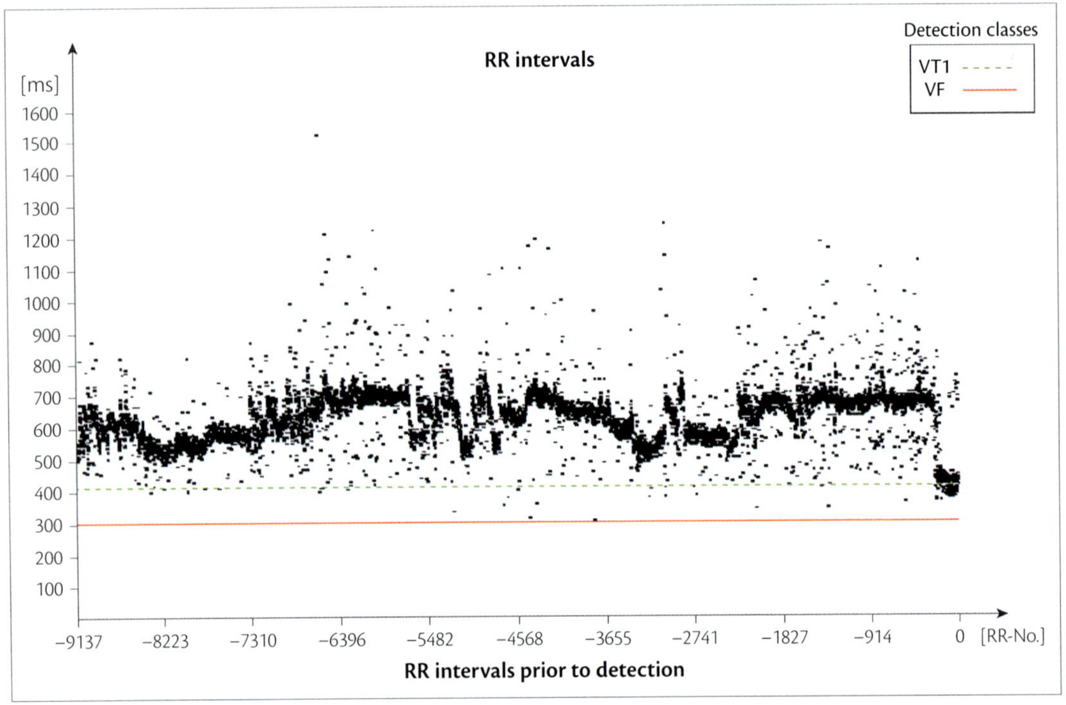

Question

Figure 38.2 EGM of the stored episode

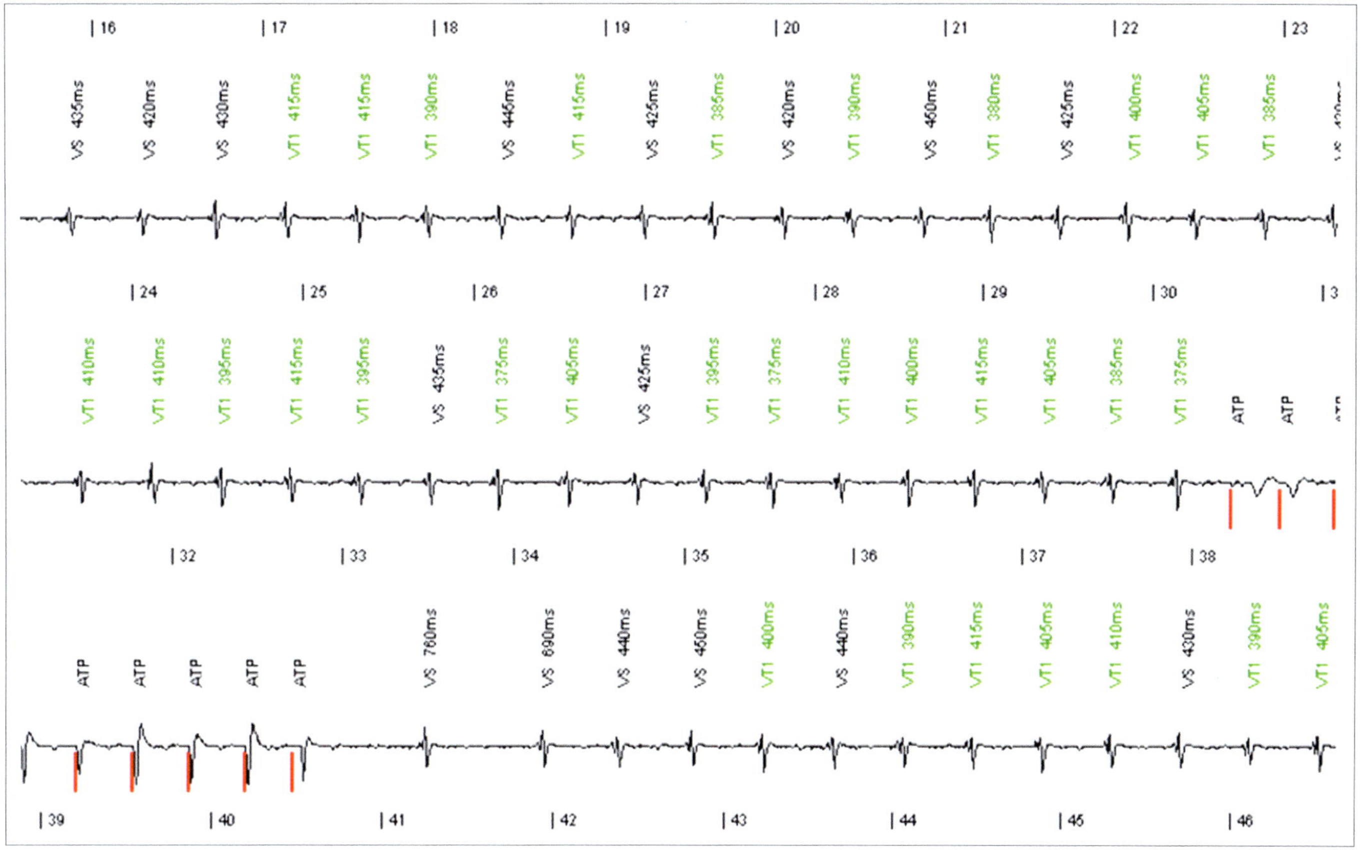

What is your diagnosis?

A Sinus rhythm with appropriate therapy for VT

B AF with appropriate therapy for VT (double tachycardia)

C Sinus rhythm with onset of AF and inappropriate therapy

D Sinus rhythm with onset of AVNRT and inappropriate therapy

Answer

C Sinus rhythm with onset of AF and inappropriate therapy

Figure 38.3 Annotated EGM of the stored episode

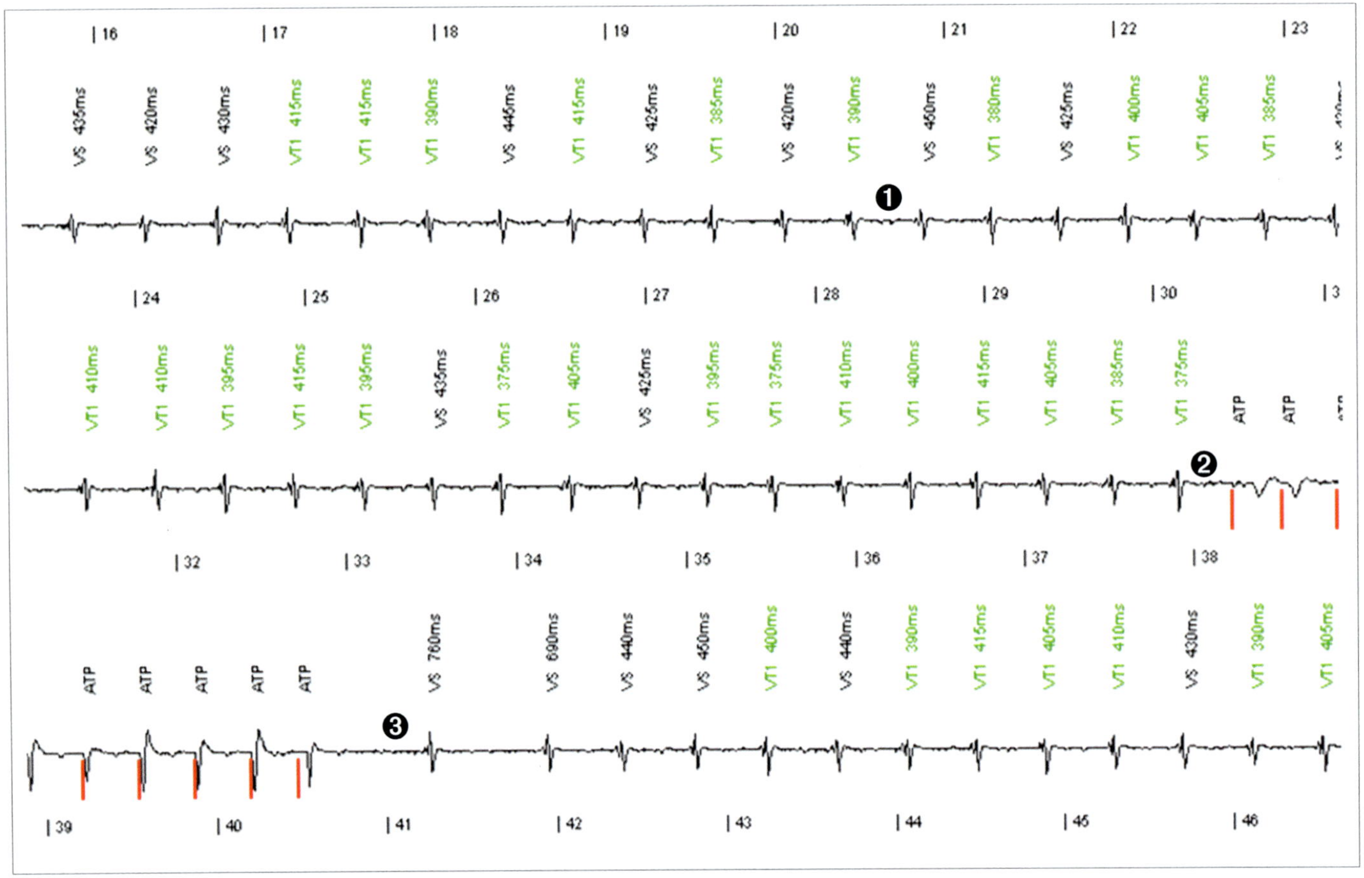

The patient was in sinus rhythm, with a sudden onset of AF, which resulted in inappropriate ICD therapy (Figure 38.3).

❶ An irregular rhythm (cycle length of 375–450ms) is observed, corresponding to AF, with rates bordering the VT detection zone of 420ms. Note that the cycles entering the VT zone (labelled 'VT1') are of identical morphology as those labelled as 'VS'. The EGM recording was not triggered when the patient was still in sinus rhythm, as VT detection only occurred about 200 RR intervals after the onset of AF.

❷ VT is classified after eight consecutive intervals in the VT zone, triggering an ATP burst sequence of eight cycles.

❸ A pause is observed after the ATP sequence, due to slowing of AV conduction by concealed retrograde conduction into the AV node. As in Case 1, this should not be interpreted as successful ICD therapy.

Comments

Sudden onset tachycardia

Inappropriate therapy would have been avoided by programming a higher treatment zone for VT (e.g. >182ms, as in the PREPARE study)[1] and with a greater number of intervals for detection (the MADIT-RIT[2] trial has validated a duration of 60s in a VT zone of 170–200bpm). A morphology discrimination algorithm (unavailable in this device) would also have been useful. Even though AF had a sudden onset (as visualized on the tachogram), the sudden onset criterion would also have avoided therapy, as conducted AF rates were just bordering the VT zone (i.e. entering and exiting the zone without great changes in cycle intervals). Sudden onset may distinguish sinus tachycardia from VT (see Figure 38.4 showing gradual onset of sinus tachycardia) but may not discriminate correctly SVT with sudden onset (such as AF or AVNRT) and may withhold therapy in rare cases of VT induced by exercise.

References

1. Wilkoff BL, Williamson BD, Stern RS, *et al.* Strategic programming of detection and therapy parameters in implantable cardioverter-defibrillators reduces shocks in primary prevention patients: results from the PREPARE (Primary Prevention Parameters Evaluation) study. *J Am Coll Cardiol* 2008; **52**: 541–50.
2. Moss AJ, Schuger C, Beck CA, *et al.* Reduction in inappropriate therapy and mortality through ICD programming. *N Engl J Med* 2012; **367**: 2275–83.

Figure 38.4 Gradual onset of sinus tachycardia

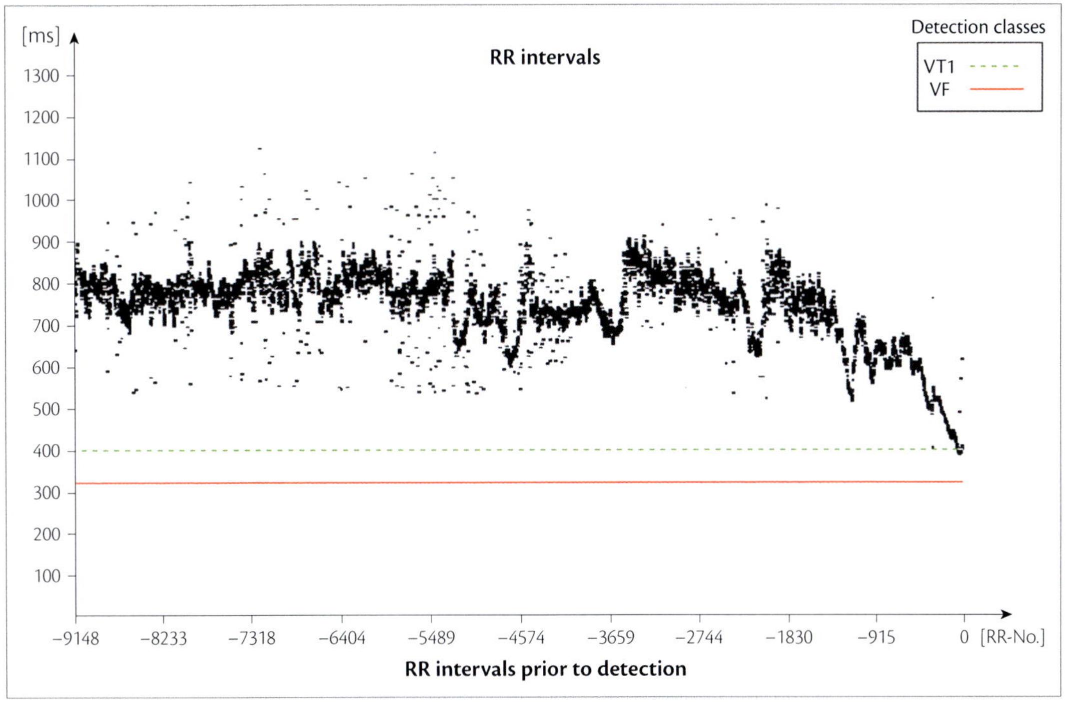

CASE 39

Introduction to the case

A patient implanted with a cardiac resynchronization therapy defibrillator (CRT-D) for ischaemic heart disease and a history of sustained VT was admitted after having received multiple shocks. He had undergone previously AV nodal ablation, due to rapidly conducted paroxysmal AF that was refractory to drug therapy. The device settings are shown in Table 39.1 and Figure 39.1. The tachogram of one of the stored episodes is displayed in Figure 39.2, with the EGM at the onset of the arrhythmia in Figure 39.3.

Table 39.1 Device settings

Zone	Slow VT	Fast VT	VF
Rate (bpm/ms)	105/570	162/370 (via VT)	222/270
Detection (intervals)	16	18/24	18/24
Redetection (intervals)	12	12/16	12/16
SVT/VT discriminators	Disabled		
Therapy	Five bursts + four ramps + shocks	One burst + one ramp + shocks	Shocks

Figure 39.1 Device settings

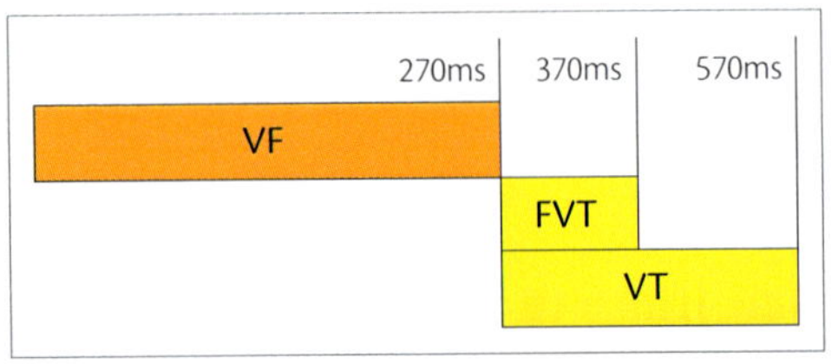

Figure 39.2 Tachogram of the stored episode

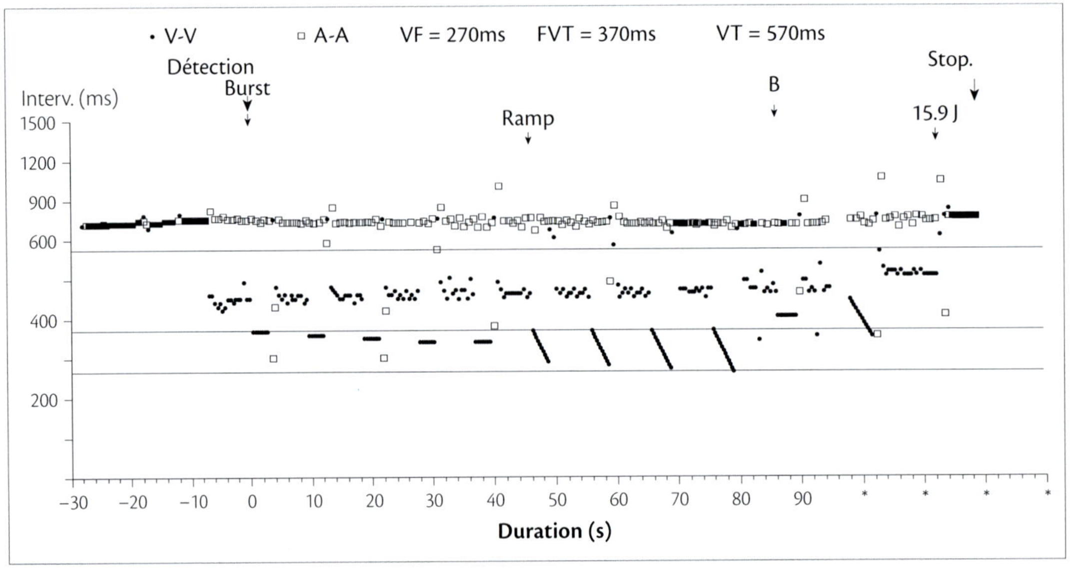

Question

Figure 39.3 EGM of the stored episode

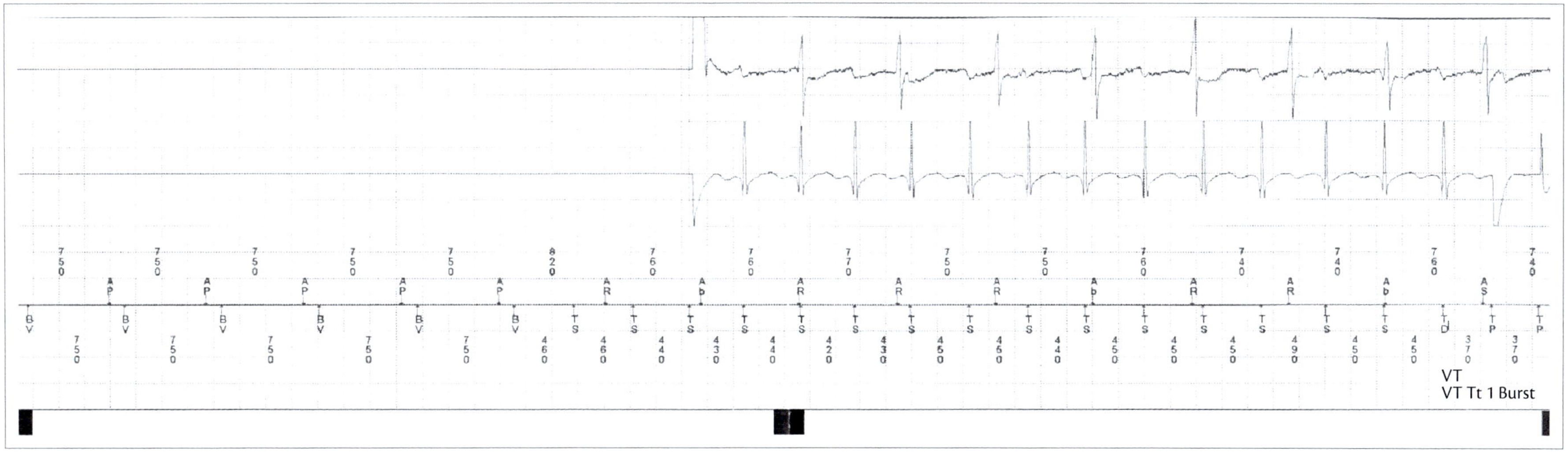

What is your diagnosis?

A Sinus rhythm with appropriate therapy for VT

B AVNRT with 2:1 retrograde conduction

C Inappropriate therapy for SVT

D Double tachycardia

Answer

A Sinus rhythm with appropriate therapy for VT

Figure 39.4 Annotated EGM of the stored episode

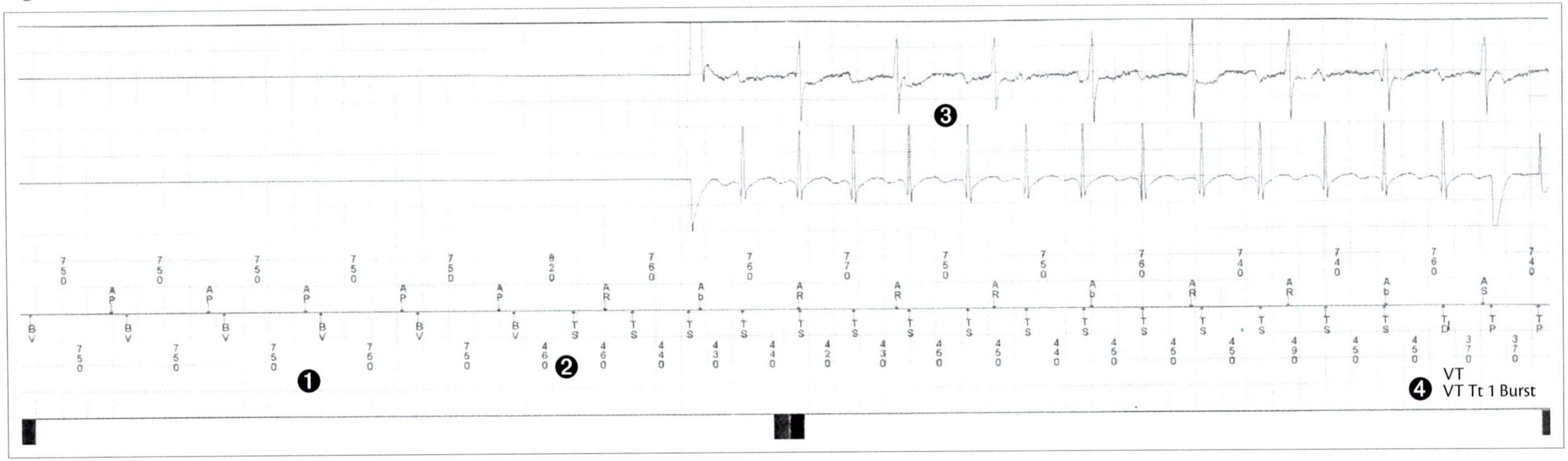

The patient had appropriate therapy for monomorphic slow VT (Figure 39.4).

❶ The rhythm is initially in atrial–biventricular pacing.

❷ The episode starts with a ventricular event that falls in the slow VT zone (TS).

❸ There are more ventricular than atrial events (V > A) with AV dissociation, confirming VT.

❹ The criteria for VT are fulfilled after 16 consecutive intervals falling in the slow VT zone, and burst ATP is delivered.

Comments

Inactivation of ventricular tachycardia/supraventricular tachycardia discrimination algorithms

The only instance where VT/SVT discrimination algorithms may be inactivated is in the case of permanent complete AV block, as in this patient who had undergone ablation of the AV node. In this case, it is impossible to have conducted SVT. The aim of these algorithms is to increase the specificity of ICD therapy, but they may reduce the sensitivity (i.e. inappropriately withhold therapy). Artefacts or T-waves may, however, be detected as rapid VS events but may be identified as such by other algorithms which should remain activated (see later cases in this book).

After delivery of the five bursts and four ramps for slow VT, the arrhythmia was reclassified as fast VT, due to a single beat (in the last eight intervals before detection) falling in the fast VT zone (❶). This then initiated therapy for fast VT with one burst (labelled as 'B' on the figure) and one ramp sequence, which resulted in a slower VT (❷), which was successfully cardioverted by a 15.9J shock (Figure 39.5).

Some VTs, despite being slow, can be difficult to overdrive with ATP. Due to recurrent VT, the patient underwent VT ablation.

Figure 39.5 Annotated tachogram of the stored episode

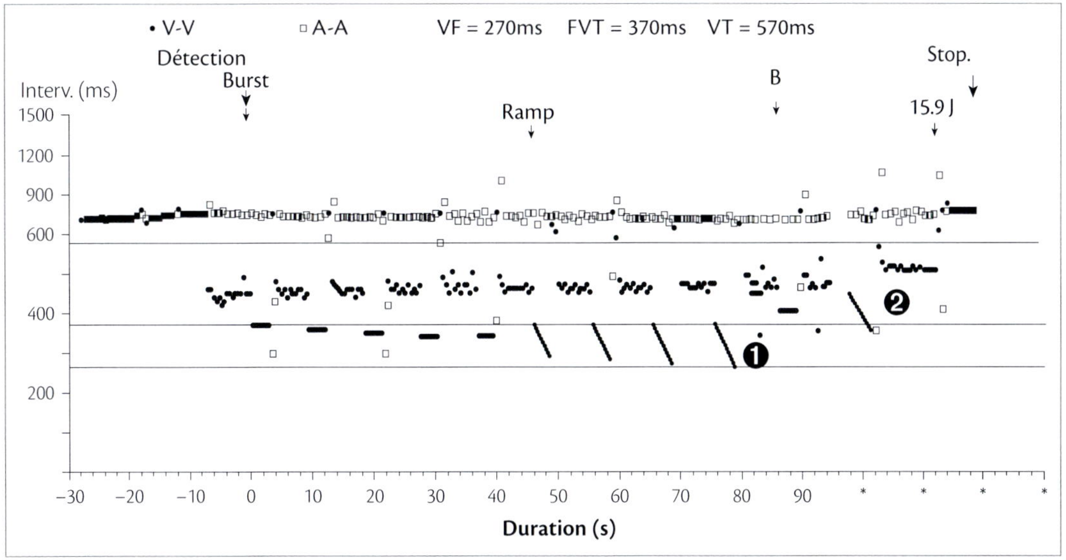

Introduction to the case

A patient, implanted with a CRT-D for secondary prevention of VT, consulted after having received a shock that was preceded by palpitations. The tachogram of the retrieved episode is shown in Figure 40.1, and the EGM in Figure 40.2. The device settings are displayed in Table 40.1 and Figure 40.3.

Figure 40.1 Tachogram of the stored episode

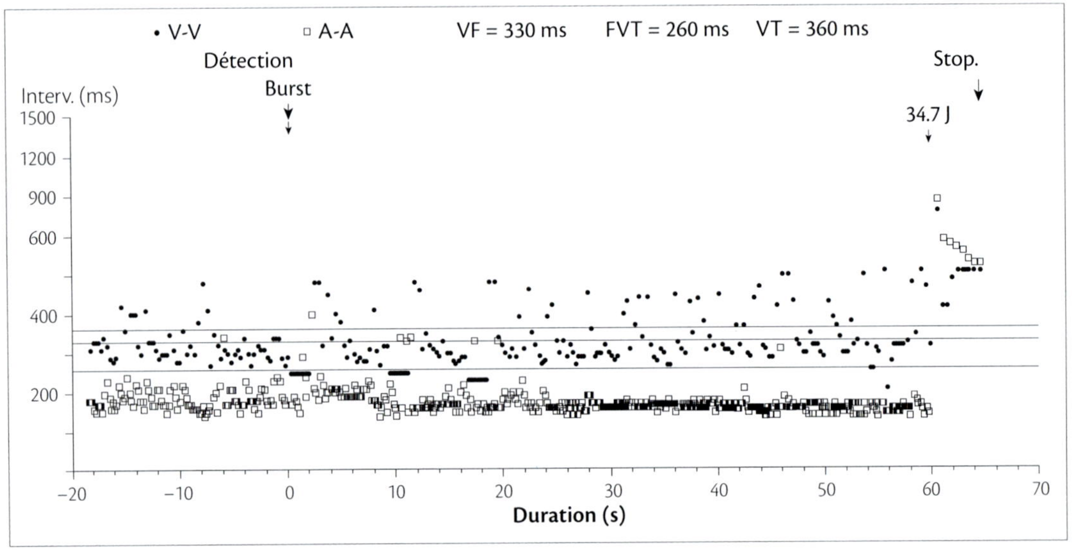

Table 40.1 Device settings

Zone	Slow VT	Fast VT (via VF)	VF
Rate (bpm/ms)	167/360	231/260	182/330
Detection	100	30/40	30/40
Redetection	12	12/16	12/16
SVT/VT discriminators	PR logic on; stability off; sudden onset and morphology 'monitor'		Therapy
ATP + shocks	ATP + shocks	Shocks	

Figure 40.3 Device settings

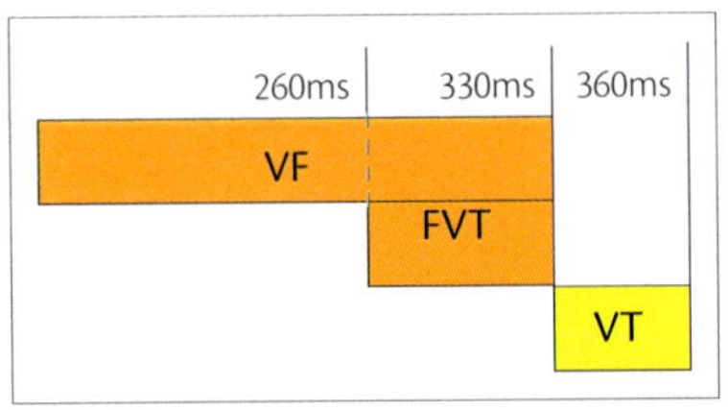

Question

Figure 40.2 Stored EGM of the episode

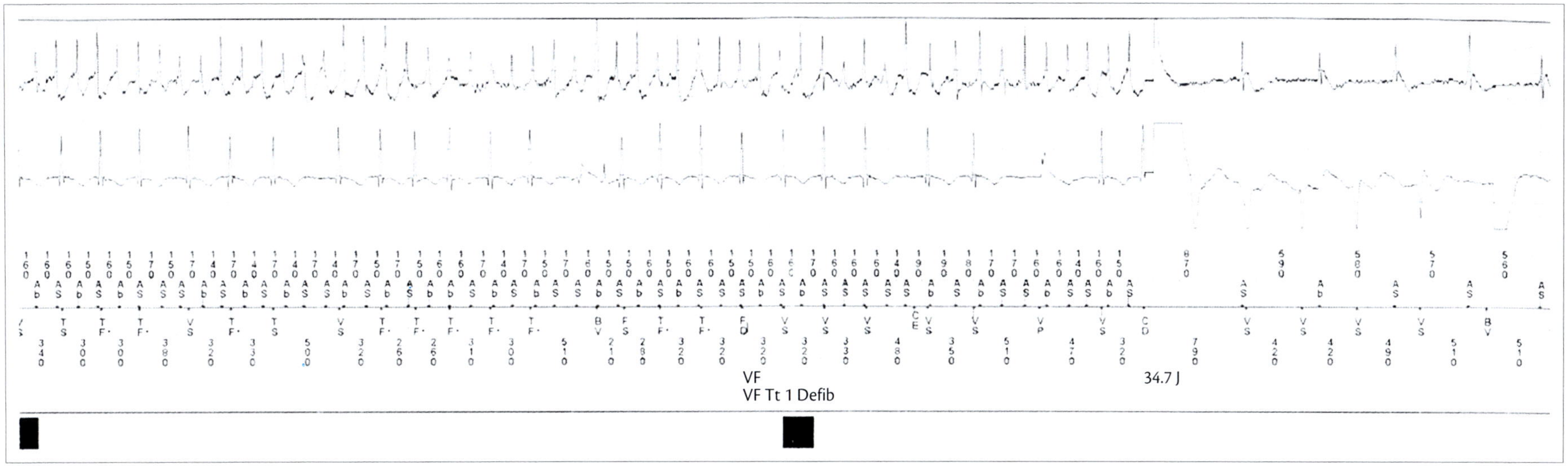

What is your diagnosis?

A Sinus rhythm with appropriate therapy for VT

B AF with appropriate therapy for VT

C Sinus rhythm with inappropriate therapy for SVT

D AF with inappropriate therapy for SVT

Answer

D AF with inappropriate therapy for SVT

Figure 40.4 Annotated stored EGM of the episode

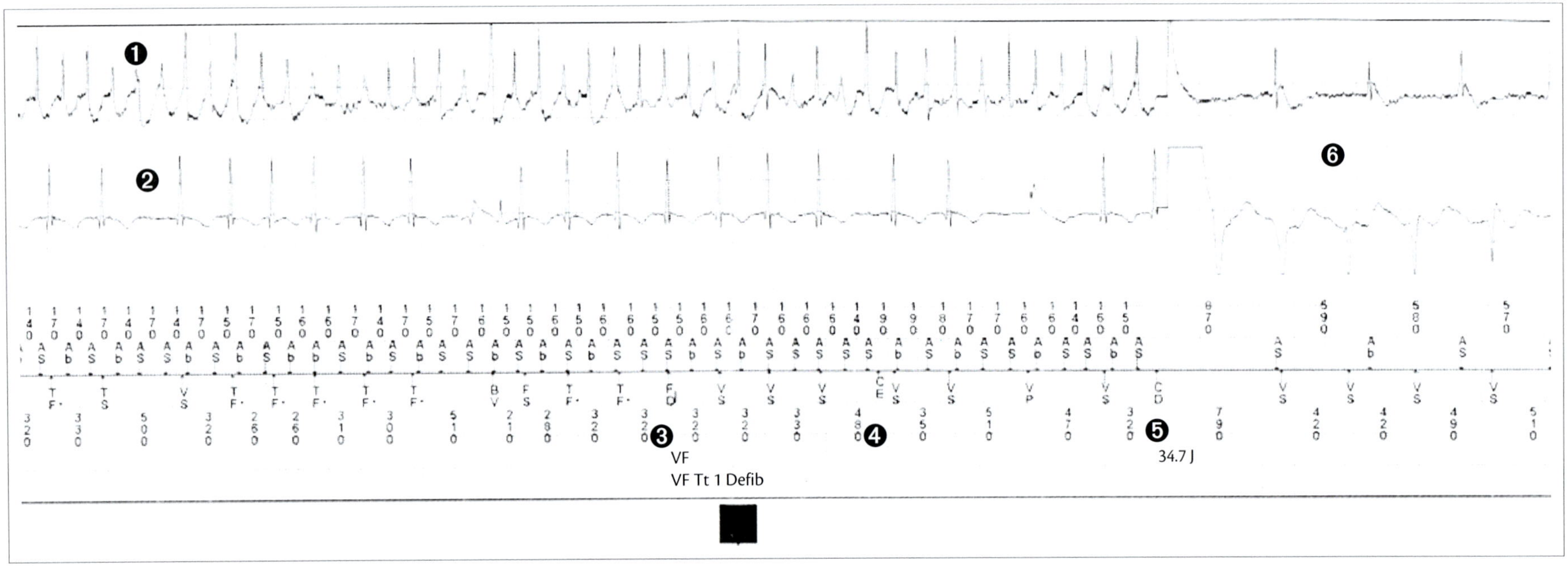

This is a case of an inappropriate ICD shock due to rapidly conducted AF, which cardioverted the AF to sinus rhythm (Figure 40.4).

❶ The atrial EGM shows AF.

❷ The ventricular channel shows an irregular monomorphic rhythm, corresponding to rapidly conducted AF that enters the tachycardia zones.

❸ The criteria for VF are fulfilled, as ≥1 of the last eight intervals is in the VF zone (FS 210ms) and VF is detected (FD). Note that the detection counters are shared between the VF and 'FVT via VF' zones in Medtronic devices. At detection (i.e. when the counter is full), the device will detect either FVT (if *all* the last eight intervals were inside the FVT zone, in this case between 330ms and 260ms) or VF (if ≥1 of the last eight intervals fall in the VF zone, in this case shorter than 230ms).

❹ The capacitor has reached the end of its charge (CE).

❺ Ventricular arrhythmia is reconfirmed at the end of the capacitor charge (≥2/5 intervals faster than the VT zone + 60ms for this model, corresponding to 420ms in this case, i.e. cycles labelled as 350ms and 320ms), resulting in the delivery of a shock.

❻ The shock results in cardioversion of AF to sinus rhythm. The ventricular channel shows a short run of ventricular beats (V > A) directly after the shock. Ventricular pacing was resumed thereafter.

Comments

Implantable cardioverter–defibrillator capacitor charge durations

The ICD transformers multiply the battery voltage (which is approximately 3V) to charge capacitors, in order to be able to deliver shocks of approximately 750V. The charge duration of ICDs reflect the battery status and are usually within 6–10s for a capacitor full-energy charge. In this case, the charge time was very short (<2s), confirmed by the episode details shown in Figure 40.5.

In Figure 40.5a, it can be seen that the arrhythmia was classified initially as fast VT (FVT), for which three bursts were delivered (Figure 40.5b, arrows on the tachogram) with persistence of the arrhythmia, resulting in a charge of the capacitors to 35J in 8.07s. As the first shock of all ICDs are 'non-committed', verification of the rhythm after the end of the charge had resulted in the abortion of shock delivery (the criterion in this model being <2/5 cycles within the VT/VF zone + 60ms). Rhythm reconfirmation should not be confounded with redetection, which refers to whether an arrhythmia is terminated or not after therapy delivery. Short cycles were then detected again, with the arrhythmia being classified as VF this time and reconfirmed, leading to delivery of a 34.7J shock, which at least had the favourable effect of cardioverting the AF back to sinus rhythm. The charge duration was only 1.33s this time, as the capacitors were still charged at 28J. The entire sequence was classified as being a single episode, as there were never >8 consecutive cycles that were outside the VT/VF zone (each manufacturer has its own specific criterion).

Figure 40.5 Episode details

Therapies		Delivered	Charge	Ohms	Energy
Confirmation		VT/VF			
FVT	Tt 1 Burst	Seq. 1 to seq. 3			
FVT	Tt 2 CV	Abandon.	8.07 s		0.0 - 35 J
VF	Tt 1 Defib	34.7 J	1.33 s	50 ohms	28 - 35 J
Stop					

(a)

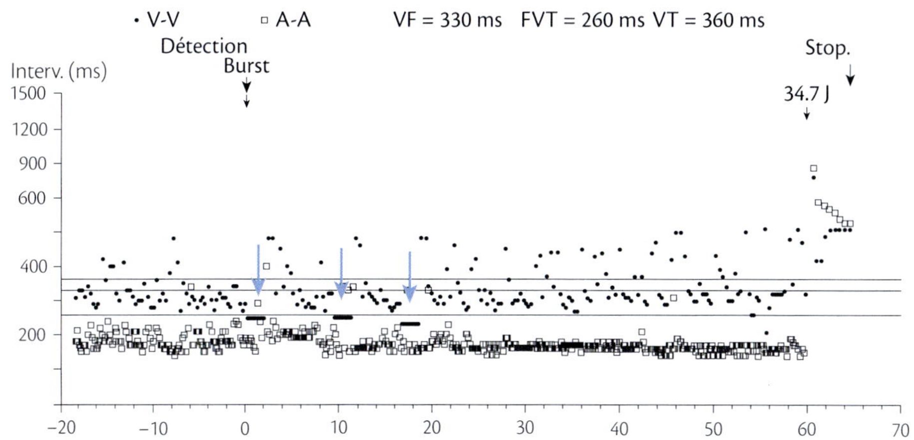

(b)

Introduction to the case

A patient implanted with a dual-chamber ICD for ischaemic cardiomyopathy and a history of VT presented for routine follow-up, without any complaints. An arrhythmic episode was retrieved from the device memory and is shown in Figure 41.1. The device settings are shown in Table 41.1.

Table 41.1 Device settings

Zone	VT	VF
Rate (bpm/ms)	171/350	214/280
Detection (intervals)	16	12
Therapy	ATP + shocks	Shocks

Pacing mode	DDD
Lower rate	40bpm
Upper rate	120bpm
Atrial output (bipolar)	2.5V@0.4ms
Atrial sensitivity (bipolar)	0.3mV
RV output (bipolar)	2.5V@0.4ms
RV sensitivity (bipolar)	0.4mV
Discrimination algorithm (dual-chamber)	A:V ratio, onset, stability, morphology

Question

Figure 41.1 EGM of the stored episode

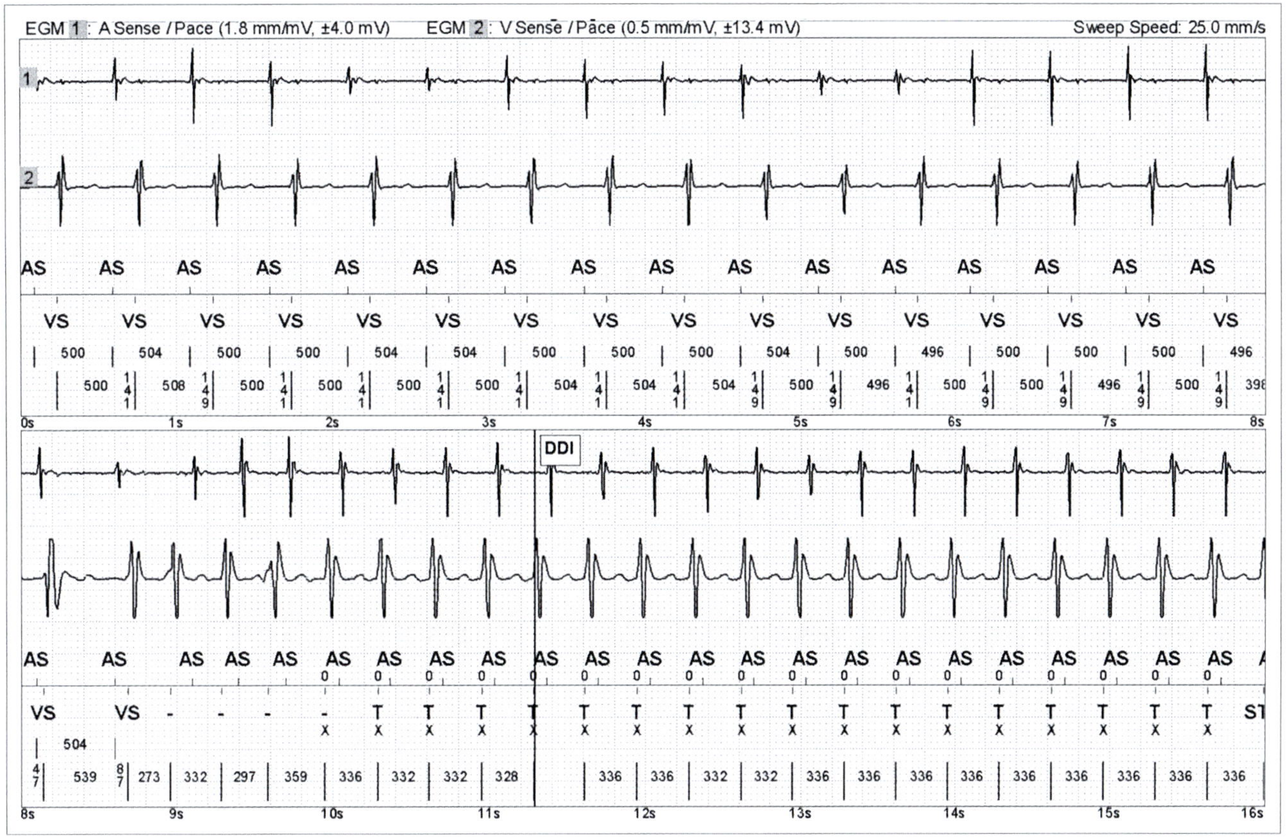

What is your diagnosis?

A Atrial tachycardia

B AVNRT

C AVRT

D VT

Answer

D **VT**

Figure 41.2 Annotated EGM of the stored episode

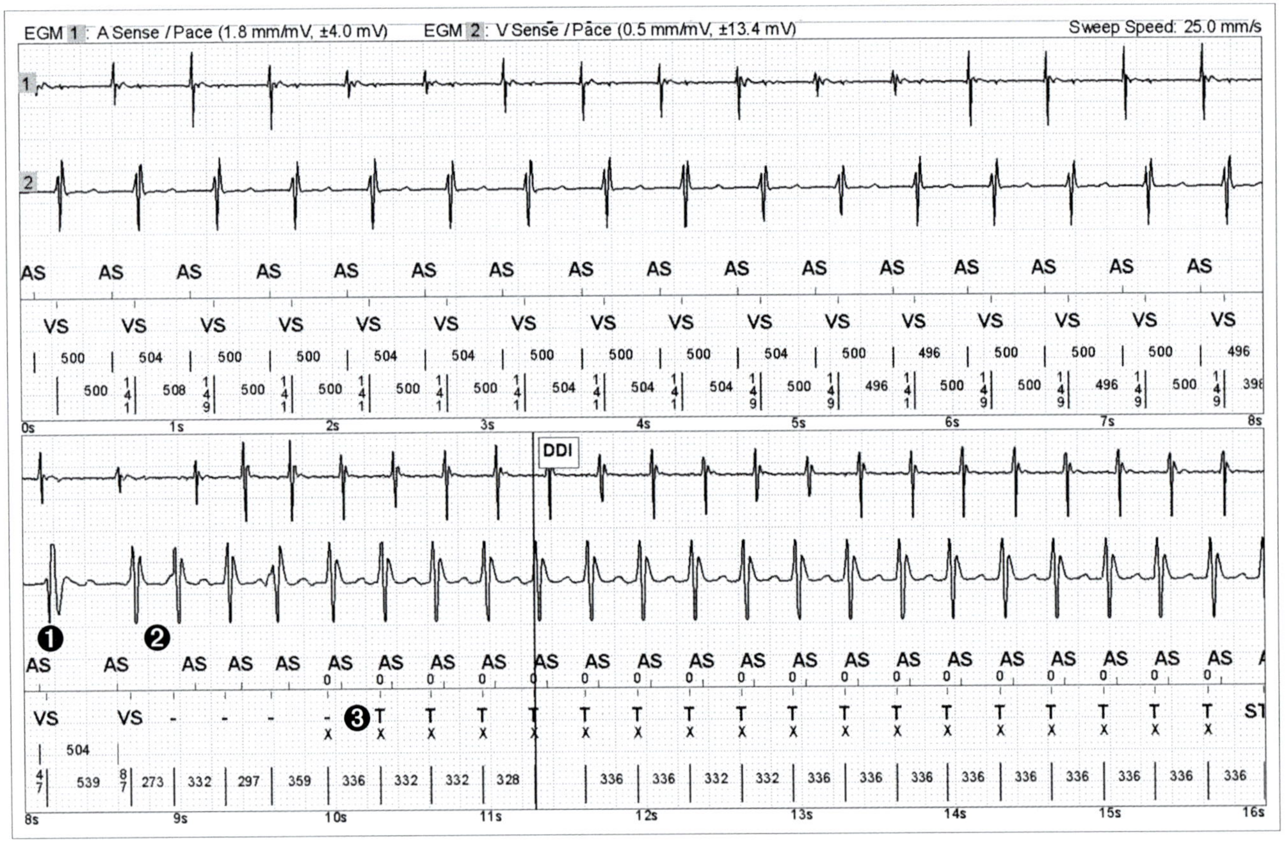

There are several criteria that identify this arrhythmia as being VT (Figure 41.2).

❶ A first VPB precedes (and probably triggers) the arrhythmia. The AS–VS interval is shorter (47ms) than the interval in sinus rhythm on the top of the strip (141–147ms), implying that this is not intrinsic AV conduction. Furthermore, the morphology of the ventricular EGM is different, compared to that in sinus rhythm.

❷ The 1st beat of the tachycardia is also of different morphology, compared to the ventricular EGM in sinus rhythm, and again is ventricular in origin, as the AS–VS interval is too short (87ms) for AV conduction. An initial V > A ratio can be observed, confirming VT.

❸ The tachycardia later has a 1:1 AV ratio, due to retrograde VA conduction. The morphology discrimination algorithm indicates 0% resemblance with the stored EGM template in sinus rhythm, which is below the match threshold (and the complexes are therefore labelled as 'X'). Each rapid cycle (labelled as 'T') is then binned in the VT zone.

Comments

Morphology criterion for rhythm discrimination

The arrhythmia was classified correctly as VT, and burst ATP was delivered, resulting in a return to sinus rhythm (Figure 41.3).

Morphology discrimination algorithms are used by several manufacturers, using either the far-field EGM (e.g. can to RV coil), the near-field EGM (RV tip to RV ring), or a combination of the two. The EGM during tachycardia is compared to the stored template in normal rhythm (which is usually updated automatically; Figure 41.4). Errors in rhythm classification may be induced by rate-dependent aberration, inaccurate template, alignment errors, EGM truncation, and post-shock EGM distortion.[1]

Reference

1. Swerdlow CD, Friedman PA. Advanced ICD troubleshooting: Part I. *Pacing Clin Electrophysiol* 2005; **28**: 1322–46.

Figure 41.4 Morphology discrimination algorithm

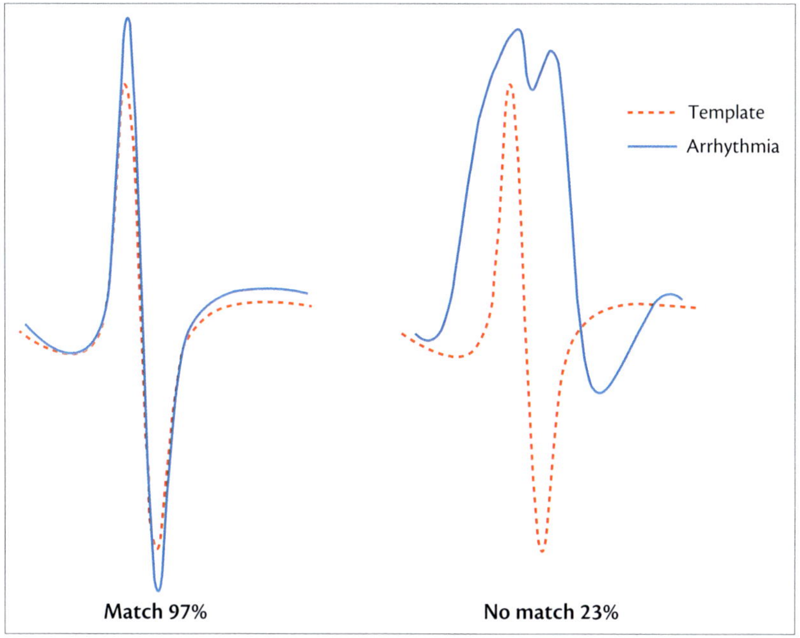

Figure 41.3 Burst ATP, with return to sinus rhythm. After the ATP sequence, morphology discrimination shows a match of 74–97% (labelled with a ✓), compared to the stored template, which exceeds the programmed threshold of 60%.

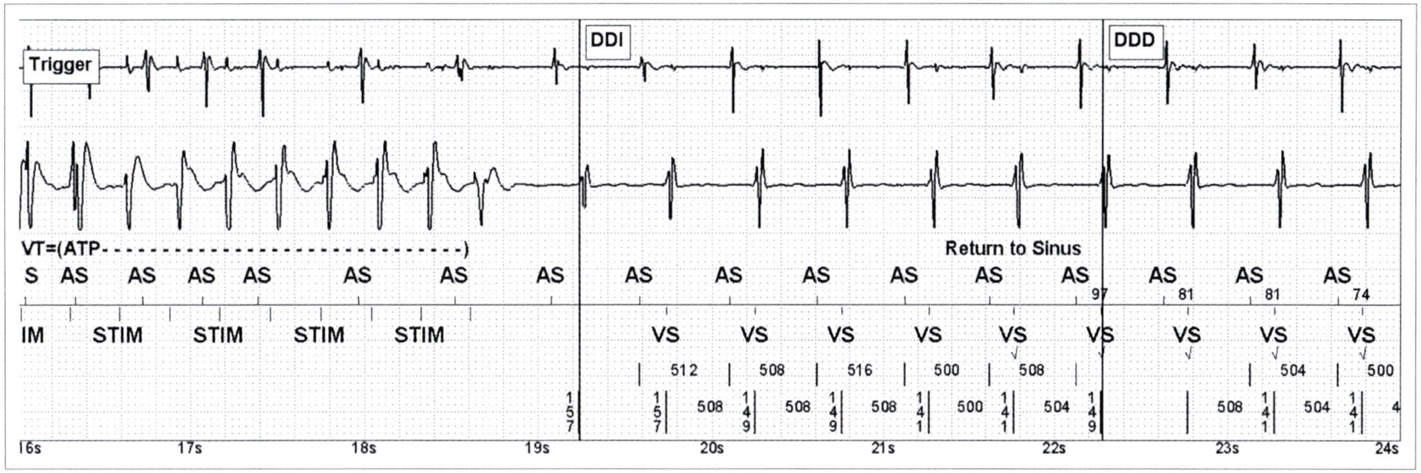

CASE 42

Introduction to the case

A 76-year-old patient with a CRT-D implanted for the primary prevention of sudden death presented for routine follow-up. He had no complaints. An episode classified as non-sustained VT was retrieved from the device memory and is shown in Figure 42.1. The device settings are shown in Table 42.1.

Table 42.1 Device settings

Zone	Slow VT	Fast VT (via VF)	VF
Rate (bpm/ms)	Off	240/250	188/320
Detection (intervals)		30/40	30/40
Redetection (intervals)		12/16	12/16
Therapy		2× bursts + shocks	Shocks

Question

Figure 42.1 EGM of the stored episode

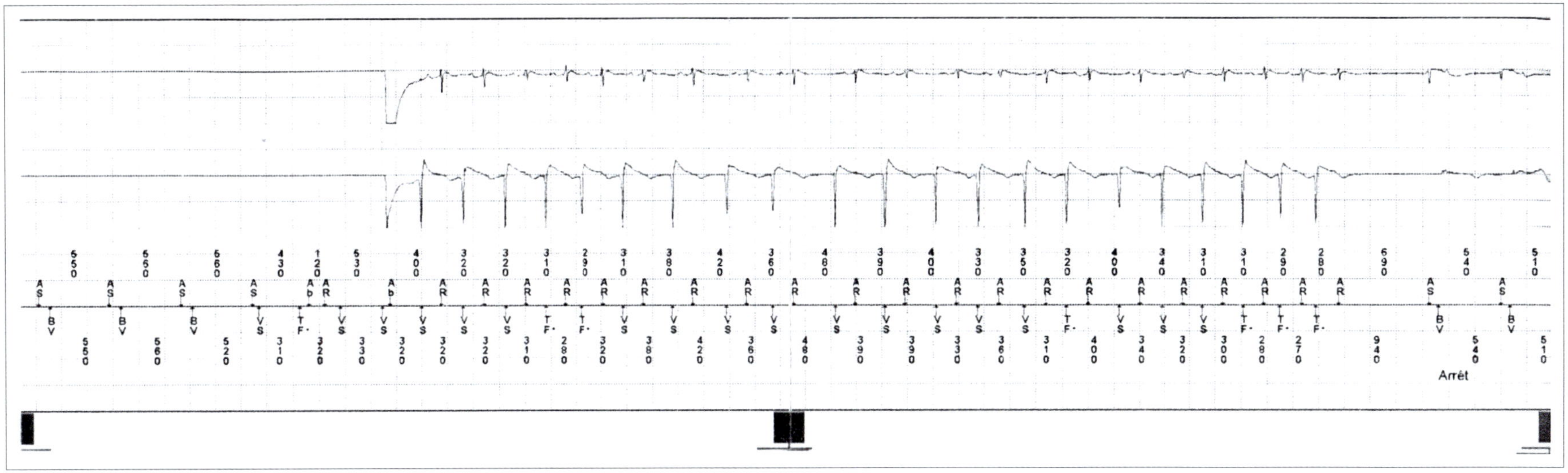

What is the most likely diagnosis?

A Non-sustained VT

B AVNRT

C Atrial tachycardia

D AVRT

Answer

A Non-sustained VT

Figure 42.2 Annotated EGM of the stored episode

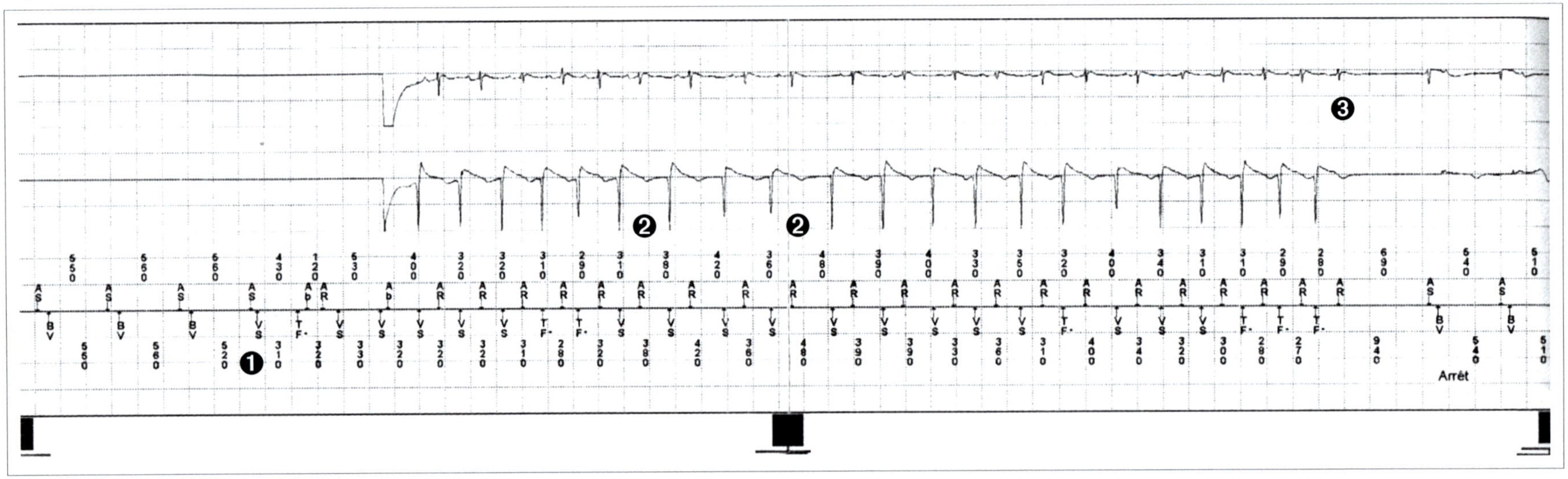

This case (Figure 42.2) illustrates several criteria which indicate non-sustained VT and speaks against atrial tachycardia. AVNRT or AVRT initiated by VPBs are not ruled out but are unlikely, given the cycle length irregularity.

❶ The event is initiated by a VPB (the AS–VS interval is too short for intrinsic AV conduction).

❷ Longer VV intervals *precede* longer AA intervals, with relatively constant VA intervals (VA linking).

❸ The episode ends with an atrial event.

Comments

Clues to differentiate supraventricular tachycardia from ventricular tachycardia

A summary of the clues that discriminate VT from SVT (several of which have been covered in the previous examples) are shown in Table 42.2.

Many ICDs use criteria that are in Table 42.2 as discriminatory algorithms. Details of how these algorithms function for each manufacturer are beyond the scope of this book and can be found in the device technical manuals, as well as in review articles.[1, 2]

Table 42.2 Differentiating VT from SVT on EGM tracings

VT	SVT
• Complete AV block • V > A • Very rapid (e g. >240bpm) and not artefacts • EGM morphology very different (! aberration) • Starts with V • V–V irregularities precede A–A irregularities (! may also be seen with AVNRT) • Ends with A (! may also be seen with AVNRT or AVRT) • ATP is effective (! SVT that can be stopped by ATP: AVNRT, AVRT, AT if VA conduction; ! AF with post-ATP pause)	• Gradual onset (! VT induced by exercise) • Irregular rhythm (! some VTs may be irregular) • Starts with A • EGM is *identical* to normal rhythm (use all EGMs, also 'can–RV coil'; ! EGM may change after shock) • A–A irregularities *precede* V–V irregularities • 'VAAV' sequence after ineffective ventricular ATP and atrial reset (→ AT/atypical AVNRT)

AT, atrial tachycardia; AF, atrial fibrillation; ATP, antitachycardia pacing; AVNRT, atrioventricular nodal re-entrant tachycardia; AVRT, atrioventricular re-entrant tachycardia; EGM, electrogram; caveats are indicated by '!'.

References

1. Swerdlow CD, Friedman PA. Advanced ICD troubleshooting: Part I. *Pacing Clin Electrophysiol* 2005; **28**: 1322–46.
2. Swerdlow CD, Friedman PA Advanced ICD troubleshooting: Part II. *Pacing Clin Electrophysiol* 2006; **29**: 70–96.

Introduction to the case

A 65-year-old male with dilated cardiomyopathy was implanted with a dual-chamber ICD, following an aborted sudden death with documented VF. Follow-up of the patient over the next 6 months revealed 46 episodes of asymptomatic tachycardia at a rate of 140/min, interpreted as VT, which were interrupted by ATP. An EGM at the onset of one of these episodes is shown in Figure 43.1.

Question

Figure 43.1 EGM at onset of the tachycardia

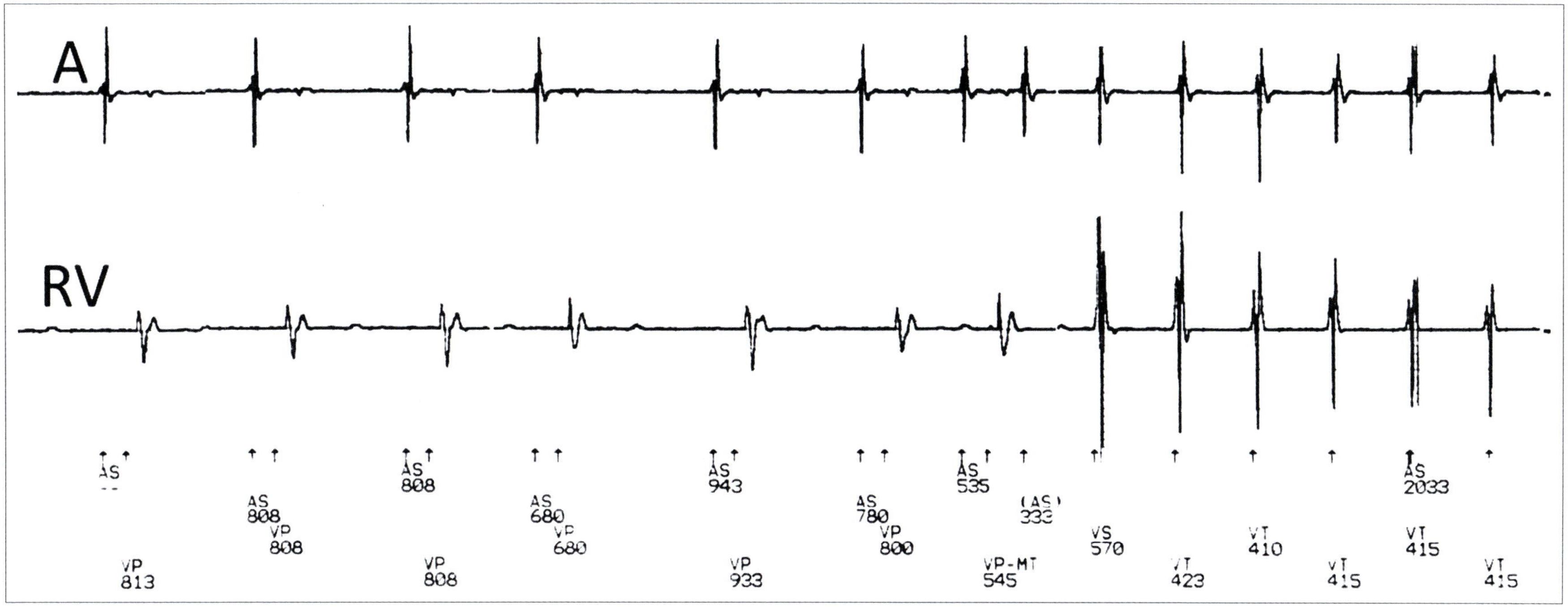

What is the most likely diagnosis?

A Atrial tachycardia

B AVNRT

C AVRT

D VT

Answer

B AVNRT

Figure 43.2 Annotated EGM at onset of the tachycardia

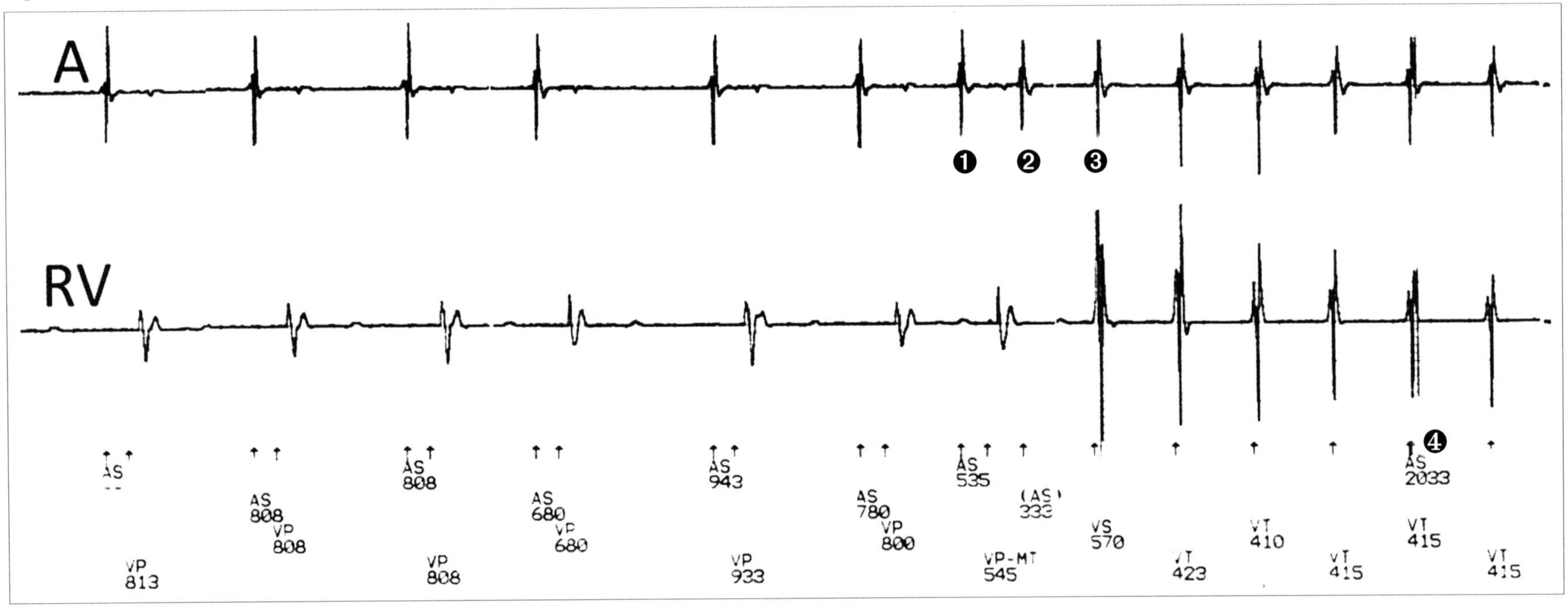

This is an example (Figure 43.2) of how ventricular ATP may interrupt SVT successfully.

❶ The arrhythmia is initiated by atrial premature beats, which suggests SVT. The 1st atrial premature beat is tracked to the ventricle by the ICD at the maximum tracking interval and results in ventricular pacing (indicated by the VP–MT 545 marker).

❷ The 2nd atrial premature beat falls within the PVARP, which is indicated by the (AS) marker, and therefore is not tracked to the ventricle and results in intrinsic AV conduction with a prolonged AS–VS interval, indicating conduction by the slow pathway.

❸ Atrial events thereafter occur almost simultaneously with every ventricular event, indicating retrograde conduction by the fast pathway. In case of AVRT, the VA interval would have been longer.

❹ Atrial sensing occurs intermittently, as most events are hidden in the ventricular blanking period. The V > A criterion then leads to the (erroneous) diagnosis of VT by the ICD, leading to the delivery of therapy.

Comments

Atrioventricular nodal re-entrant tachycardia masquerading as ventricular tachycardia

A rhythm strip was recorded during patient monitoring and is shown in Figure 43.3.

The patient, in this case example, underwent an electrophysiological study, which confirmed AVNRT with successful radiofrequency ablation of the slow pathway.

Figure 43.3 Rhythm strip recorded during patient monitoring. (A) Initiation of AVNRT (an atrial premature beat is shown by *). (B) Termination of the tachycardia by ventricular ATP

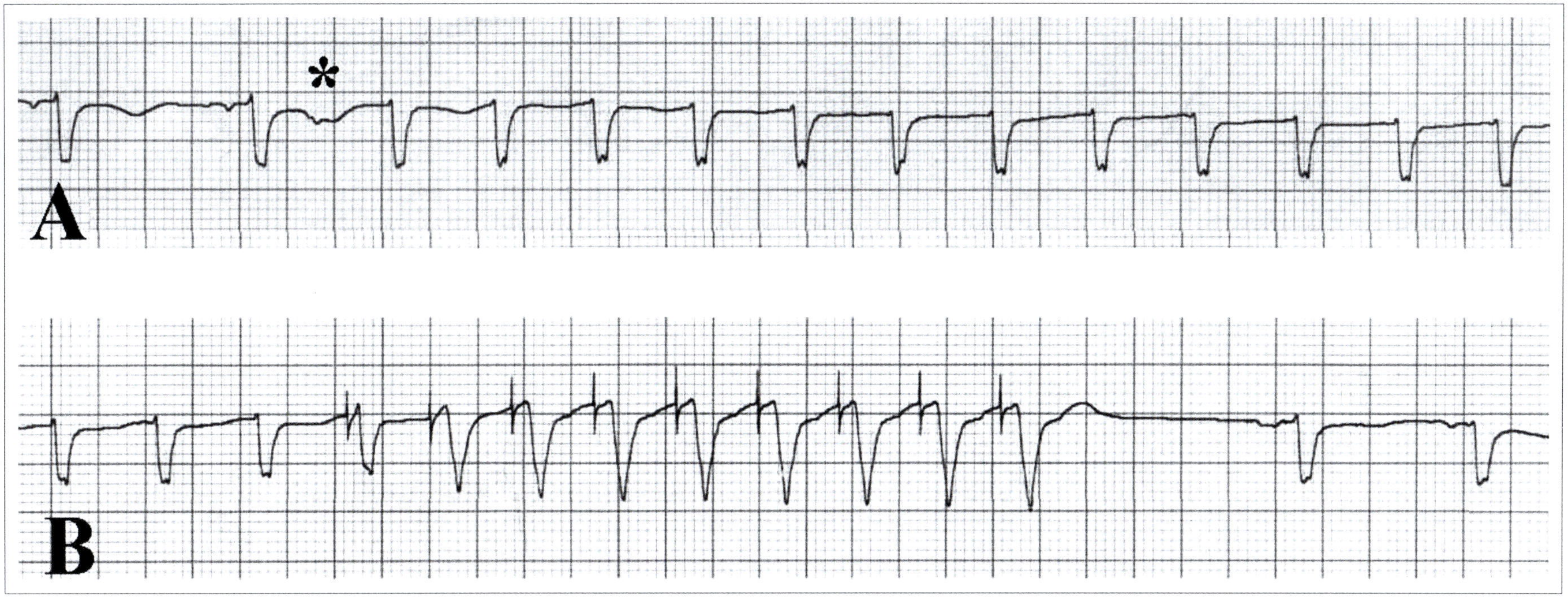

Introduction to the case

A 74-year-old patient with ischaemic heart disease had a single-chamber ICD implanted 3 years ago for resuscitated VF. He was admitted after having received multiple shocks. The tachogram is shown in Figure 44.1. The EGM strip preceding one of the shocks is displayed in Figure 44.2.

Figure 44.1 Tachogram of the stored episode

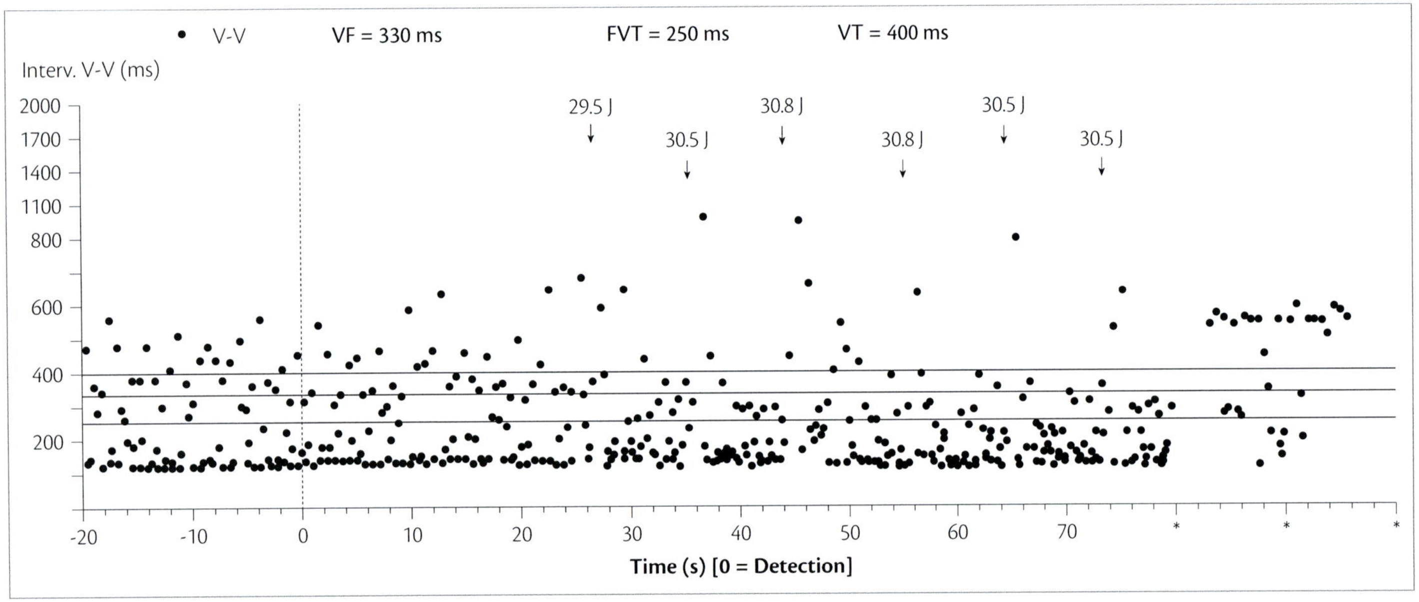

Question

Figure 44.2 EGM of the 3rd shock of the stored episode

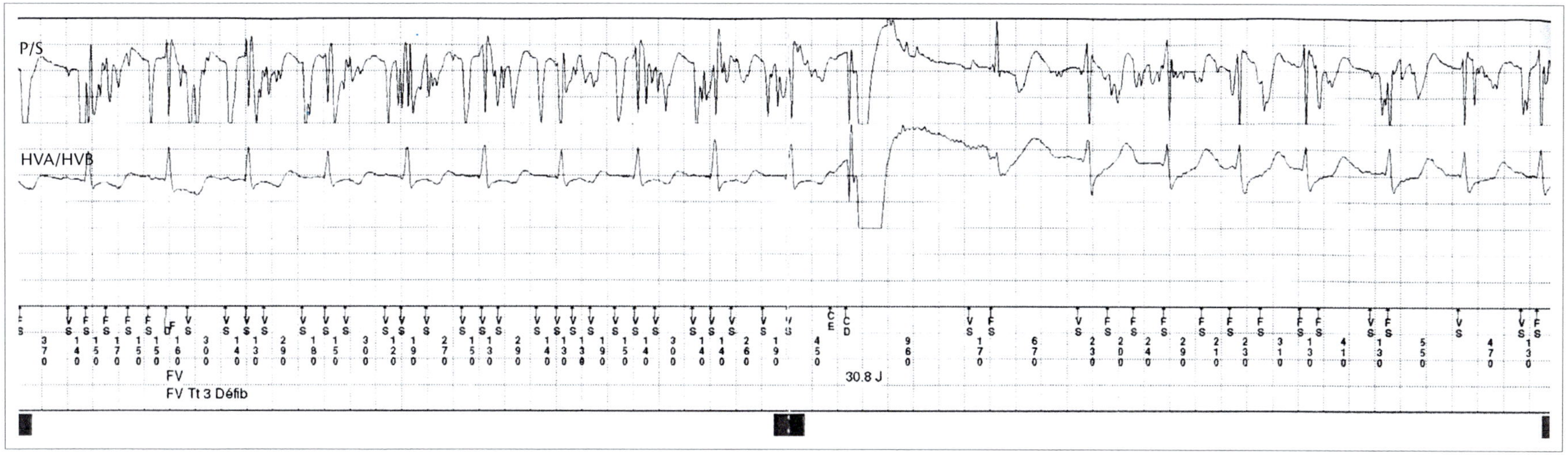

What is your diagnosis?

A Fast VT

B VF

C Lead fracture

D Electromagnetic interference

Answer

C Lead fracture

Figure 44.3 Annotated EGM of the 3rd shock of the stored episode

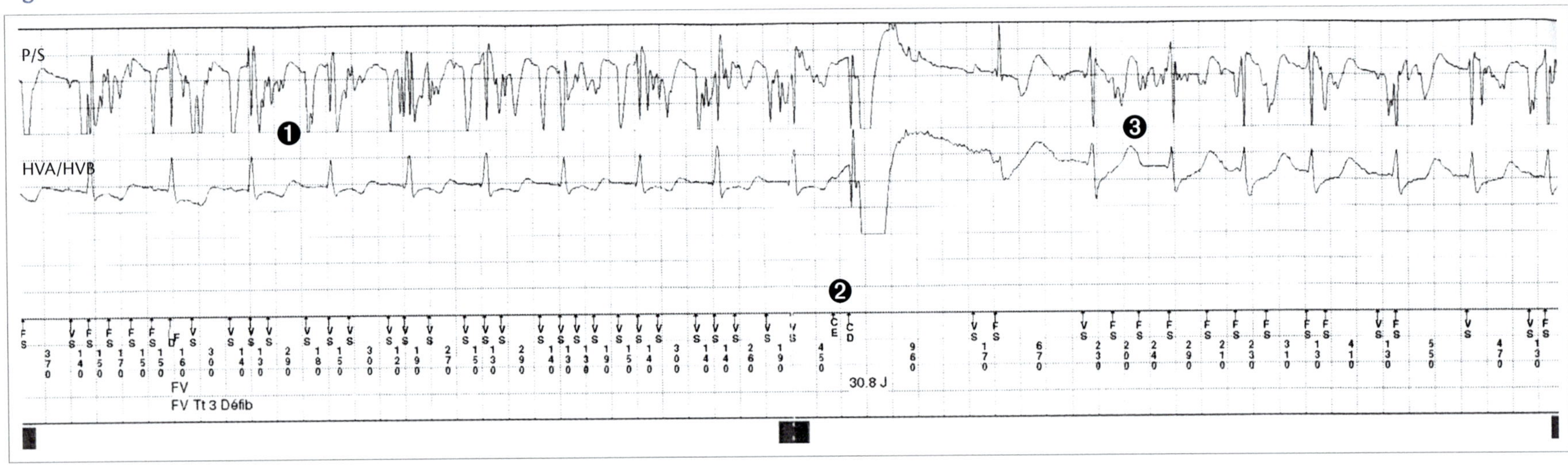

This patient (Figure 44.3) had been implanted with a Medtronic Sprint Fidelis lead, which was prone to fracture and has been subject to a recall in 2007.

❶ High-amplitude, erratic artefacts, which suggest lead fracture, are observed on the pace–sense (P/S) channel and are absent on the far-field can–RV coil (HVA/HVB) channel, ruling out electromagnetic interference. The far-field EGM shows a regular rhythm at 100bpm which rules out fast VT or VF.

❷ A shock is delivered (CD) directly after the charge end (CE) of the capacitor. This indicates that this was not the 1st shock of this episode, as the shock was 'committed', i.e. the rhythm was not reconfirmed before delivery of the shock. The first shock is always 'non-committed', i.e. tachyarrhythmia needs to be reconfirmed before the shock is delivered, whereas subsequent shocks of the same episode are committed.

❸ Artefacts continue to be present after the shock, leading to further shocks.

Comments

Recognizing lead fracture

Lead impedance had risen to abnormal levels (Figure 44.4), triggering an audible alert that had not been heard by the patient. Remote monitoring would have been useful and may have allowed medical intervention before the delivery of inappropriate shocks.

Lead impedance may, however, be normal, despite lead fracture. Algorithms have also been developed to recognize fracture potentials, based upon their very high frequency and also by comparing near-field and far-field EGM channels. Fracture artefacts may not always be as easy to recognize, as shown in Figure 44.5.

Fluoroscopy and X-rays are seldom useful for diagnosing fracture. If the fracture occurs near the generator, manipulation of the pocket or pressing the lead at the clavicular region may trigger artefacts (Figure 44.6).

This manoeuvre may also be useful for diagnosing lead connection problems (e.g. a loose setscrew or an incompletely inserted lead in the header).

Figure 44.4 Lead impedance graph

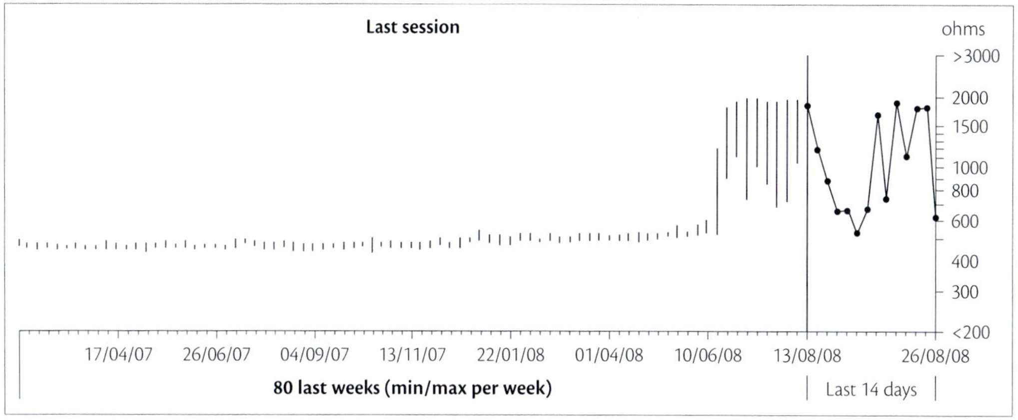

Figure 44.5 Lead fracture artefacts (indicated by *)

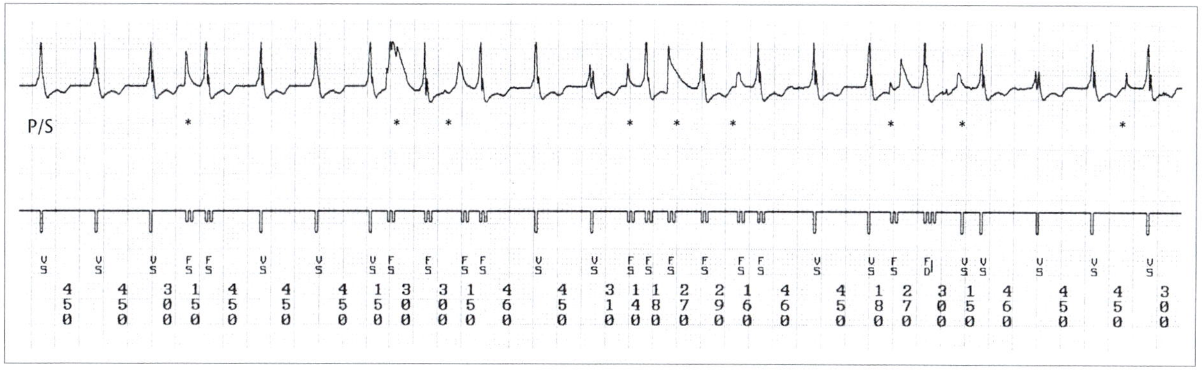

Figure 44.6 Lead fracture artefacts reproduced by manipulation of the generator pocket

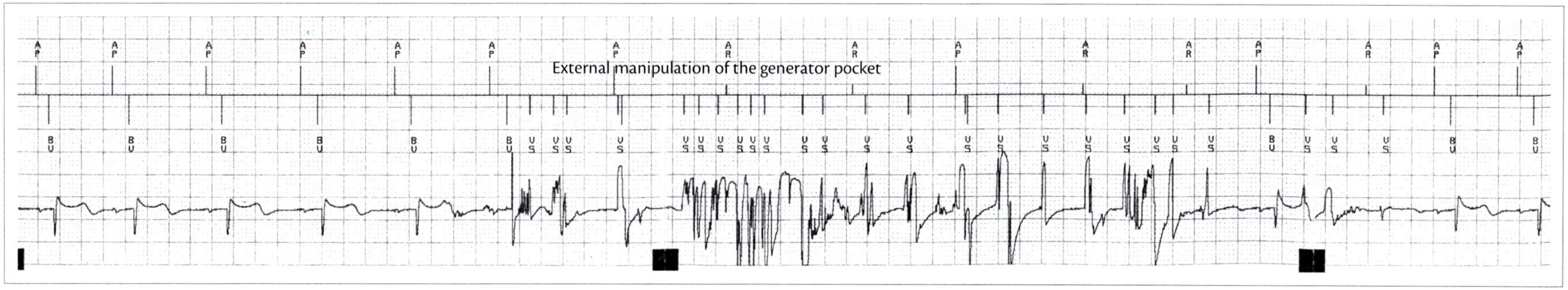

Introduction to the case

A 67-year-old patient with dilated cardiomyopathy was implanted with a CRT-D for the primary prevention of sudden death. The control on the day following the implant was normal, apart from an R-wave sensing amplitude of 4.2mV in the true bipolar configuration, which increased to 8mV when the sensing configuration was programmed to integrated bipolar (RV tip to RV coil). At 1-month follow-up, 68 episodes of asymptomatic non-sustained ventricular arrhythmia were recorded. The EGM of one of these episodes is shown in Figure 45.1, and the device settings are displayed in Table 45.1.

Table 45.1 Device settings

Zone	Slow VT	Fast VT (via VF)	VF
Rate (bpm/ms)	160/375	250/240	200/300
Detection (intervals)	24	30/40	30/40
Redetection (intervals)	12	9/12	9/12
Therapy	None	ATP + shocks	Shocks

Pacing mode	DDDR
Lower rate	60bpm
Upper rate	140bpm
Atrial output (bipolar)	Auto@0.4ms
RV output (bipolar)	Auto@0.4ms
LV output (LV tip–RV coil)	Auto@0.4ms
Atrial sensitivity (bipolar)	0.3mV
RV sensitivity (RV tip–RV coil)	0.45mV

Question

Figure 45.1 EGM of a stored non-sustained high ventricular rate episode

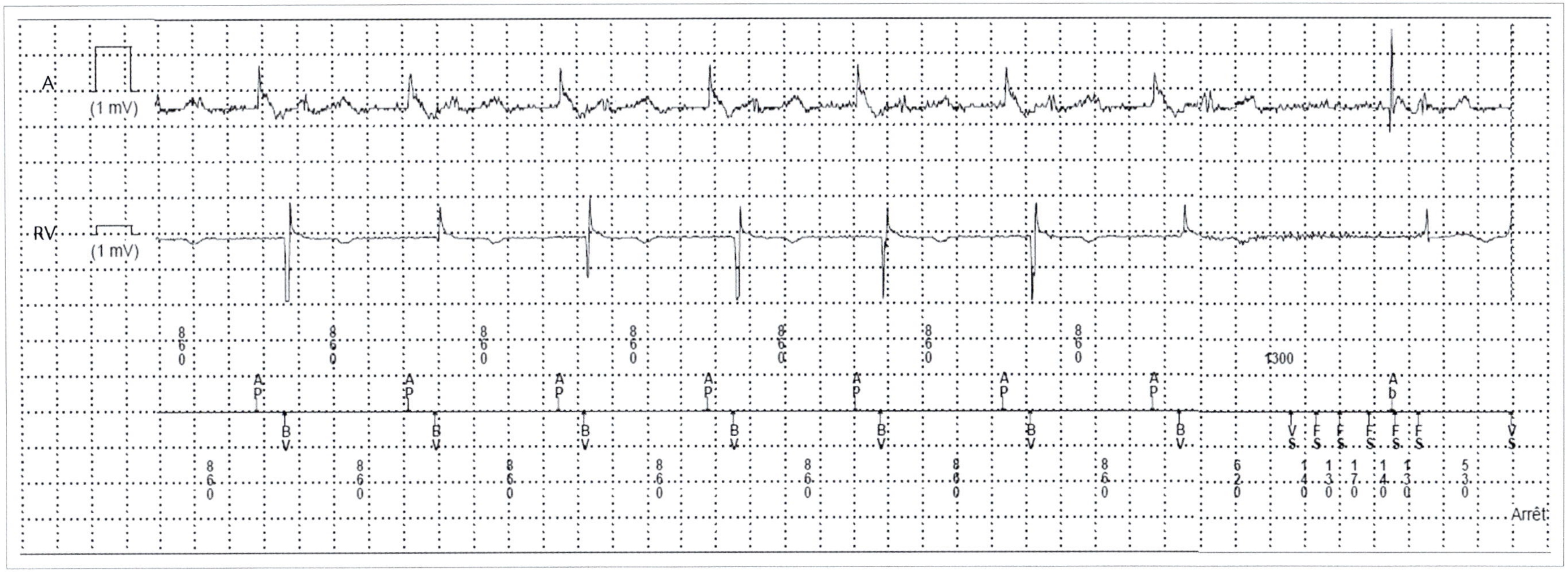

What is your diagnosis?

A Lead fracture

B Pectoral muscle oversensing

C Diaphragmatic muscle oversensing

D Electromagnetic interference

Answer

C Diaphragmatic muscle oversensing

Figure 45.2 Annotated EGM of a stored non-sustained high ventricular rate episode

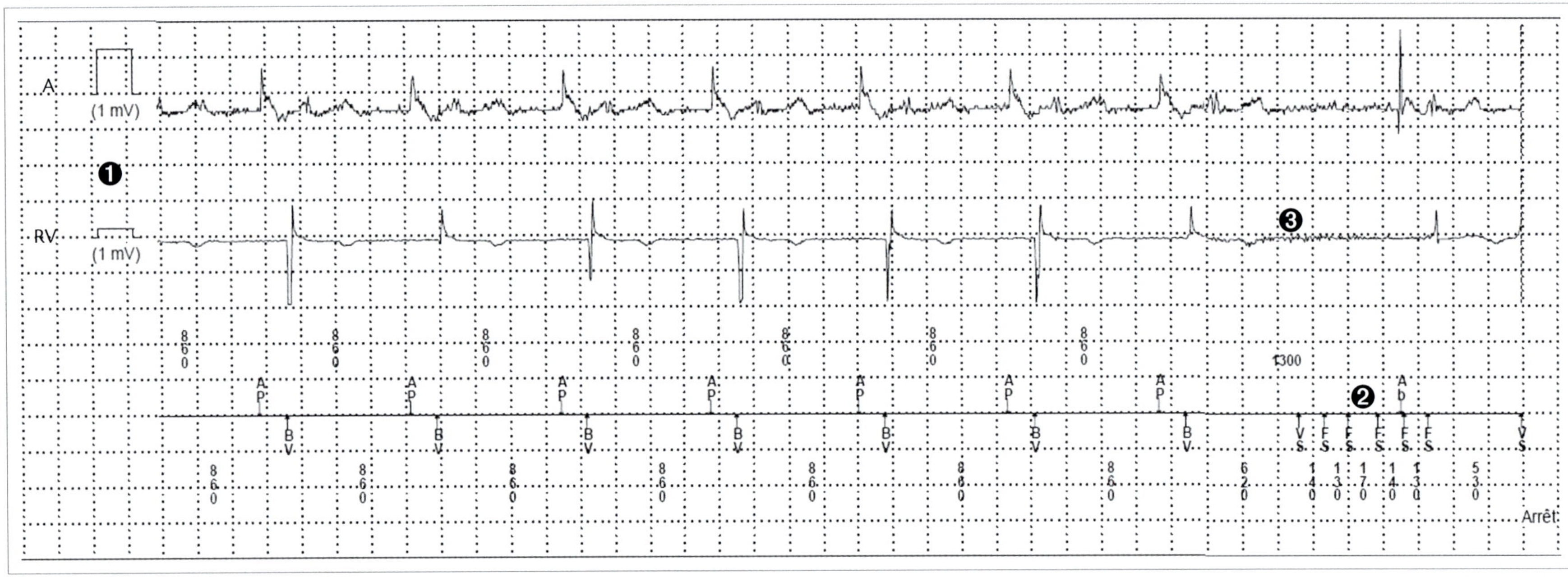

Diaphragmatic myopotential oversensing resulted from the extended bipolar ventricular sensing configuration (Figure 45.2) and was confirmed at follow-up by reproducing the artefacts during a Valsalva manoeuvre.

❶ The automatic scale is larger for the atrial channel, resulting in the visualization of background noise that is constant throughout the tracing (and is not sensed). The scale for the right ventricular (RV) channel is however small, and should be taken into account when interpreting the EGM.

❷ A ventricular high-rate episode is detected by the ICD, according to the marker channel.

❸ Upon close inspection, low-amplitude high-rate artefacts are visible on the ventricular channel (note the scale), which are absent on the tracing to the left of the event. There is no simultaneous increase in artefacts in the atrial channel, which speaks against electromagnetic interference. Pectoral myopotentials would not be sensed by the bipolar sensing configuration. The potentials are of very low amplitude, speaking against fracture artefacts (see Case 44). These artefacts correspond to diaphragmatic myopotentials.

Comments

True bipolar and integrated bipolar implantable cardioverter–defibrillator leads

True bipolar ICD leads have a separate ring electrode that acts as the anode, whereas integrated bipolar leads use the RV coil as the anode (Figure 45.3).

This patient had a true bipolar ICD lead, which was programmed to an integrated bipolar configuration, because of a greater sensed R-wave amplitude. Due to the wider inter-electrode spacing of the integrated bipolar configuration, there is an increased risk of diaphragmatic myopotential oversensing. The problem was confirmed at follow-up by reproducing the phenomenon during a Valsalva manoeuvre. It was resolved easily by reprogramming the lead to a true bipolar sensing configuration.

Figure 45.3 Differences between true bipolar and integrated bipolar ICD leads

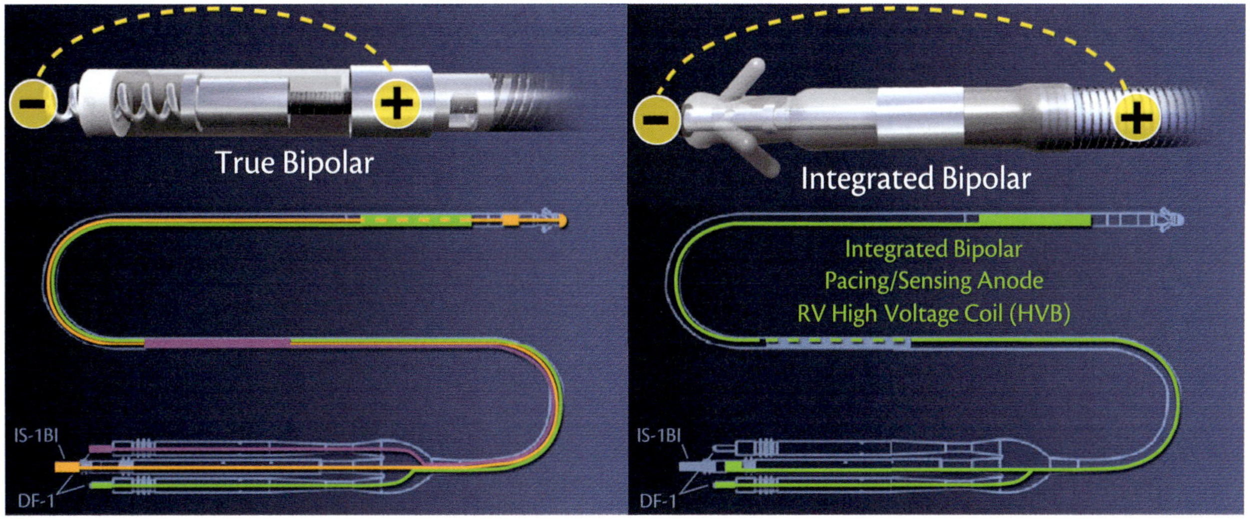

Adapted from Medtronic Core ICD

Introduction to the case

A patient was implanted with a dual-chamber ICD for the primary prevention of sudden death. An episode of non-sustained ventricular arrhythmia was retrieved at routine device follow-up and is shown in Figure 46.1.

Question

Figure 46.1 EGM of non-sustained ventricular high-rate episode

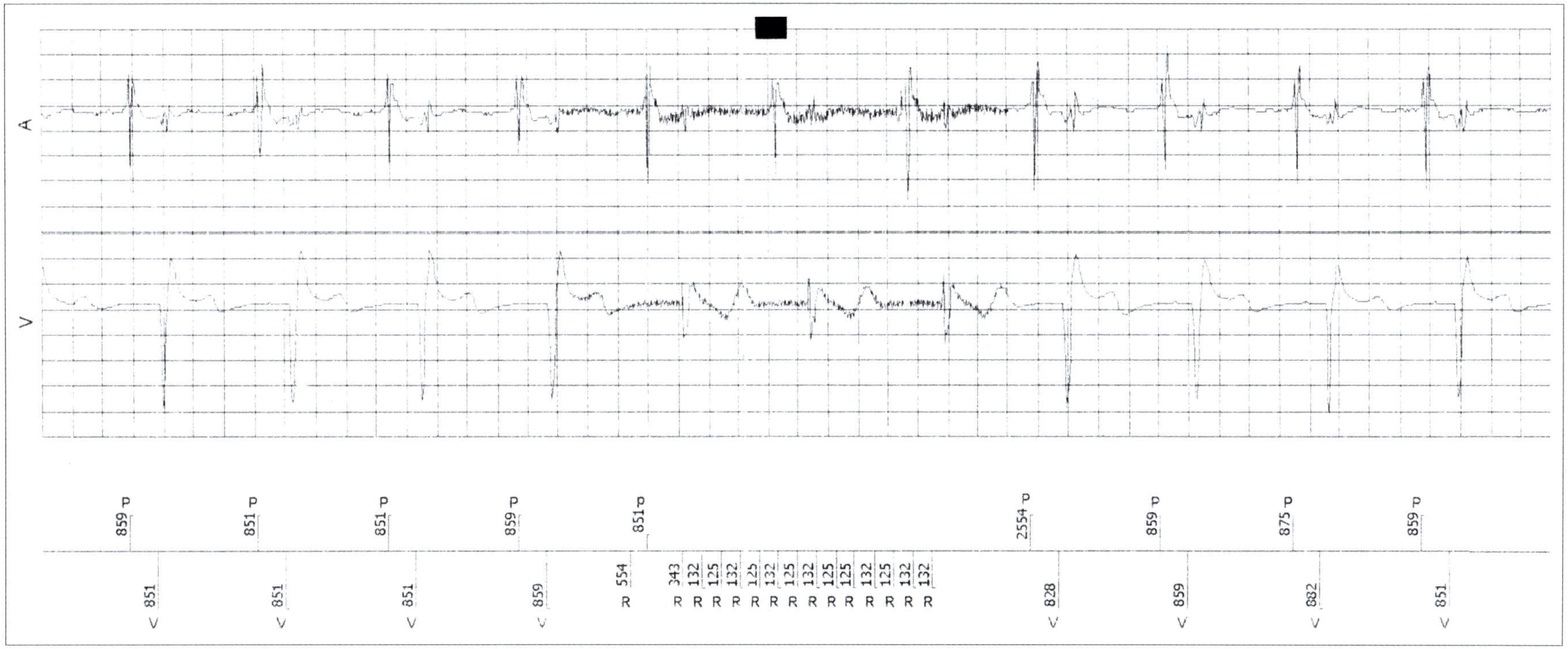

What is your diagnosis?

A Lead fracture

B Pectoral muscle oversensing

C Diaphragmatic oversensing

D Electromagnetic interference

Answer

D Electromagnetic interference

Figure 46.2 Annotated EGM of non-sustained ventricular high-rate episode

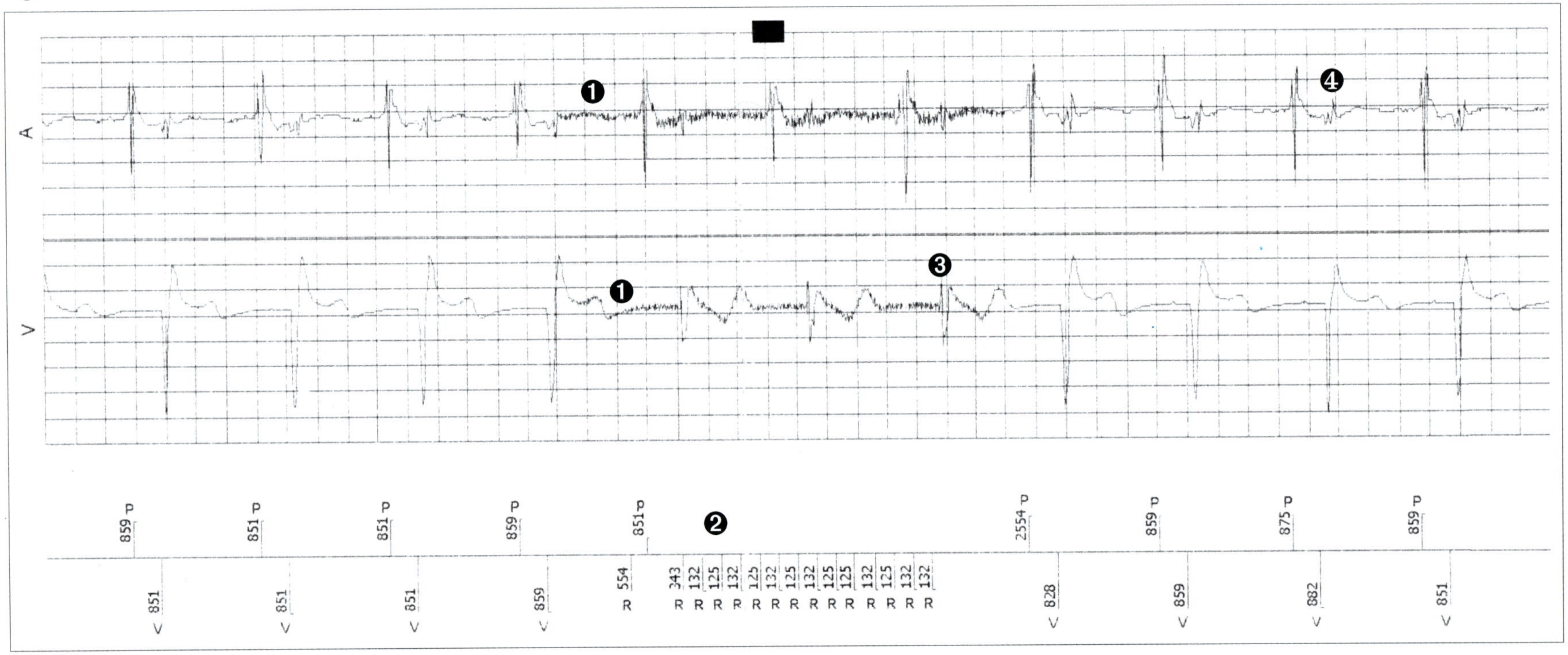

The cause of the external electromagnetic interference could not be determined in this case (Figure 46.2), as the patient did not remember his activity at the time of the event.

❶ High-rate artefacts are visible simultaneously on the atrial and ventricular channels, which indicates electromagnetic interference. Another possibility would be pectoral myopotentials in a device programmed to unipolar sensing for both the atrial and ventricular channels, but ICDs only sense in the bipolar mode in these channels.

❷ Electromagnetic interference is detected as ventricular events in the VF zone but is too short in duration to lead to a capacitor charge. Note that the electromagnetic signals are not sensed in the atrium, probably due to low amplitude and also to PVAB.

❸ Preserved AV conduction is visible during the inhibition of ventricular pacing by the electromagnetic interference. The pacing mode of the device should be changed to minimize ventricular pacing (from DDD to, e.g. DDI or ADI/DDD mode).

❹ FFRWs are visible on the atrial channel but are not sensed, as they fall in the PVAB period.

Comments

Electromagnetic interference

Most modern ICDs have band filters which reduce the risk of detecting external electromagnetic interference emitted by devices such as household appliances, cell phones, etc. The risk of interference will depend upon factors such as:

- the frequency of the signal (which will determine attenuation by the band filters)
- the signal amplitude
- the proximity of the source to the device (amplitude decreases with the square of the distance)
- the orientation of the source with respect to that of the electrode dipole
- the sensing polarity
- the inter-electrode spacing
- the programmed sensitivity.

Atrial leads have been shown to be more susceptible to electromagnetic interference than ventricular leads.[1] Interference detected by the atrial channel may lead to an inappropriate mode switch or to tracking of the signals with rapid ventricular pacing. If interference is detected by the ventricular channel, pacing may be inhibited or inappropriate therapy may be delivered. Electromagnetic interference may also result in noise reversion with asynchronous pacing at the baseline rate.

Elements which allow distinguishing between different types of artefacts are shown in Table 46.1.

Table 46.1 Distinguishing artefacts on EGM tracings

Electromagnetic interference	• Usually repetitive and of high rate (e.g. 50Hz) • Artefacts visible simultaneously on all channels • Amplitude on far-field EGM > near-field EGM*
Lead fracture artefacts	• Usually of erratic morphology and high amplitude (channel saturation) • Only observed on a single EGM channel (or on the channels of all fractured leads, but usually not perfectly simultaneously) • May be associated with elevated lead impedance or abnormal thresholds (! electrical parameters may be normal!) • May sometimes be provoked by manipulation of the pocket (if the fracture is in the extrathoracic portion of the lead)
Myopotentials	• Usually of high rate, with sometimes crescendo/decrescendo amplitude • Diaphragmatic myopotentials are only observed on the ventricular channel, with amplitude on the near-field EGM > far-field EGM* • Pectoral myopotentials may be observed in any lead programmed to unipolar sensing • May be reproduced by provocative manoeuvres (Valsalva manoeuvre, cough; prayer manoeuvre, etc.)

*The far-field EGM (e.g. generator can to RV coil) may be recorded for morphology recognition; the near-field EGM corresponds to the true or integrated bipolar EGM. Caveats are indicated by '!'.

Reference

1. Napp A, Joosten S, Stunder D, *et al*. Electromagnetic interference with implantable cardioverter defibrillators at power frequency: an in vivo study. *Circulation* 2014; **129**: 441–50.

Introduction to the case

A 69-year-old patient with ischaemic heart disease and a history of VT was implanted with a dual-chamber ICD. He was seen at routine device follow-up, without any cardiac complaints. An episode classified as SVT was retrieved from the device memory and is shown in Figure 47.1. The device settings are shown in Table 47.1.

Table 47.1 Device settings

Zone	Slow VT	Fast VT	VF
Rate (bpm/ms)	130/462	185/324	240/250
Detection (intervals)	20	12	6
Therapy	ATP + shock	ATP + shock	Shock

Pacing mode	ADI/DDD
Lower rate	40bpm
Upper rate	120bpm
Atrial output	2.5V@0.5ms (bipolar)
RV output	2.5V@0.5ms (bipolar)
Atrial sensitivity	0.2mV (bipolar)
RV sensitivity	0.4mV (bipolar)

Question

Figure 47.1 EGM of SVT episode

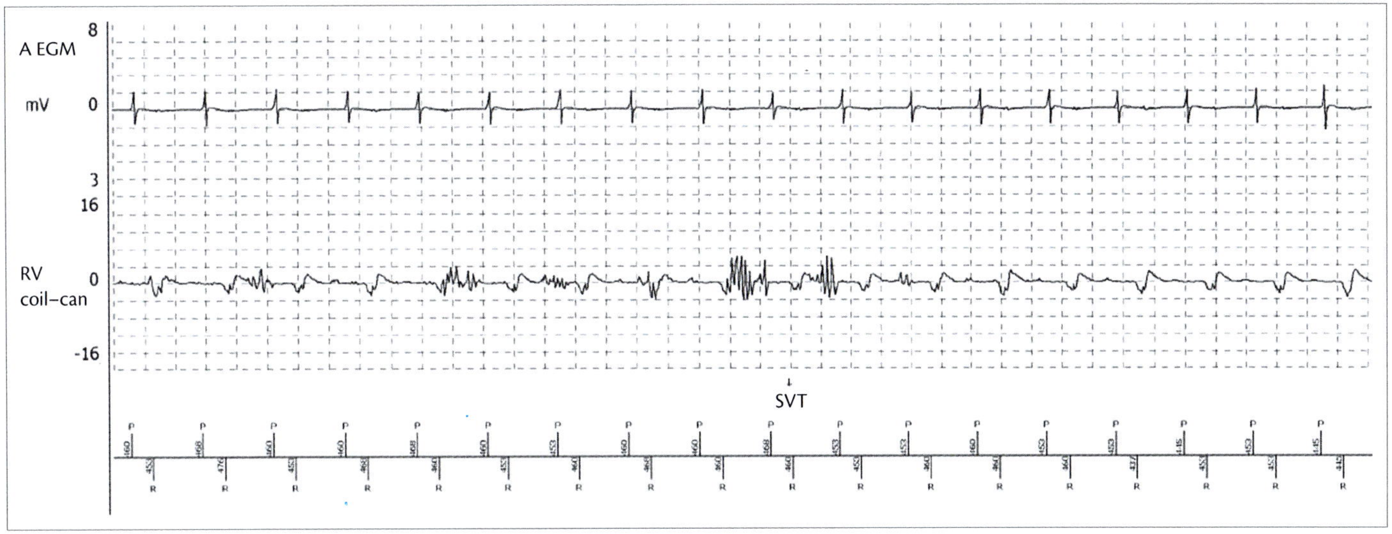

What is your diagnosis?

A Lead fracture

B Myopotential oversensing

C Electromagnetic interference

D Normal device function

Answer

D **Normal device function**

Figure 47.2 Annotated EGM of SVT episode

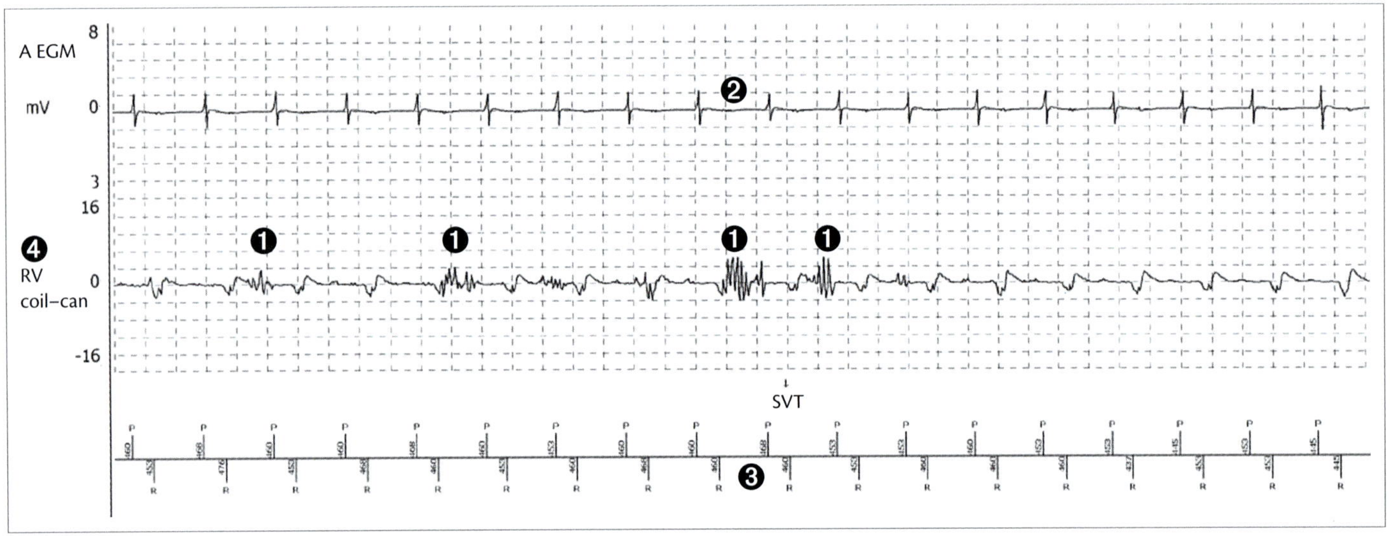

This episode had been stored, due to the detection of SVT while the patient was exercising, and the artefacts on the ventricular channel are an incidental finding (Figure 47.2).

❶ High-rate artefacts are visible on the ventricular channel.

❷ The atrial channel shows no artefacts, pointing against electromagnetic interference.

❸ The artefacts are not sensed by the device, even though they are of higher amplitude than the R-wave.

❹ The artefacts are due to pectoral myopotentials recorded by the far-field RV coil-can EGM. This 'unipolar' EGM is displayed to facilitate the interpretation of tracings (as it resembles a surface ECG). It is, however, the near-field pace/sense (RV tip-RV ring) EGM that is used by the device for detection, but this channel is not displayed on the recorded EGM.

Comments

Bipolar sensing in implantable cardioverter-defibrillators

Atrial and RV sensing (and pacing) can only be programmed in the bipolar mode in ICDs, in order to avoid oversensing of myopotentials, electromagnetic interference, T-waves, FFRWs, etc. Many ICD models display a 'far-field' EGM, which is usually the can-RV coil EGM, as this resembles an ECG signal which facilitates the evaluation of QRS morphology (and may be used by the device for the morphology discrimination algorithm). The device model shown in this example is unusual, as only the far-field EGM is displayed (although only the bipolar EGM is used for rate sensing).

Biventricular devices may have LV sensing programmed to either a unipolar, bipolar, or to an extended bipolar (LV electrode-RV ring or coil) configuration, but this channel is not used for VT/VF detection, due to the risk of oversensing (e.g. myopotential oversensing in the unipolar mode or P-wave oversensing in the case of LV lead dislodgement into the coronary sinus).

Introduction to the case

A 28-year-old patient with arrhythmogenic RV dysplasia had a single-chamber ICD implanted for the secondary prevention of sudden death. During physical exertion, he received 42 ICD shocks and presented to the emergency room. The tachogram is shown in Figure 48.1, and the stored EGM of one of the shocks is shown in Figure 48.2.

Figure 48.1 Tachogram of one of the stored events

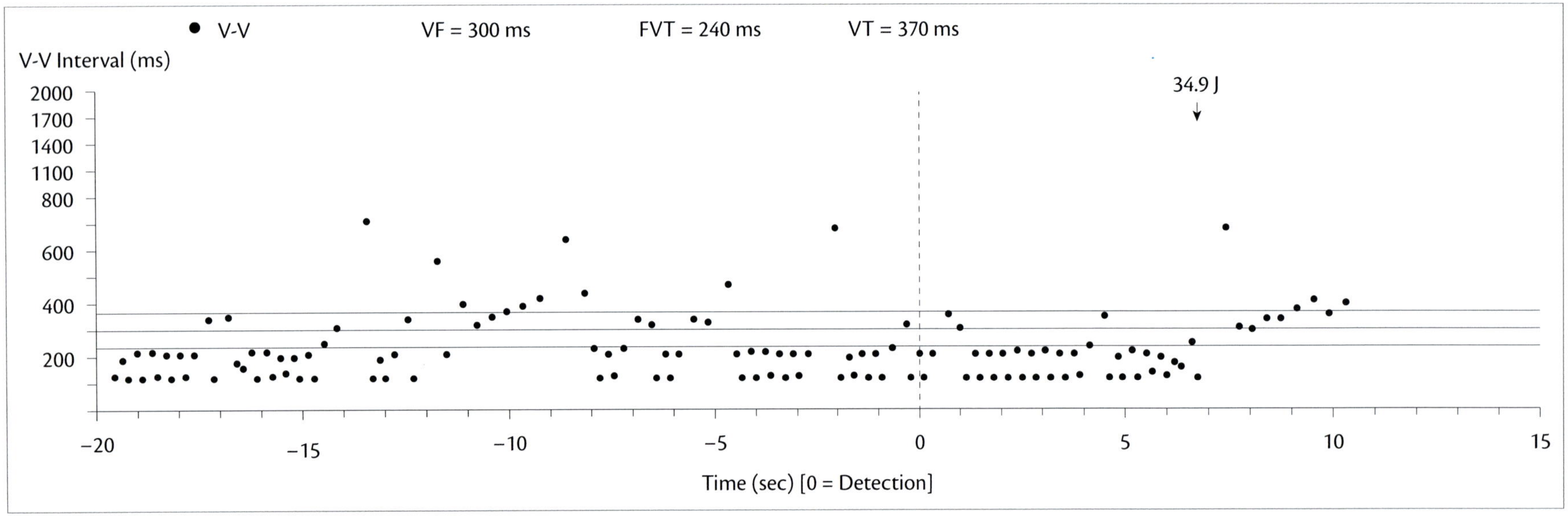

Question

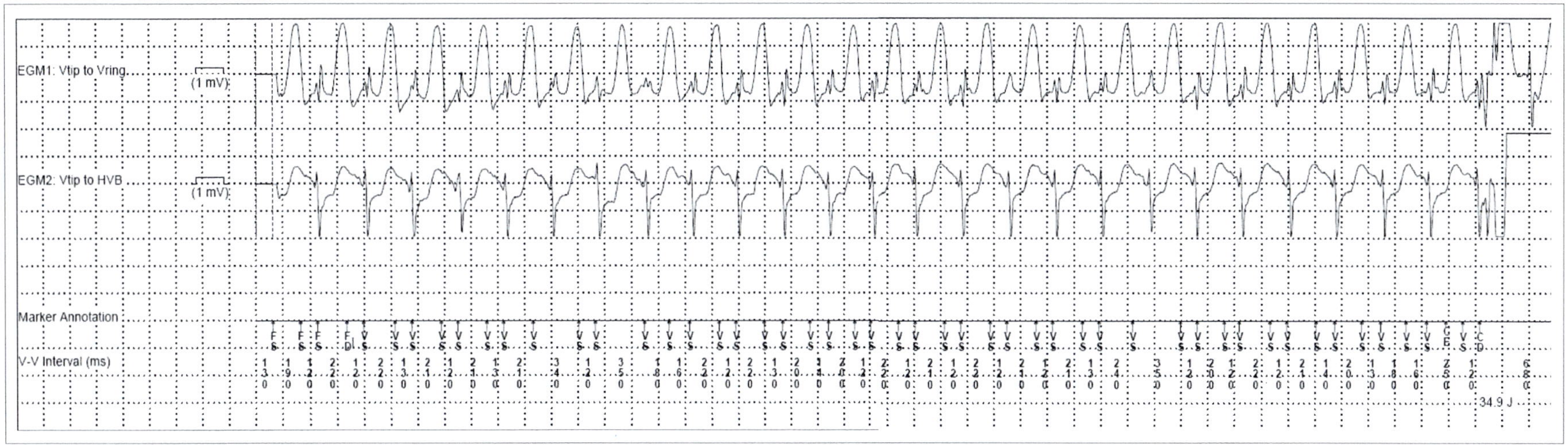

Figure 48.2 EGM of the stored event

What is your diagnosis?

A VT

B SVT

C R-wave double-counting

D T-wave oversensing

Answer

D **T-wave oversensing**

Figure 48.3 Annotated EGM of the stored event

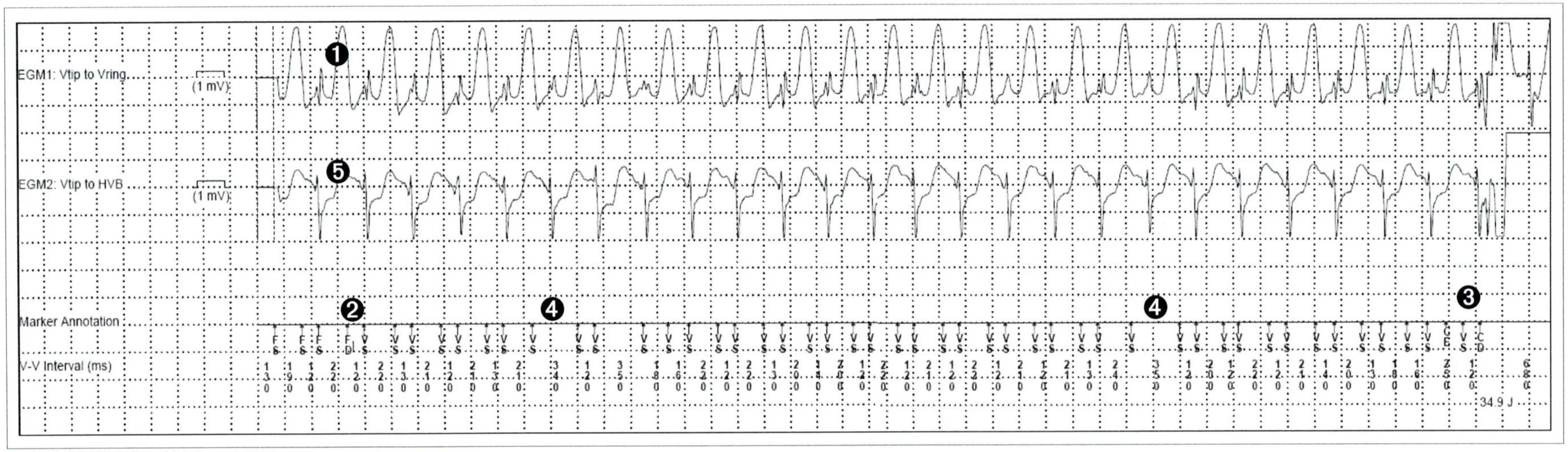

The T-waves had increased in amplitude during physical exertion and were sensed by the ventricular channel, leading to double-counting of the cycles and multiple inappropriate shocks (Figure 48.3).

❶ The T-waves are of high amplitude in this channel which is used for rate sensing.

❷ VF is detected (FD), resulting in capacitor charge.

❸ A full-energy shock is delivered.

❹ The R-waves are sometimes undersensed after sensing of the high-amplitude T-wave, due to the adaptive sensitivity.

Comments

Avoiding T-wave oversensing

T-wave oversensing may occur in patients who have low R-wave amplitude (resulting in sensitive value of the sensing threshold start) or high-amplitude T-waves (e.g. patients with Brugada syndrome, hyperkalaemia, etc.). It can be recognized on the tachogram by the classical 'railroad track' appearance of the RR intervals (Figure 48.1). The consequences may be dramatic, with multiple inappropriate shocks, as in this patient.

Simply reducing the maximum sensitivity would not have solved the problem in this case, due to the amplitude of the T-waves that were even higher than the R-waves. The issue was solved by programming sensing to an integrated bipolar configuration, as the T-waves were of low amplitude (as seen on the stored EGM 2 'V tip to HVB' in Figure 48.3).Recent devices have algorithms that avoid T-wave oversensing (Figure 48.4).

Figure 48.4 Algorithms to avoid T-wave oversensing. (a) Increasing the threshold start level and/or prolonging the decay delay. (b) Recognizing the characteristic patterns of sensing ('TW')

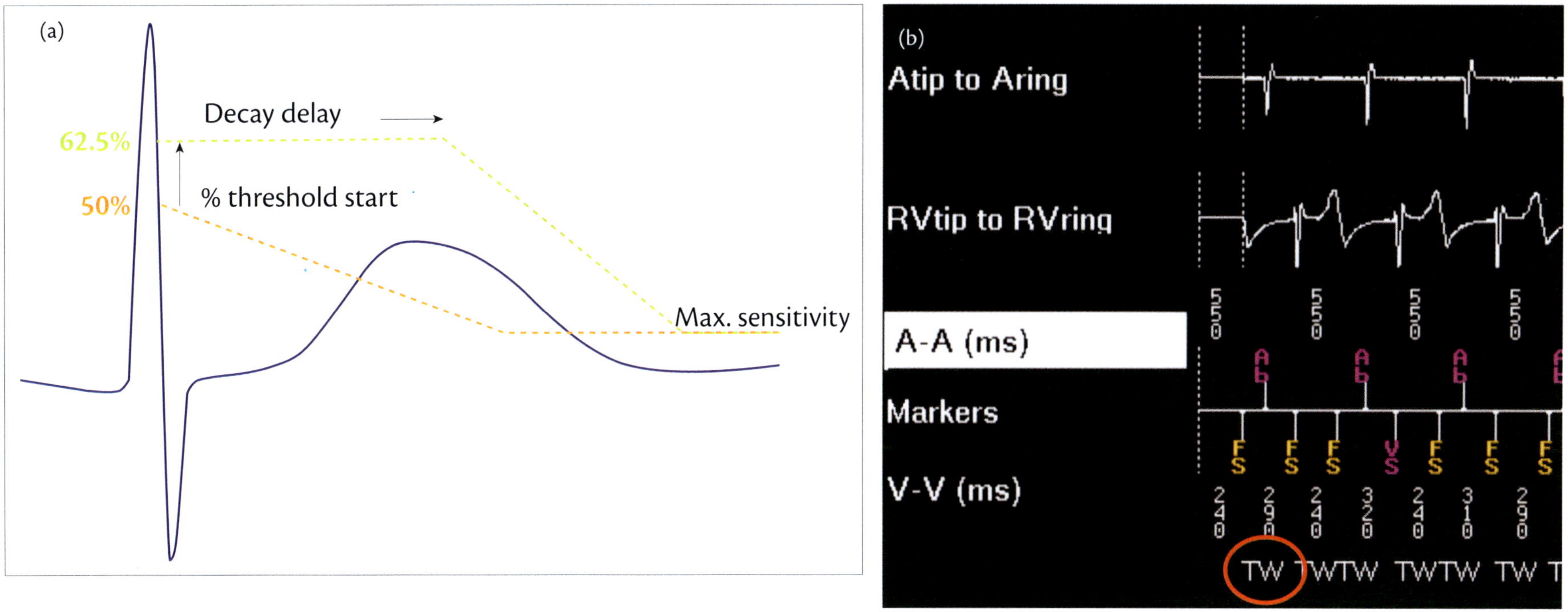

Courtesy of Marta Roca

Introduction to the case

A patient implanted with a CRT-D presented for routine follow-up. He had no complaints. Device interrogation revealed 11% RV sensing; the device settings are shown in Table 49.1, and the rate histogram in Figure 49.1. A real-time EGM was printed during the follow-up and is shown in Figure 49.2.

Table 49.1 Device settings

Zone	Slow VT	VT	VF
Rate (bpm/ms)	170/353	220/273	240/250
Detection (s)	4s	2.5s	2s
Therapy	ATP + shocks	ATP + shocks	Shocks

Pacing mode	DDDR
Lower rate	60bpm
Upper rate	120bpm
AV delay (paced/sensed)	160/140ms
Atrial output	2.5V@0.4ms
RV output (bipolar)	2.5V@0.4ms
LV output (LV tip–RV coil)	2.5V@0.4ms
Atrial sensitivity (bipolar)	0.3mV
RV sensitivity (integrated bipolar)	0.4mV
LV sensitivity (LV tip–RV coil)	2.5mV

Figure 49.1 Rate histogram

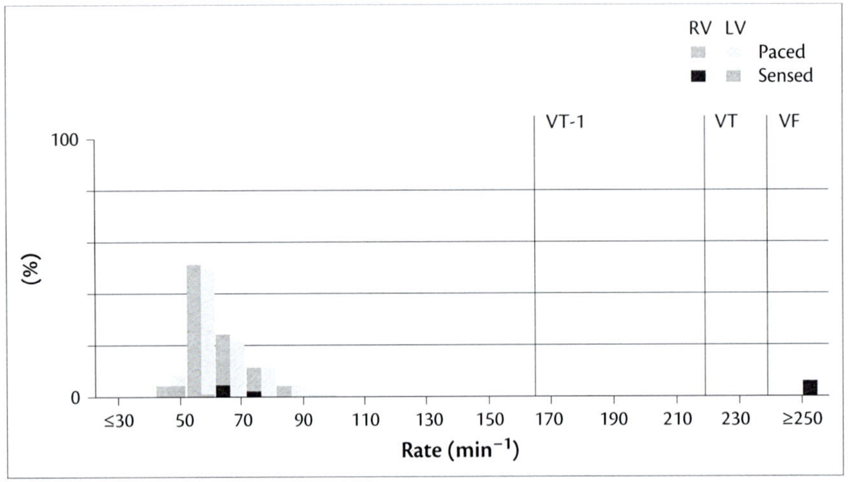

Question

Figure 49.2 Real-time EGM recorded at follow-up

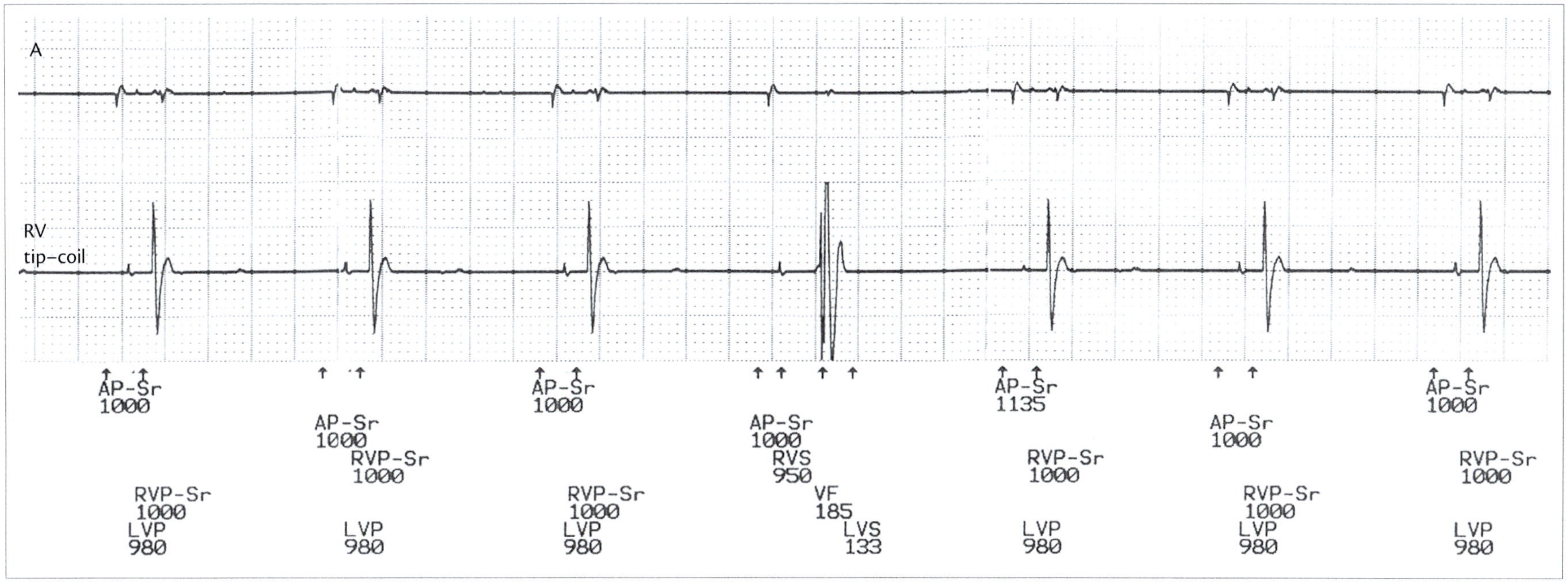

What do you observe?

A Atrial non-capture

B Crosstalk

C Far-field P-wave oversensing

D R-wave double-counting

Answer

C Far-field P-wave oversensing

Figure 49.3 Annotated real-time EGM recorded at follow-up

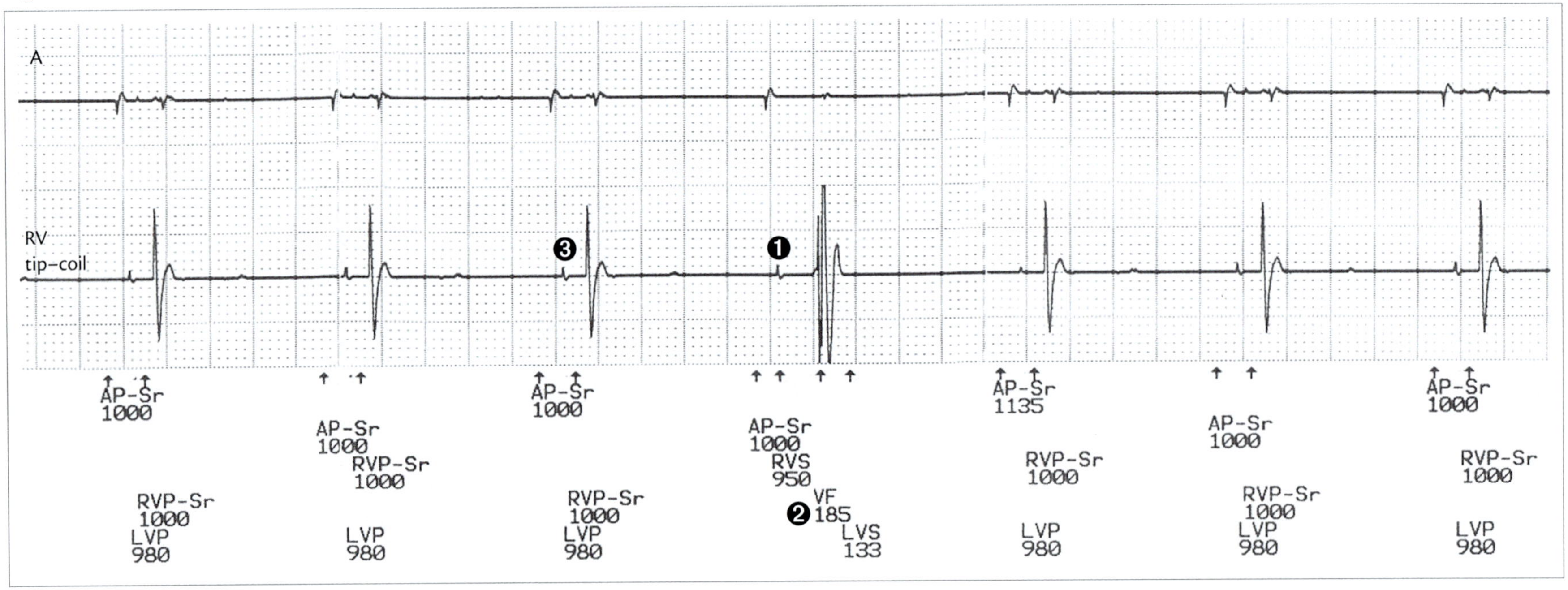

This is one of the rare instances of far-field P-wave oversensing by a ventricular lead, due to the integrated bipolar RV sensing configuration (Figure 49.3).

❶ A low-amplitude signal is observed in the RV channel at about 100ms after atrial pacing (which is too long for crosstalk), corresponding to the far-field P-wave which is sensed by the RV coil straddling the tricuspid annulus.

❷ The far-field P-wave is sensed in the RV channel (RVS), inhibiting ventricular pacing, and is followed by sensing of the near-field RV signal which occurs after 185ms (and is labelled as VF); this is then followed by LV sensing (LVS).

❸ The far-field P-wave is visible during each cycle but is sensed intermittently, due to its low amplitude.

Comments

Far-field P-wave oversensing by integrated bipolar implantable cardioverter–defibrillator leads

Far-field P-wave oversensing by the ventricular lead is a much rarer phenomenon than FFRW oversensing by the atrial lead. It should nevertheless be evaluated at implantation of integrated bipolar leads, especially if the lead is placed in a mid-ventricular position (e.g. on the interventricular septum) which leads to the RV coil straddling the tricuspid annulus and sensing atrial signals. The PAVB period will not solve the problem entirely, as it is only applied during atrial pacing (and also may not be long enough). The issue was solved here by reducing the ventricular sensitivity from 0.4mV to 0.6mV.

Other causes of far-field P-wave oversensing by the RV lead include dislodgement of the lead to near the tricuspid annulus and accidental implantation of the RV lead in the coronary sinus.

Introduction to the case

A patient with a single-chamber ICD, implanted for the primary prevention of sudden death, presented after having received a shock. The stored EGM of the event is shown in Figure 50.1. The device settings are shown in Table 50.1 and Figure 50.2.

Table 50.1 Device settings

Zone	Slow VT	VT (via VF)	VF
Rate (bpm/ms)	160/375	240/250	187/320
Detection (intervals)	20	24/30	24/30
Redetection (intervals)	12	9/12	9/12
Therapy	None	ATP + shocks	Shocks

Figure 50.2 Device settings

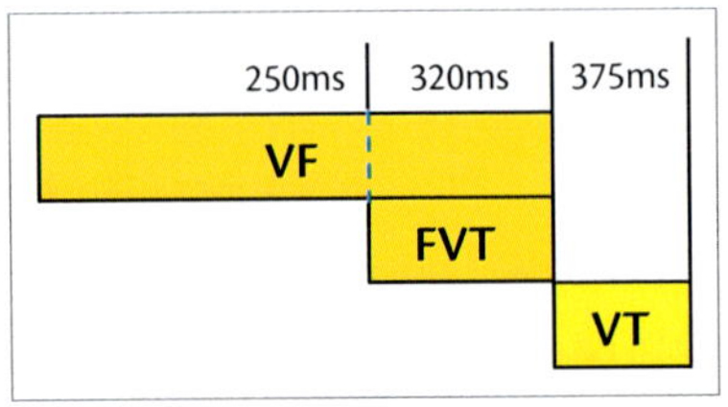

Question

Figure 50.1 EGM of the stored event

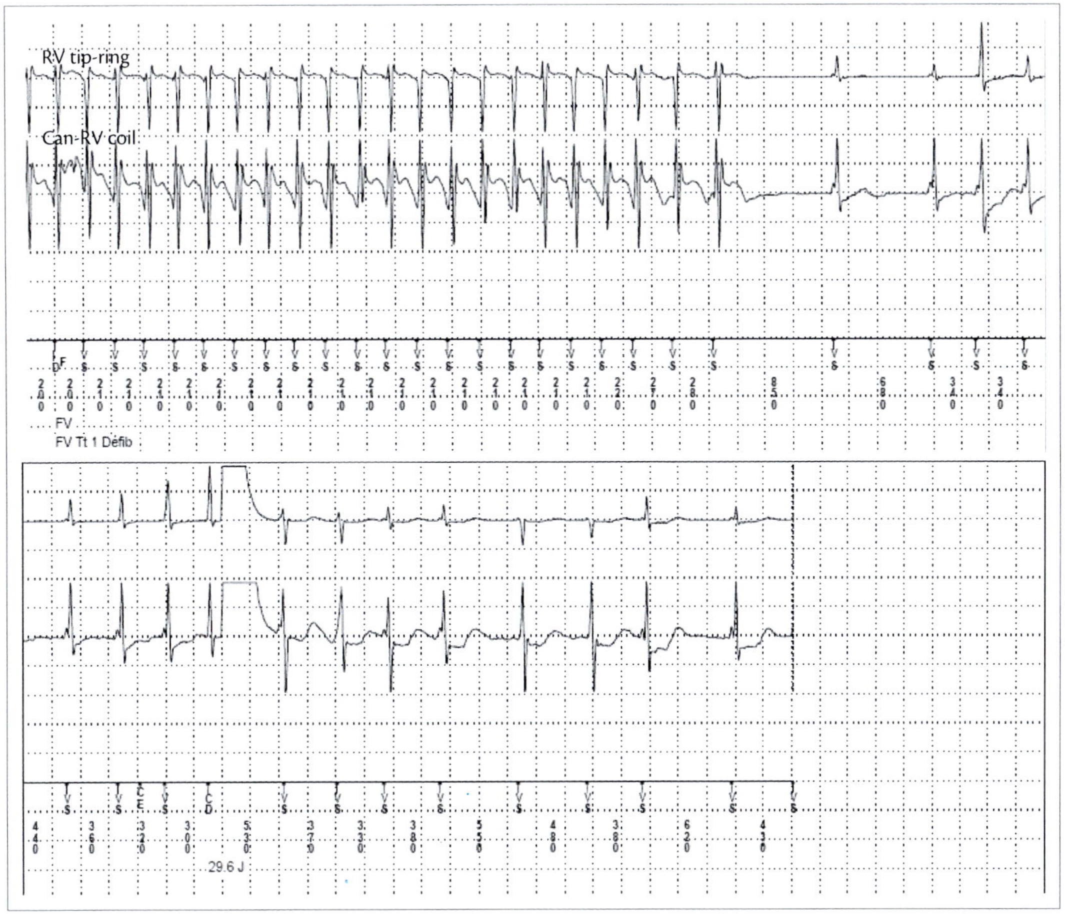

What do you observe?

A Normal device function

B T-wave oversensing

C R-wave double-counting

D Committed shock

Answer

A Normal device function

Figure 50.3 Annotated EGM of the stored event

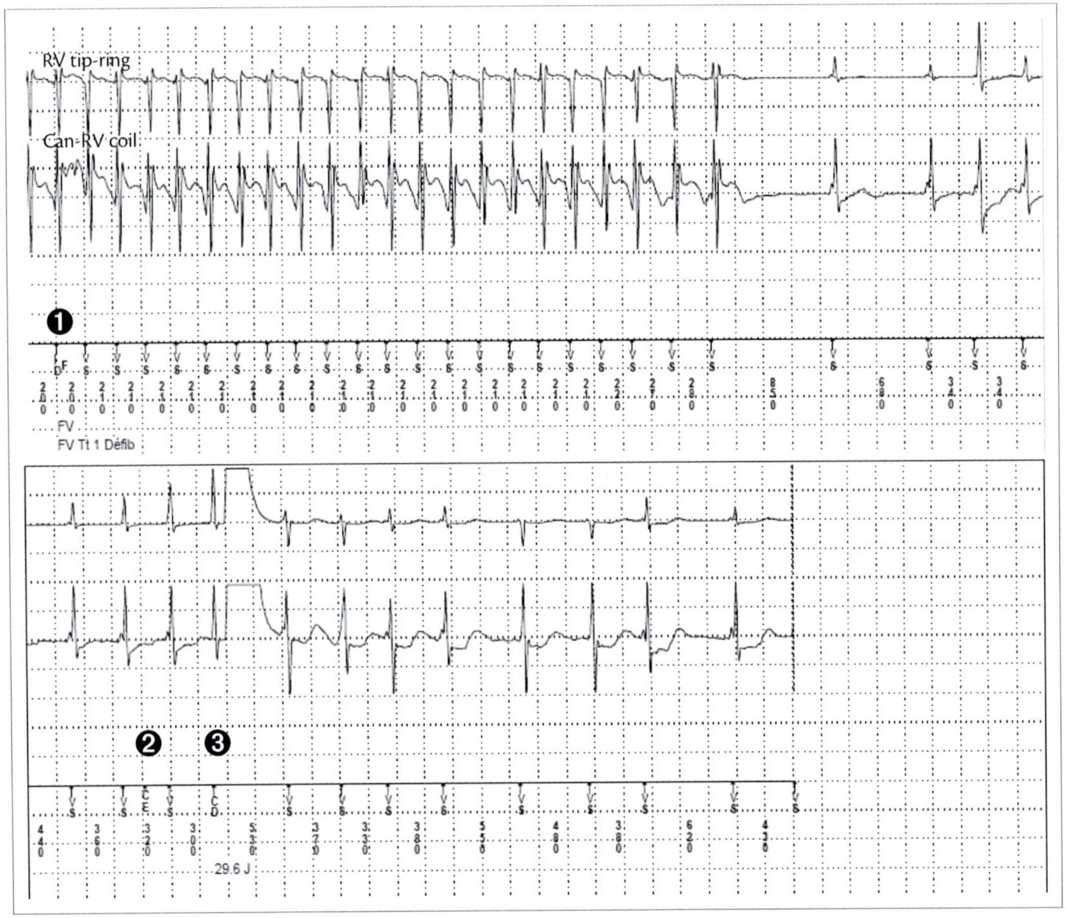

As shown in Figure 50.3, the patient received a shock after the end of non-sustained VT (SVT is unlikely because of the short cycle length and the different morphology, compared to normal rhythm).

❶ The VT fulfils the detection criteria in the VF zone, triggering capacitor charge.

❷ The VT has spontaneously stopped before the capacitor charge end (CE).

❸ The shock is non-committed, as it is not delivered immediately at the end of capacitor charge. There are two short cycles (320ms and 300ms) that fall in the VT zone, fulfilling the 2/5 fast interval criterion for reconfirmation of arrhythmia before shock delivery.

Comments

Committed and non-committed shocks

The first shock of ICDs is always 'non-committed', i.e. persistence of the arrhythmia is always reconfirmed before delivery of the shock. For the ICD model in this case, the criterion is 2/5 fast intervals that fall in the VF zone or VT zone + 60ms. Current models perform rhythm reconfirmation during capacitor charge and with other criteria, which would have avoided the unnecessary shock in this case. Aborting capacitor charges also prolongs battery life.

Arrhythmia reconfirmation should be distinguished from redetection. The latter refers to verification of termination or persistence of an arrhythmia after delivery of therapy (the criteria, in this example, are shown in Table 50.1). In case the first shock is ineffective and the arrhythmia is redetected, all subsequent shocks are 'committed', i.e. there is no reconfirmation of arrhythmia during, or at the end of, capacitor charge.

CASE 51

Introduction to the case

A patient implanted with a dual-chamber ICD presented for a shock that was not preceded by any cardiac complaints. The EGM of the episode is shown in Figure 51.1. The device settings are shown in Table 51.1.

Table 51.1 Device settings

Zone	Slow VT	VT	VF
Rate (bpm/ms)	160/375	171/350	214/280
Detection (intervals)	24	18	12
Therapy	None	ATP + shocks	Shocks

Pacing mode	DDD
Lower rate	40bpm
Upper rate	120bpm
AV delay (paced/sensed)	160/140ms
Atrial output (bipolar)	2.5V@0.4ms
RV output (bipolar)	2.5V@0.4ms
Atrial sensitivity (bipolar)	0.3mV
RV sensitivity (integrated bipolar)	0.4mV
PAVB	45ms
VRP after VS	125ms
VRP after VP	250ms

Question

Figure 51.1 EGM of the stored episode

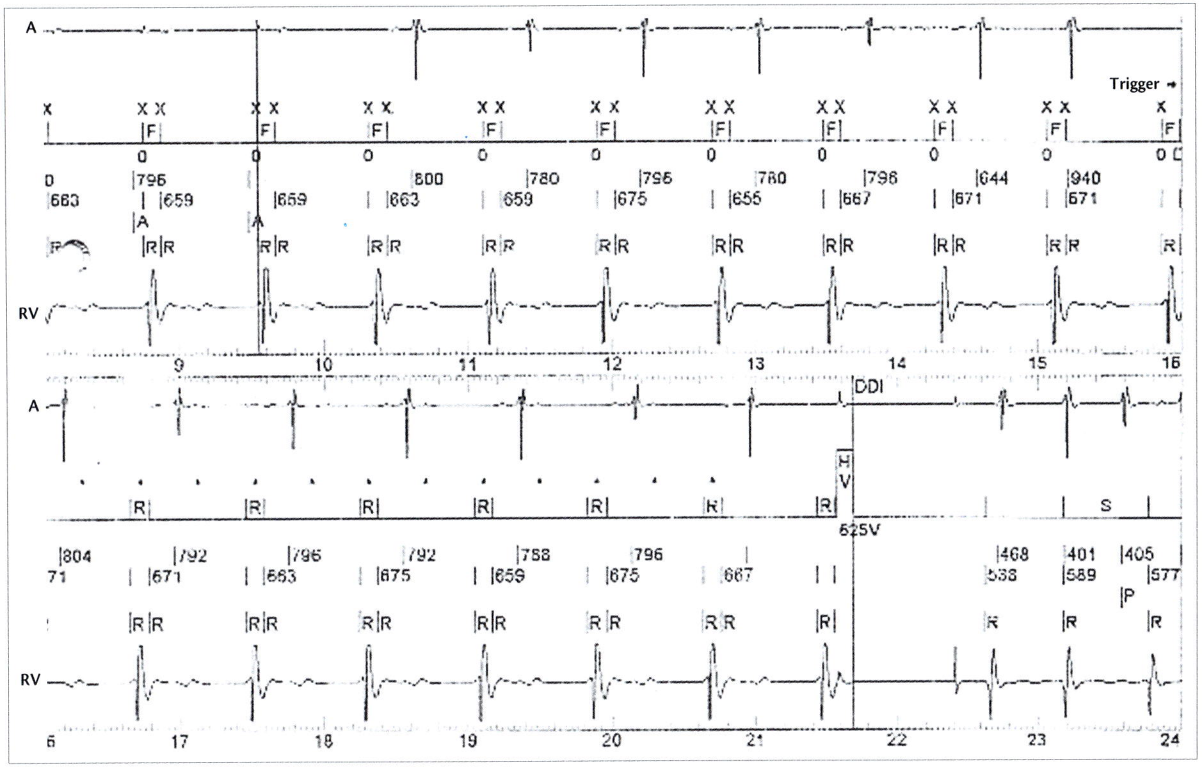

What do you observe?

A Sinus rhythm with R-wave double-counting

B Accelerated ventricular rhythm with R-wave double-counting

C T-wave oversensing

D VT

Answer

B Accelerated ventricular rhythm with R-wave double-counting

Figure 51.2 Annotated EGM of the stored episode

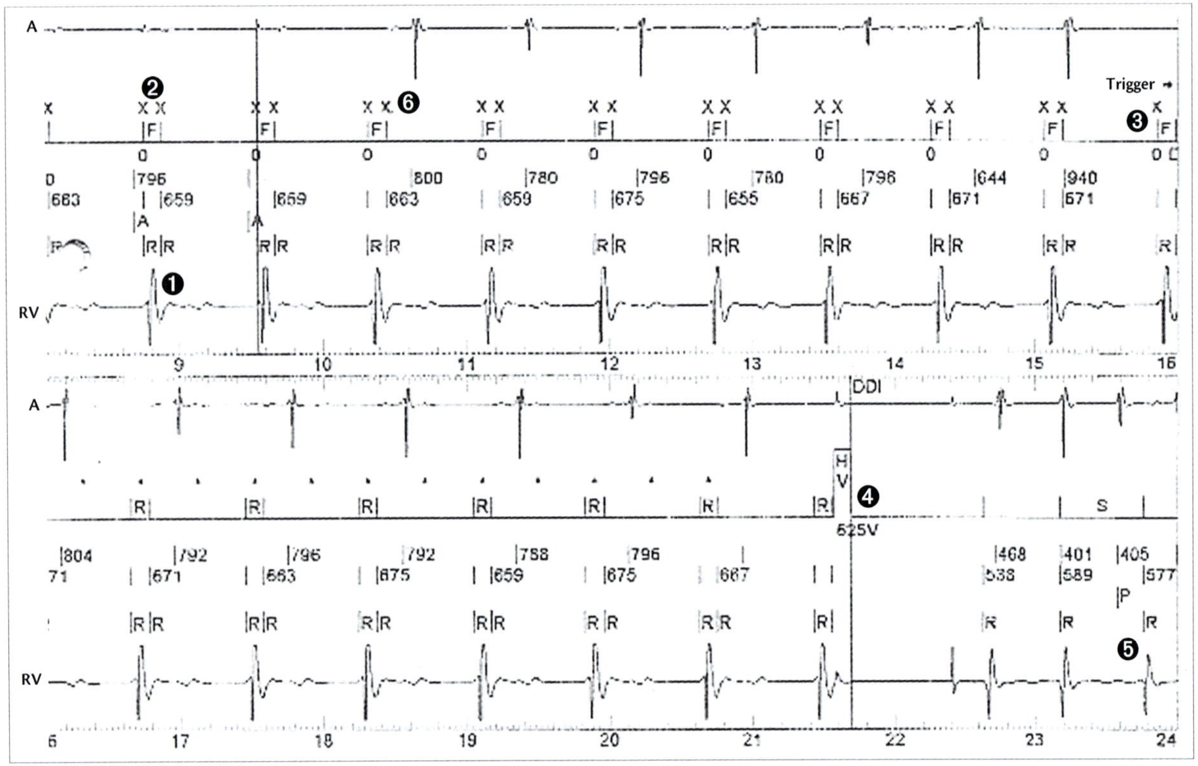

An accelerated ventricular rhythm resulted in R-wave double-counting with inappropriate shock (Figure 51.2).

❶ R-wave double-counting is seen on the marker channel.

❷ The morphology shows a mismatch with the template (0% resemblance). Due to the short RR interval, the 2nd event is binned as a VF event.

❸ The criteria for VF detection are fulfilled.

❹ A high-energy shock is delivered.

❺ The last cycle is probably sinus with AV conduction, whereas the preceding two cycles are VPBs or junctional beats (as they are not preceded by P-waves). Note that these cycles do not have R-wave double-counting.

❻ The atrial channel shows retrograde P-waves. These are detected by the device, as shown by the timing markers labelled 800, 780, 796, etc. The 1st two atrial cycles are atrial-paced (A) but are not conducted because the AR intervals are very short due the accelerated ventricular rhythm.

Comments

R-wave double-counting

This is a relatively rare cause of inappropriate shock in current devices. The R-wave double-counting interval was measured at 132ms, and the issue was resolved by increasing the VRP after ventricular sensing from 125ms to 157ms.

In case of a very wide QRS complex, the ventricular blanking may not be able to cover the full interval. If the 2nd component of the ventricular EGM is of low amplitude, the issue may be resolved by reducing sensitivity levels or by activating algorithms that avoid T-wave oversensing (such as increasing the threshold start or programming a decay delay; see Case 48).

Introduction to the case

A 71-year-old patient, implanted with a CRT-D for ischaemic heart disease and the primary prevention of sudden death, called the device clinic one afternoon, complaining of fatigue, dyspnoea, and dizziness since 3 days, without any shocks. As the patient was on remote device management, a patient-initiated interrogation was performed. The print screen of the diagnostics overview is shown in Figure 52.1, and a strip of the real-time EGM is displayed in Figure 52.2.

Figure 52.1 Diagnostics overview obtained by remote transmission

Quick Look | Current EGM | Episodes | Battery/Lead Status | More Reports | Notes | History

Device: Concerto™ C174AWK

Clinical Status	Since 27-May-2008
Treated	
VF	0
FVT	0
VT	0
AT/AF (Monitor)	
Monitored	
VT(140-158 bpm)	0
VT-NS (>4 beats, >158 bpm)	0
SVT: VT/VF Rx Withheld	0
AT/AF	0
Time in AT/AF	(0.0%)
Functional	**Last Week**
Patient Activity	2.3 hr/day

Cardiac Compass Trends (Dec-2007 to May-2008)

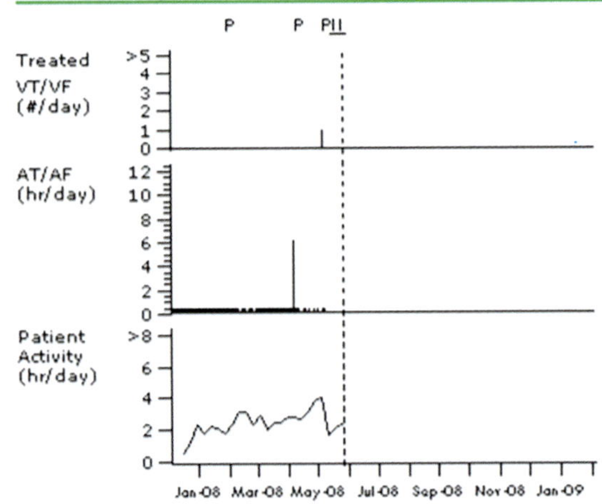

Therapy Summary	VT/VF	AT/AF
Pace-Terminated Episodes	0	0
Shock-Terminated Episodes	0	0
Total Shocks	0	0
Aborted Charges	0	0

Pacing	(% of Time Since 27-May-2008)
AS-VS	2.5%
AS-VP	28.5%
AP-VS	1.0%
AP-VP	67.9%

OBSERVATIONS (5)

- V. Pacing less than 90%.
- Longest ventricular sensing episode since the last session is greater than 60 seconds.

Question

Figure 52.2 Remotely transmitted real-time EGM

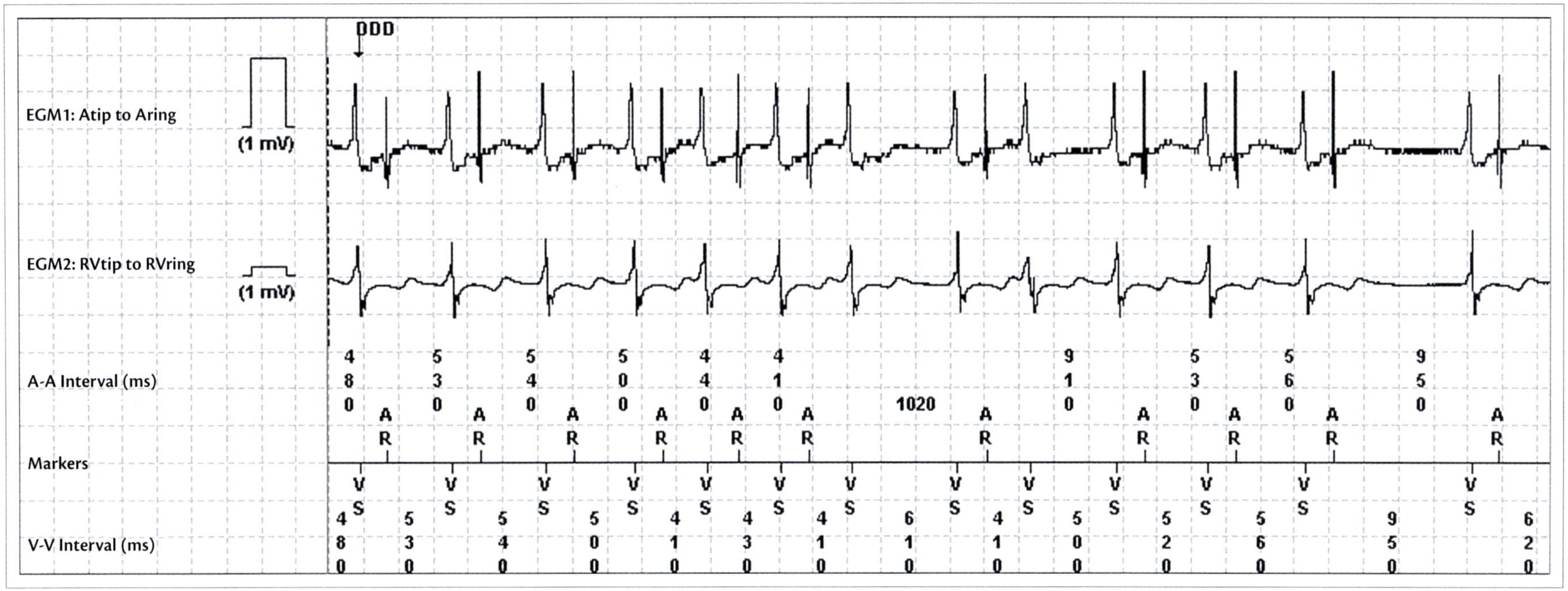

What is the patient's baseline rhythm?

A Sinus rhythm

B Atrial tachycardia

C Atrial bigeminy

D VT

Answer

D **VT**

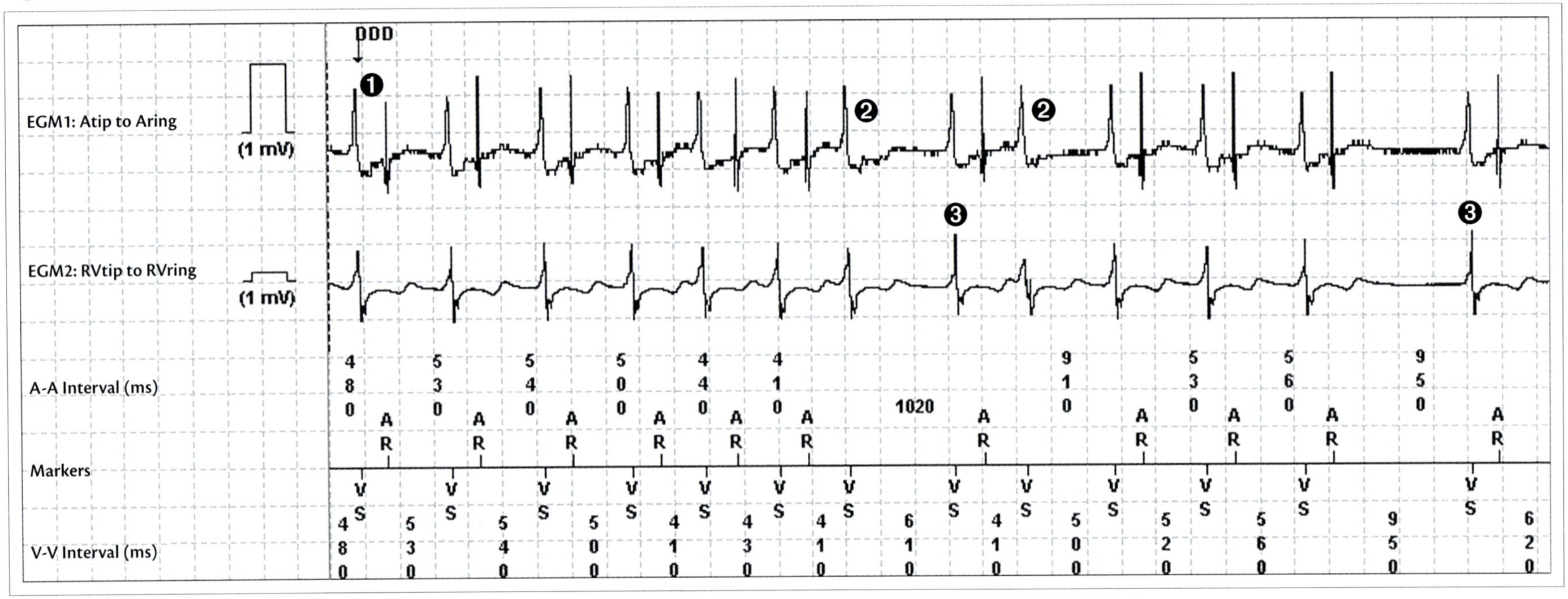

Figure 52.3 Annotated remotely transmitted real-time EGM

The device indicated that ventricular pacing was <90%, and that ventricular sensing occurred during >60s (Figure 52.1). The diagnosis of a slow irregular VT was made by analysing the real-time EGM (Figure 52.3). The VT was not detected by the ICD, because it was slower than the VT monitoring zone set at 140bpm.

❶ A large FFRW is visible on the atrial channel but is not detected by the ICD, as it falls in the PVAB period. The 2nd sharp signal is the near-field atrial signal due to retrograde VA conduction.

❷ There is intermittent VA block (that is rate-dependent). The V > A ratio confirms VT.

❸ The short runs are initiated by ventricular events, thereby also confirming VT.

Comments

Importance of real-time EGM strips for remote device management

Upon diagnosis of VT, the patient was immediately admitted to the emergency room. The VT accelerated (Figure 52.4a) with syncope and multiple shocks, with almost immediate recurrence of VT after each shock. The patient was intubated and administered intravenous amiodarone, which allowed the resumption of stable sinus rhythm (after a total of 32 shocks). Multiple organ failure developed, but the patient recovered and was discharged on amiodarone after 3 weeks. A remote device follow-up was performed after 6 months and showed no recurrence of ventricular arrhythmias, with >99% VP (Figure 52.4b). This example shows the importance of always checking the real-time EGM that is displayed with remote device transmissions.

Figure 52.4 (a) VT recorded upon admission. (b) Remote device follow-up performed at 6 months, showing the absence of recurrence of ventricular arrhythmias under amiodarone and recovered daily patient activity.

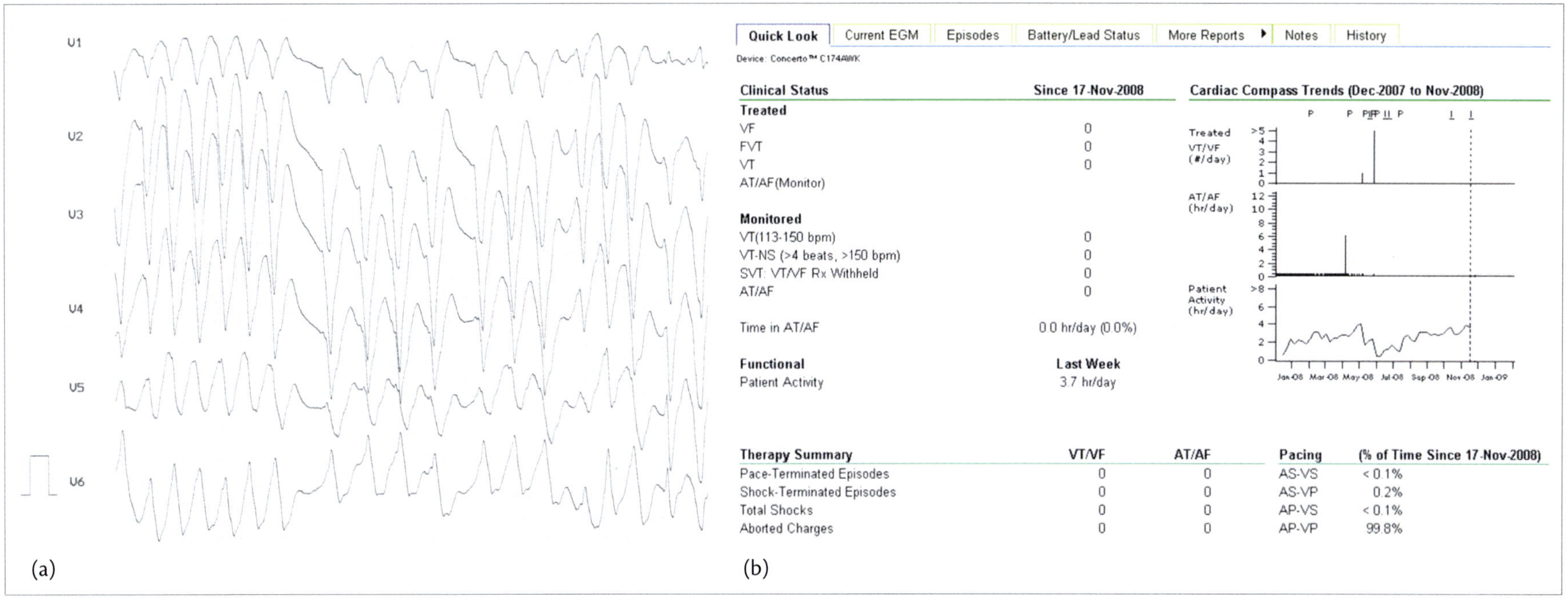

Introduction to the case

A patient with ischaemic heart disease was implanted with a dual-chamber ICD for the primary prevention of sudden death. He was seen at routine follow-up at 2 months after implantation, without any complaints. Device interrogation revealed high-rate ventricular episodes, which are shown in Figure 53.1. All electrical parameters were normal. The device settings are shown in Table 53.1.

Table 53.1 Device settings

Zone	Slow VT	VT	VF
Rate (bpm/ms)	160/375	190/316	240/250
Detection (s)	12	2.5	2
Therapy	Monitor	ATP + shocks	Shocks

Pacing mode	DDI
Lower rate	40bpm
Atrial output (bipolar)	2.5V@0.4ms
RV output (integrated bipolar)	2.5V@0.4ms
Atrial sensitivity (bipolar)	0.3mV
RV sensitivity (integrated bipolar)	0.4mV

Question

Figure 53.1 EGM of high-rate ventricular episode

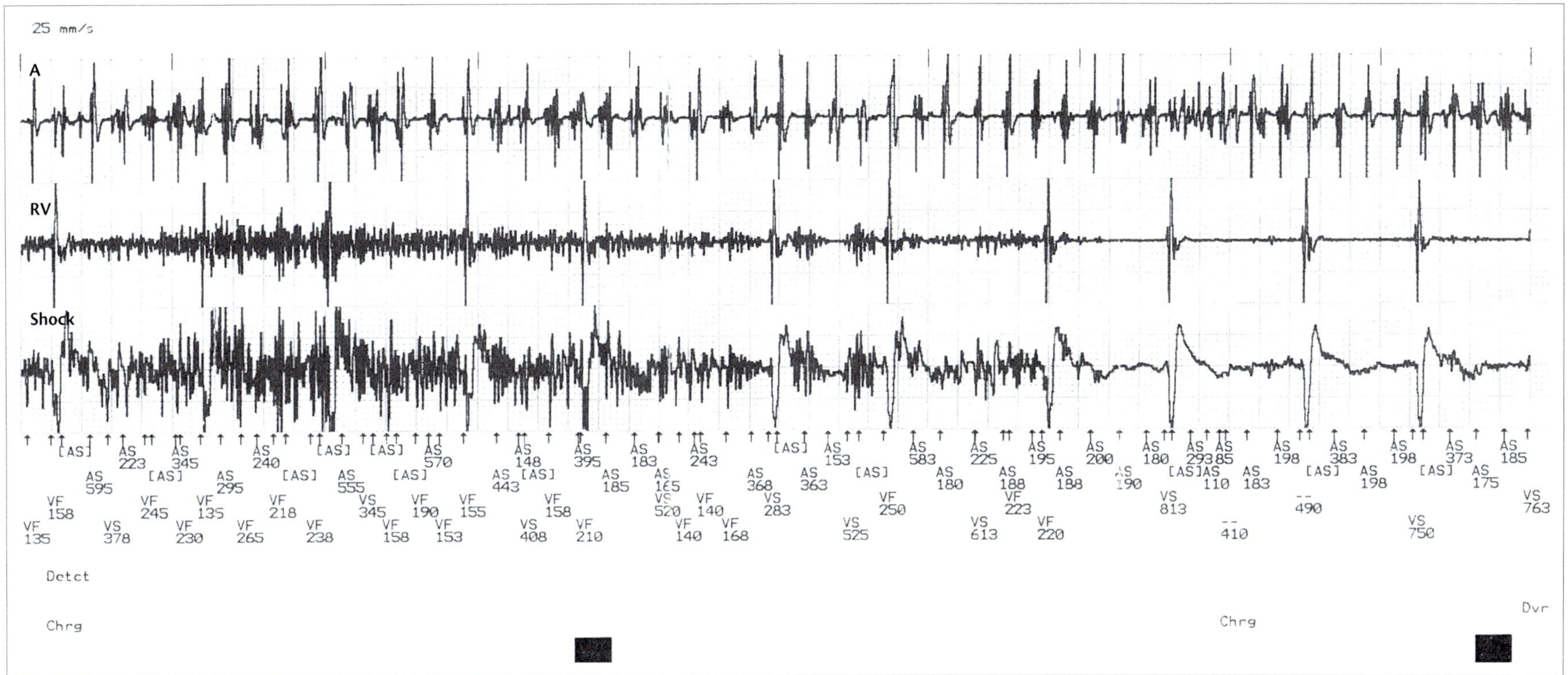

What is the most likely diagnosis?

A Electromagnetic interference

B Lead fracture

C Diaphragmatic myopotential oversensing due to integrated bipolar sensing

D Pectoral myopotential oversensing due to DF-1 switch

Answer

D Pectoral myopotential oversensing due to DF-1 switch

Figure 53.2 Annotated EGM of high-rate ventricular episode

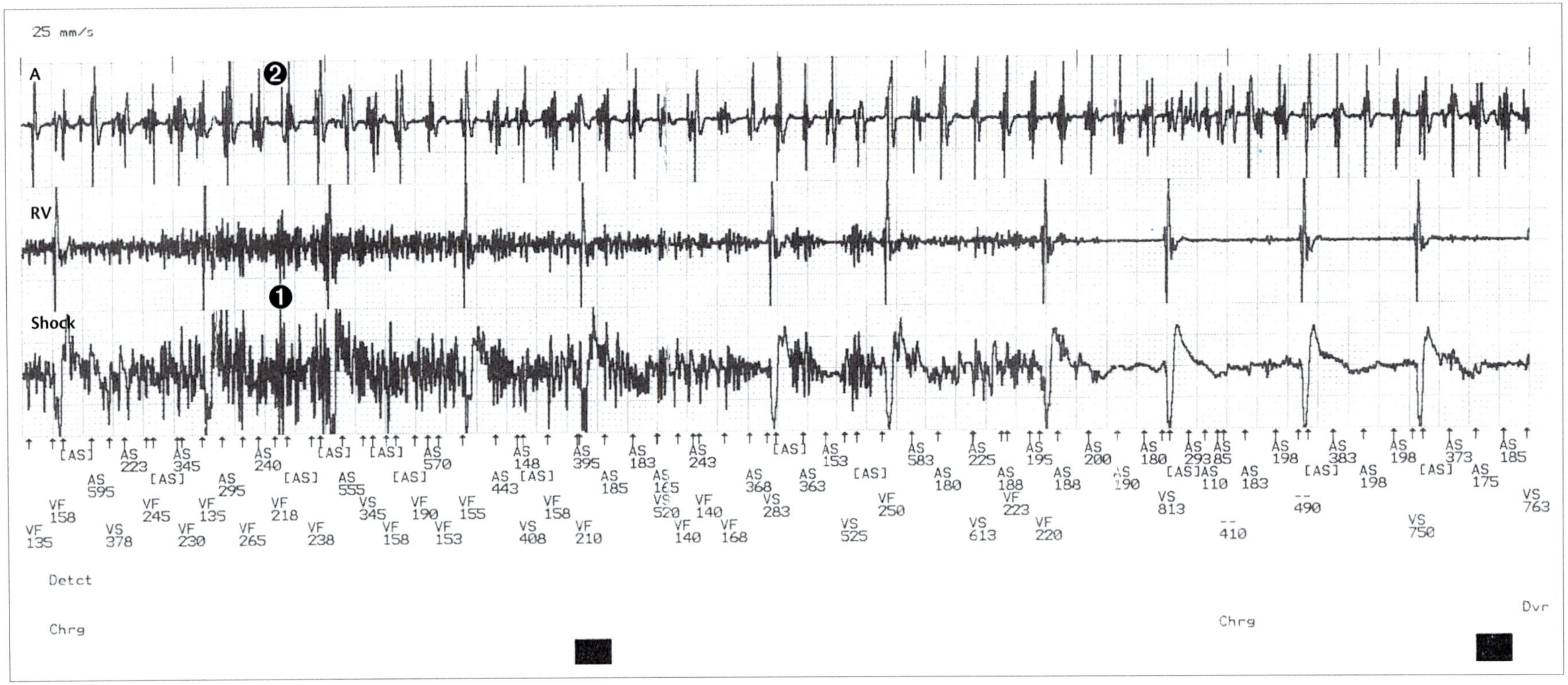

The following points from Figure 53.2 may be observed.

❶ High-frequency artefacts are visible on the RV (tip to RV coil) and shock (can to RV coil) EGMs. Lead fracture of the RV coil may produce artefacts on these two channels in an integrated bipolar lead, but fracture artefacts are usually more erratic, and the 'crescendo–decrescendo' aspect suggests myopotentials. The artefacts are of large amplitude on the shock channel, which is unusual for diaphragmatic myopotentials. A more likely explanation is pectoral myopotential oversensing due to accidental DF-1 inversion at implantation.

❷ AF is visible on the atrial channel, but there are no artefacts, which rules out electromagnetic interference.

Comments

DF-1 switch

With integrated bipolar leads, the RV coil is used as the anode in the pace/sense circuit, with an internal Y connection between the RV DF-1 connector and the IS-1 connector (Figure 53.3a). As the positive DF-1 connector is internally connected to the ICD casing, accidental inversion of the DF-1 lead terminals will result in the ICD casing becoming part of the sensing circuit (Figure 53.3d). Therefore, myopotential oversensing may be present during pectoral muscle contraction (this was confirmed in the device clinic in the present case). Not only is there a risk of inappropriate shock, but shocks may be ineffective because of shunting of the current between the SVC coil and the can (Figure 53.3e). This situation needs to be corrected by reintervening and correcting the DF-1 connections. DF-1 inversion with true bipolar leads will not result in myopotential oversensing, but the issue with the shock vectors remains. This issue is avoided with DF-4 leads.

Figure 53.3 Consequences of switching DF-1 pins with integrated bipolar ICD leads

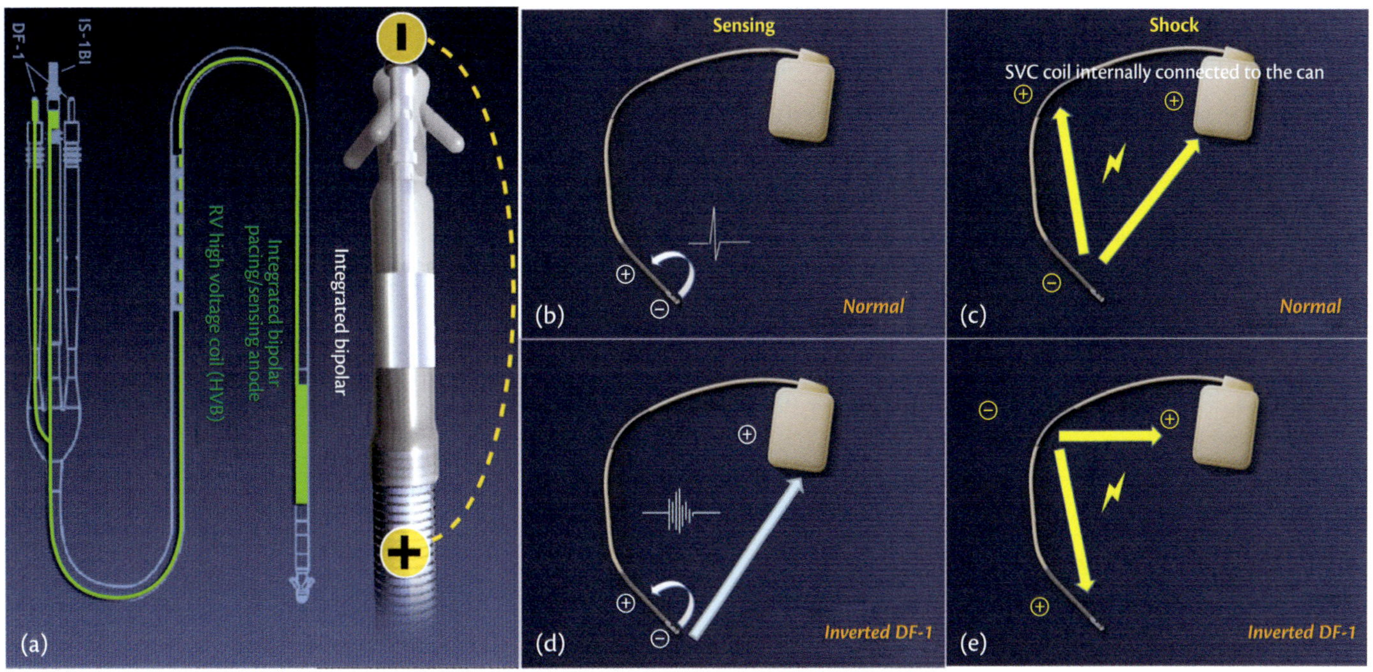

Adapted from Medtronic CorelCD

Section 3

CRT

Cases 54–70

Introduction to the case

A 76-year-old patient with ischaemic cardiomyopathy was implanted with a CRT-D and followed up 1 month after device implantation. He had no new cardiac complaints, and electrical parameters were normal. The counters indicated biventricular pacing in 66.6% of the time only (Figure 54.1). A real-time EGM is shown in Figure 54.2.

Figure 54.1 Ventricular rate histogram (left panel) and pacing counters (right panel)

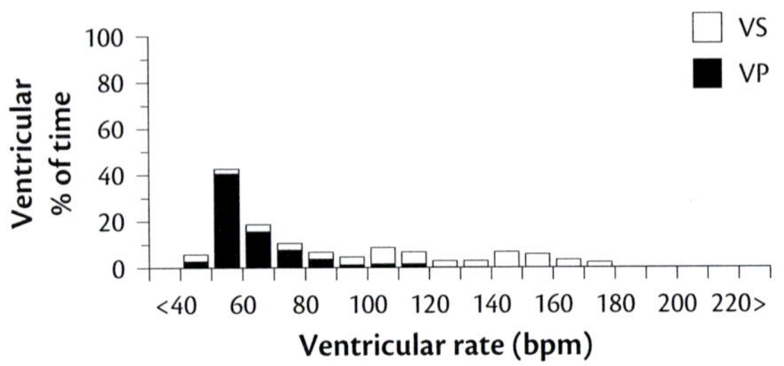

AS–VS	2.5%
AS–VP	57.9%
AP–VS	0.4%
AS–VP	39.2%
VP	66.6%
VSR pace	1.8%
VS	31.6%

Question

Figure 54.2 Real-time EGM

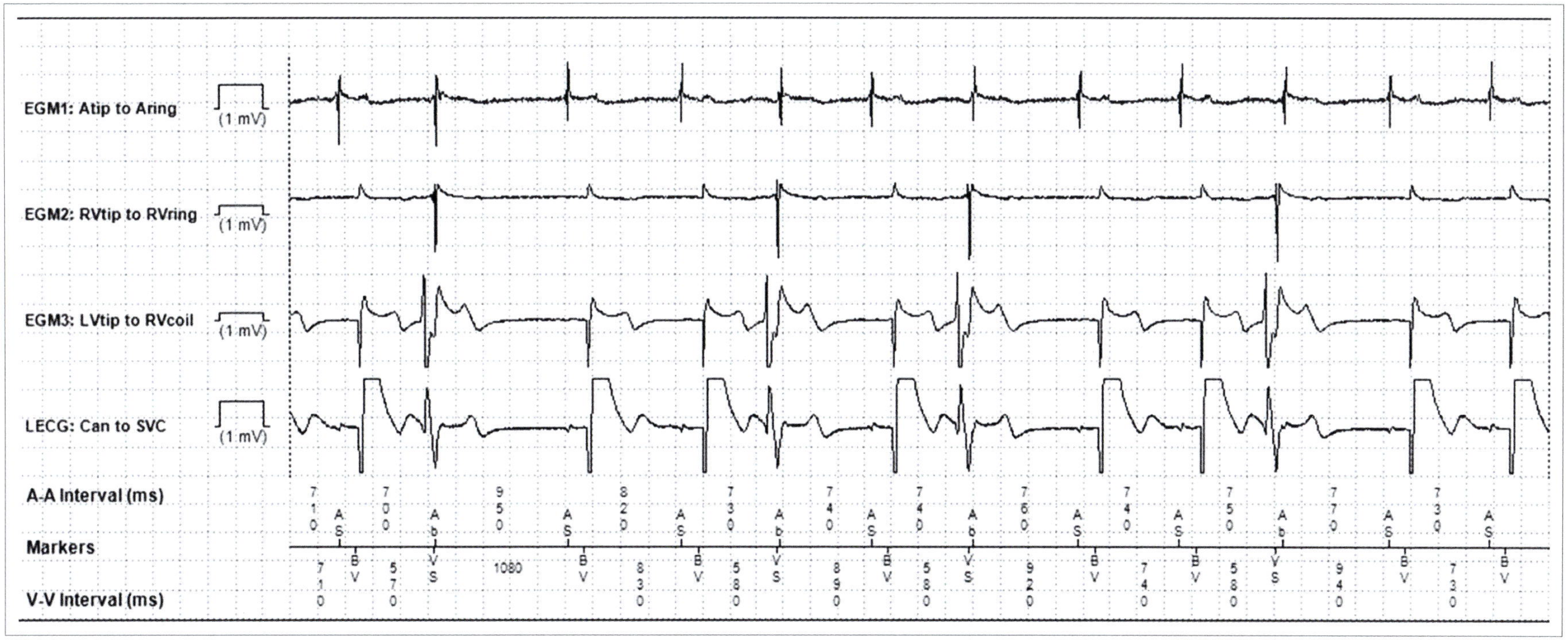

What is the cause for non-delivery of cardiac resynchronization therapy (CRT)?

A Premature atrial beats

B Premature ventricular beats

C Junctional beats

D Atrial undersensing

Answer

B Premature ventricular beats

Figure 54.3 Annotated real-time EGM

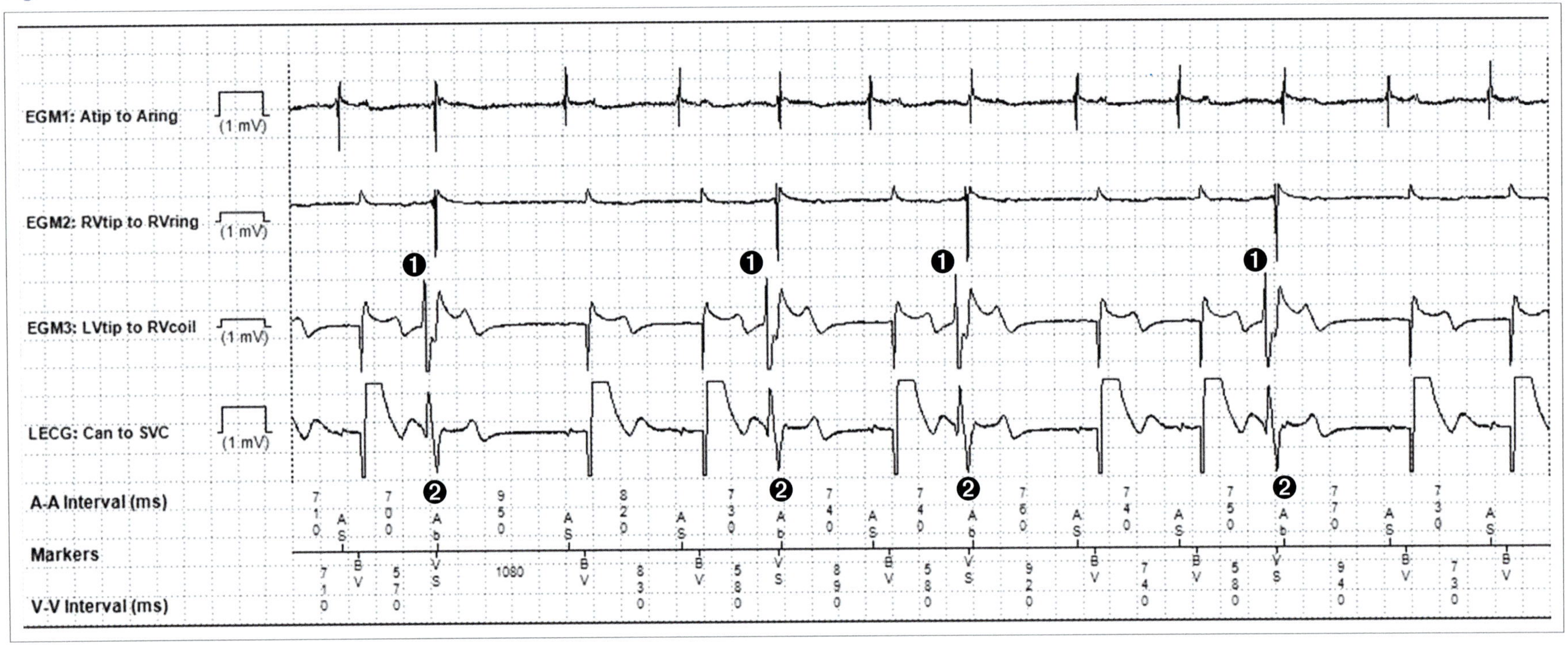

❶ Monomorphic premature beats can be visualized in the ventricular channels (Figure 54.3). These beats are earlier in the LV channel (EGM3) than the RV channel (EGM2) and also occur early with respect to the leadless ECG channel (LECG: can to SVC), implying an LV origin.

❷ The atrial events fall in the blanking period but are displayed as 'Ab' (few manufacturers currently use this denomination). The VS–Ab intervals are slightly variable, which speaks against junctional beats.

Comments

Loss of cardiac resynchronization therapy delivery due to ventricular premature beats

Note that the sum of percentages of AS–VP and AP–VP (57.9% + 39.2% = 97.1%) does not reflect the total percentage of ventricular pacing which is only 66.6%. This is due to the Vx–VS sequences (i.e. VPBs) which reduce the percentage of ventricular pacing.

The patient refused radiofrequency ablation of the VPBs and was placed on amiodarone (in addition to the beta-blocker therapy that had been introduced previously). The number of premature beats fell considerably, with delivery of CRT in 97% of the time.

Frequent VPBs may induce ventricular dysfunction and are also a cause for non-delivery of CRT. Radiofrequency ablation of VPBs in CRT non-responders has been shown to improve LVEF in these patients.[1]

Reference

1. Lakkireddy D, Di Biase L, Ryschon K, *et al.* Radiofrequency ablation of premature ventricular ectopy improves the efficacy of cardiac resynchronization therapy in nonresponders. *J Am Coll Cardiol* 2012; **60**: 1531–9.

Introduction to the case

A patient, equipped with a CRT-D, was followed by remote monitoring. An alert message was received to indicate that biventricular pacing occurred in <85% of the time. The transmission included the graphs in Figure 55.1, which indicate biventricular pacing as 78% of events and VPBs (Vx–Vx sequences) as 21% of events. An extract of the 30s real-time periodic EGM is shown in Figure 55.2.

Figure 55.1 Event counter graphs transmitted by remote monitoring

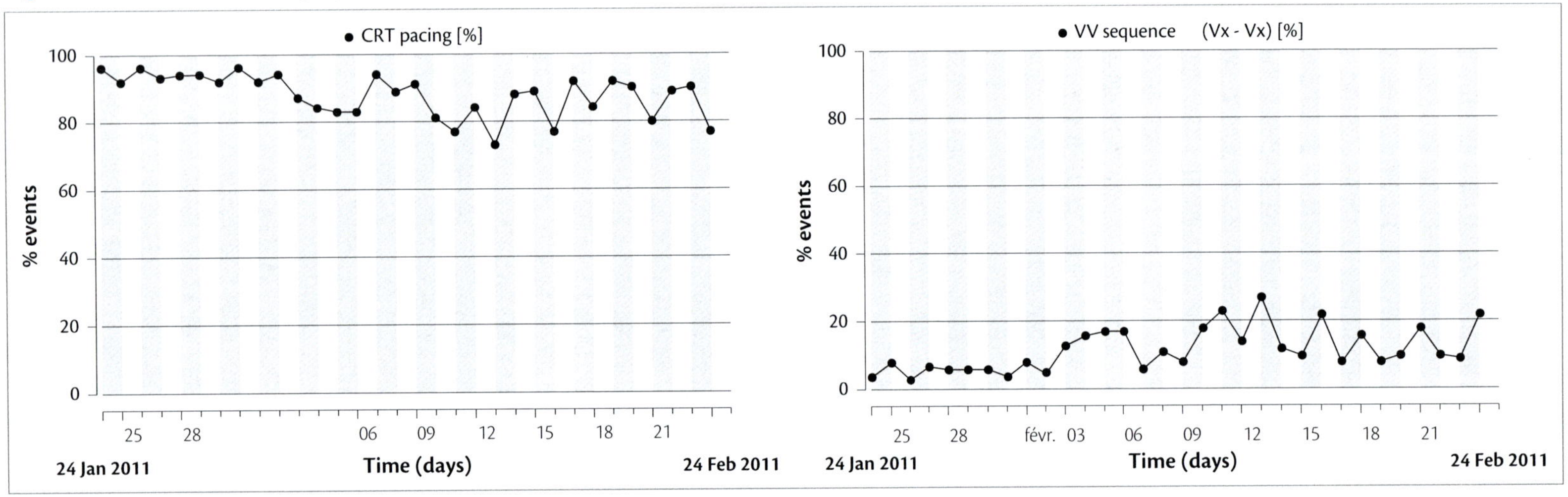

Question

Figure 55.2 Real-time EGM obtained by remote transmission

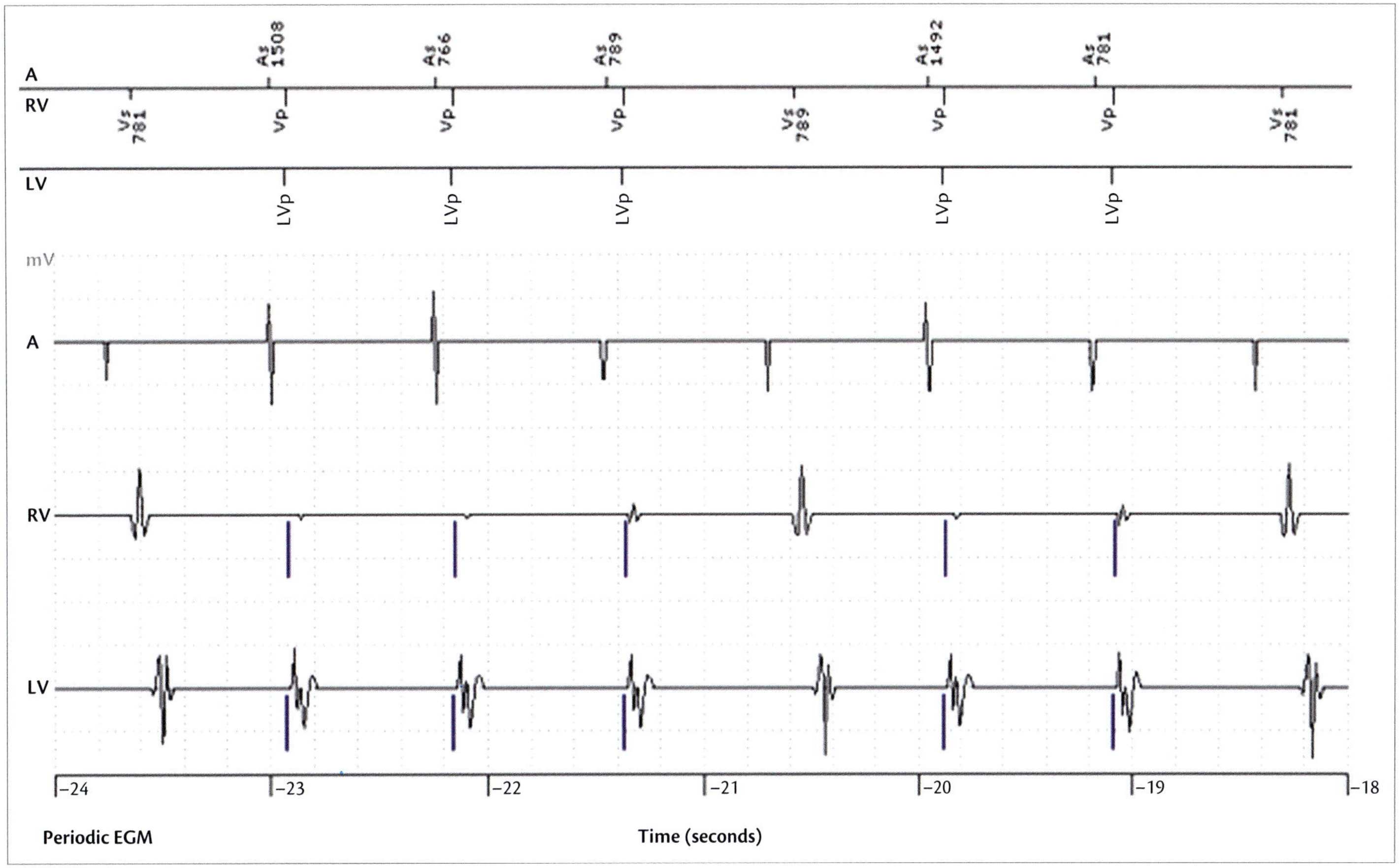

What is the reason for the reduction in CRT delivery?

A Frequent VPBs

B Ventricular non-capture

C Prolonged AVI

D Atrial undersensing

Answer

D Atrial undersensing

Figure 55.3 Annotated real-time EGM obtained by remote transmission

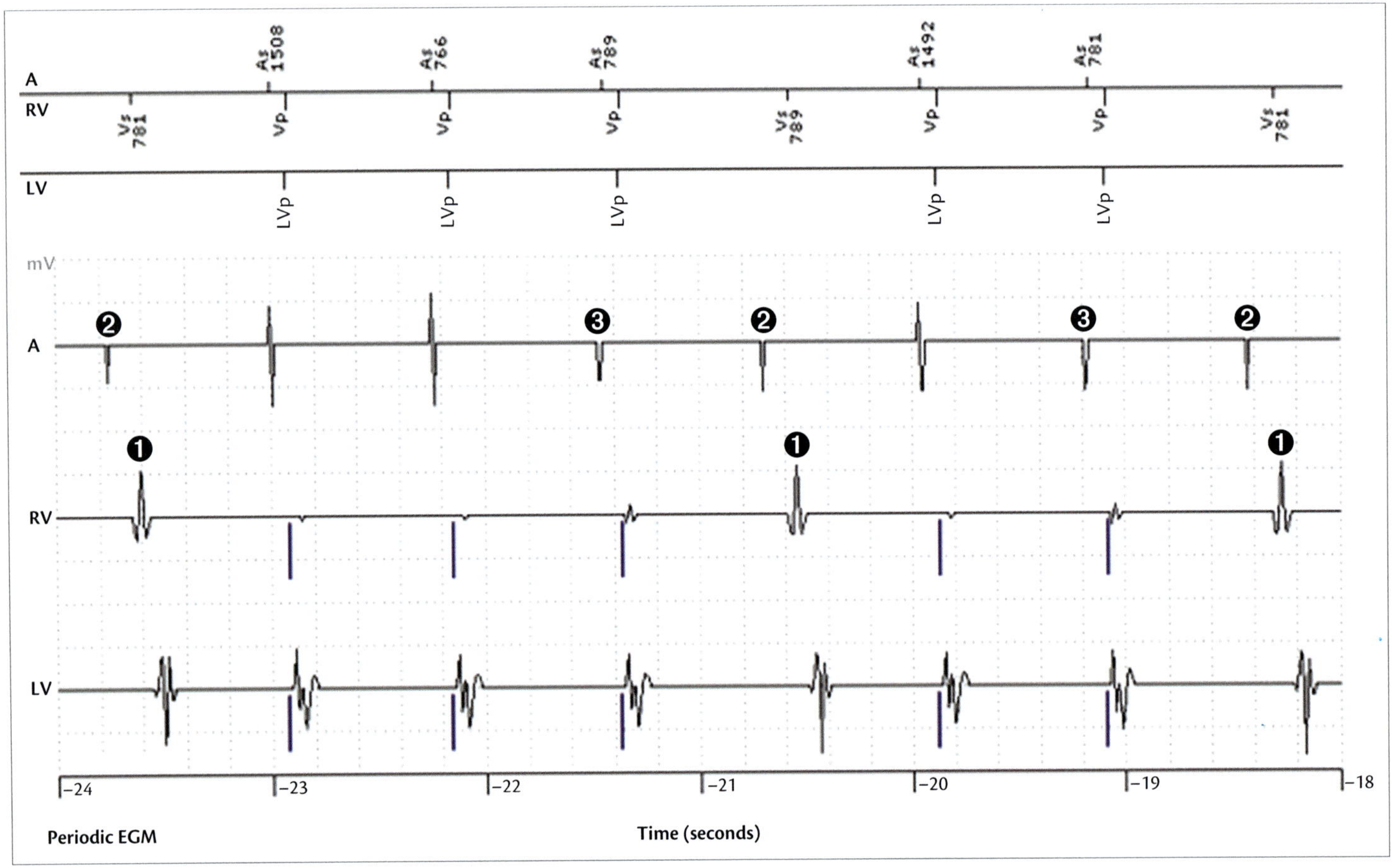

Atrial undersensing led to the absence of tracking of the P-waves by the device and resulted in intrinsic AV conduction (Figure 55.3).

❶ Intrinsic ventricular activity is visible on the ventricular channels (note the interventricular conduction delay and the difference in EGM morphology with the paced/captured ventricular events which are displayed as being of low amplitude due to the automatic gain). These events will be counted as VPBs (as there are no AS or AP events preceding them).

❷ An intrinsic atrial event is, however, visible on the atrial channel before each of these beats, but these events are not sensed.

❸ The EGM of the atrial events are sometimes clipped, due to digital processing.

Comments

Loss of cardiac resynchronization therapy delivery due to atrial undersensing

The remotely transmitted data showed that measured P-wave amplitude bordered the set sensitivity level of 0.5mV (Figure 55.4).

The patient was summoned to the device clinic where the sensitivity was set to the maximum level at 0.2mV, with an increase of CRT delivery to >95% thereafter.

Atrial undersensing should be suspected in case of a high count of VPBs by a pacemaker or ICD, as these are defined by the device as VS events that are not preceded by AS or AP events (or AR events in some devices). Atrial undersensing may then be confirmed by evaluating the trends in P-wave sensing amplitudes and by analysing real-time EGM tracings.

Figure 55.4 Evolution of P-wave detection amplitude

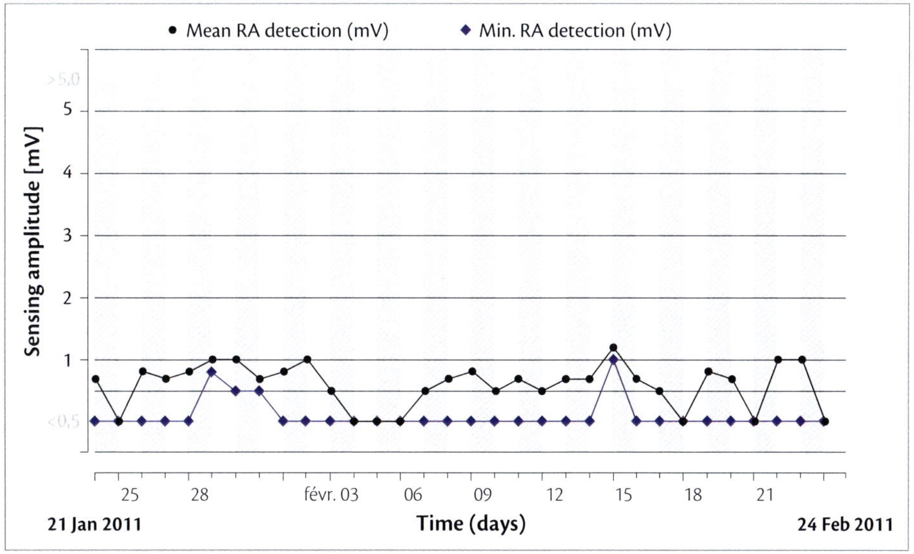

Introduction to the case

A patient with ischaemic heart disease implanted with a biventricular ICD was placed on remote device management. An alert message was received by the device clinic. The patient was contacted by phone and complained of increased dyspnoea. He was subsequently admitted to the hospital for decompensated heart failure. Elements of the device interrogation are shown in Figure 56.1.

Question

Figure 56.1 Data from device interrogation after hospital admission

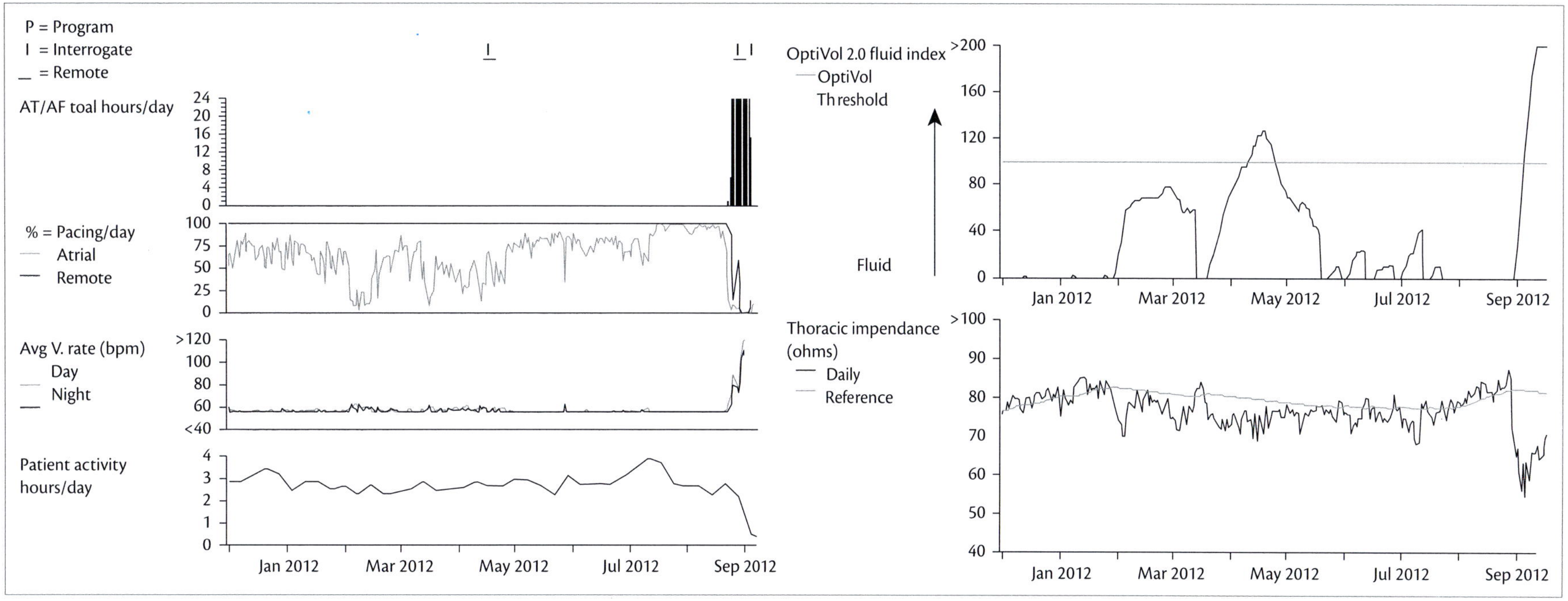

What does the device indicate?

A Rapidly conducted atrial arrhythmia with non-delivery of CRT

B Reduction in daily patient activity

C Increased lung fluid

D All of the above

Answer

D All of the above

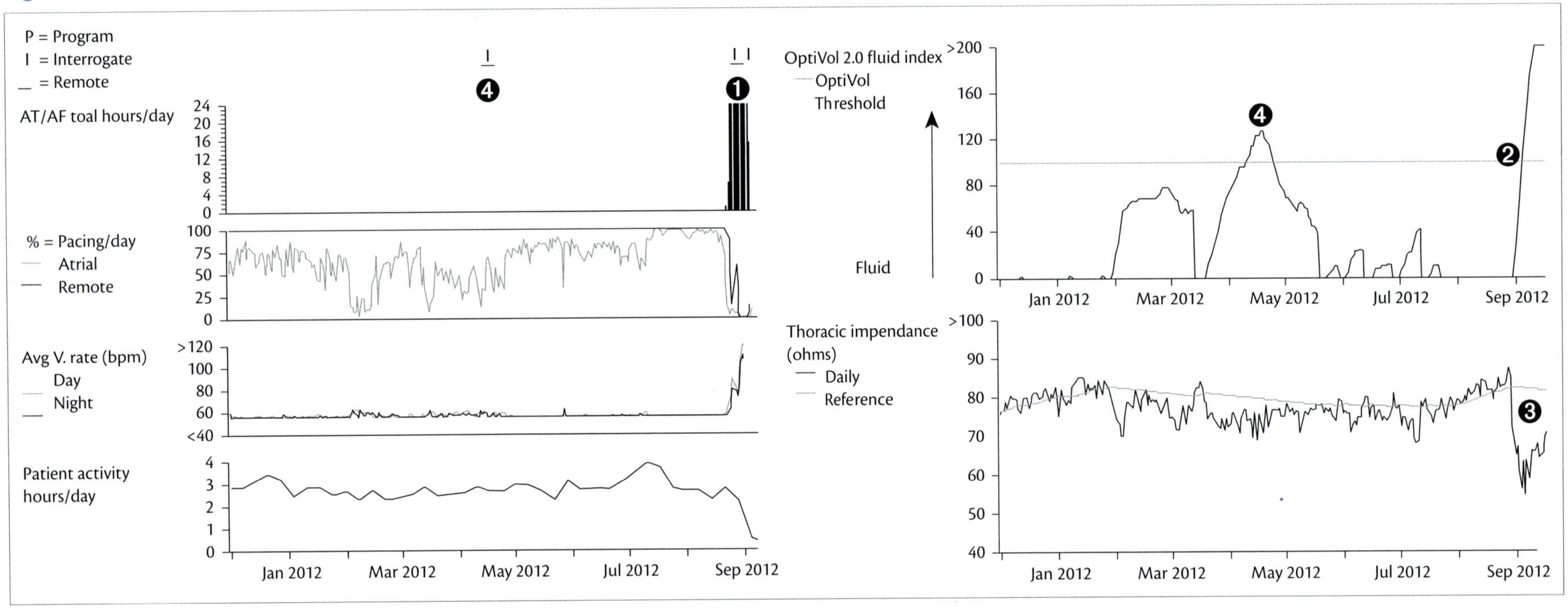

Figure 56.2 Annotated data from device interrogation after hospital admission

This example (Figure 56.2) shows device parameters that may be analysed to help manage heart failure patients.

❶ Onset of AF is accompanied by a fall in CRT delivery, increase in heart rates, and a reduction in daily patient activity.

❷ The lung fluid indicator (Optivol index of Medtronic) crossed the predefined threshold of 100 ohm.days. The threshold had been increased previously from the default value of 60 ohm.days, due to 'false positive' alerts.

❸ The Optivol threshold crossing is due to the accumulation of differences between daily transthoracic impedances and the moving average values.

❹ An Optivol 'false positive' alert had previously been triggered but had not been accompanied by changes in other risk indicators (AF, heart rate, daily activity, etc.).

Comments

Integrated heart failure diagnostic tools

Current CRT devices record a wealth of information that may be used to help manage heart failure patients. These parameters may be used to risk-stratify patients and are particularly useful in the setting of remote device and patient management, as they allow the device specialist to get a better picture of the patient being followed remotely. Parameters that may be used for remote heart failure management in device patients include: body weight, blood pressure, heart rate, heart rate variability, respiratory rate, daily activity, atrial and ventricular arrhythmias, percentage of ventricular pacing and lung fluid overload. Combining these parameters is of interest,[1] as this strategy allows to increase the specificity of risk stratification and to reduce 'false positive' lung fluid alerts (which are probably subclinical events).

Reference

1. Whellan DJ, Ousdigian KT, Al-Khatib SM, *et al.* Combined heart failure device diagnostics identify patients at higher risk of subsequent heart failure hospitalizations: results from PARTNERS HF (Program to Access and Review Trending Information and Evaluate Correlation to Symptoms in Patients With Heart Failure) study. *J Am Coll Cardiol* 2010; **55**: 1803–10.

CASE 57

Introduction to the case

Remote device management was performed in a patient implanted with a CRT-D. The device counters showed 100% atrial sensing and biventricular pacing. A periodic real-time EGM was transmitted and is shown in Figure 57.1.

Question

Figure 57.1 Periodic real-time EGM obtained by remote transmission

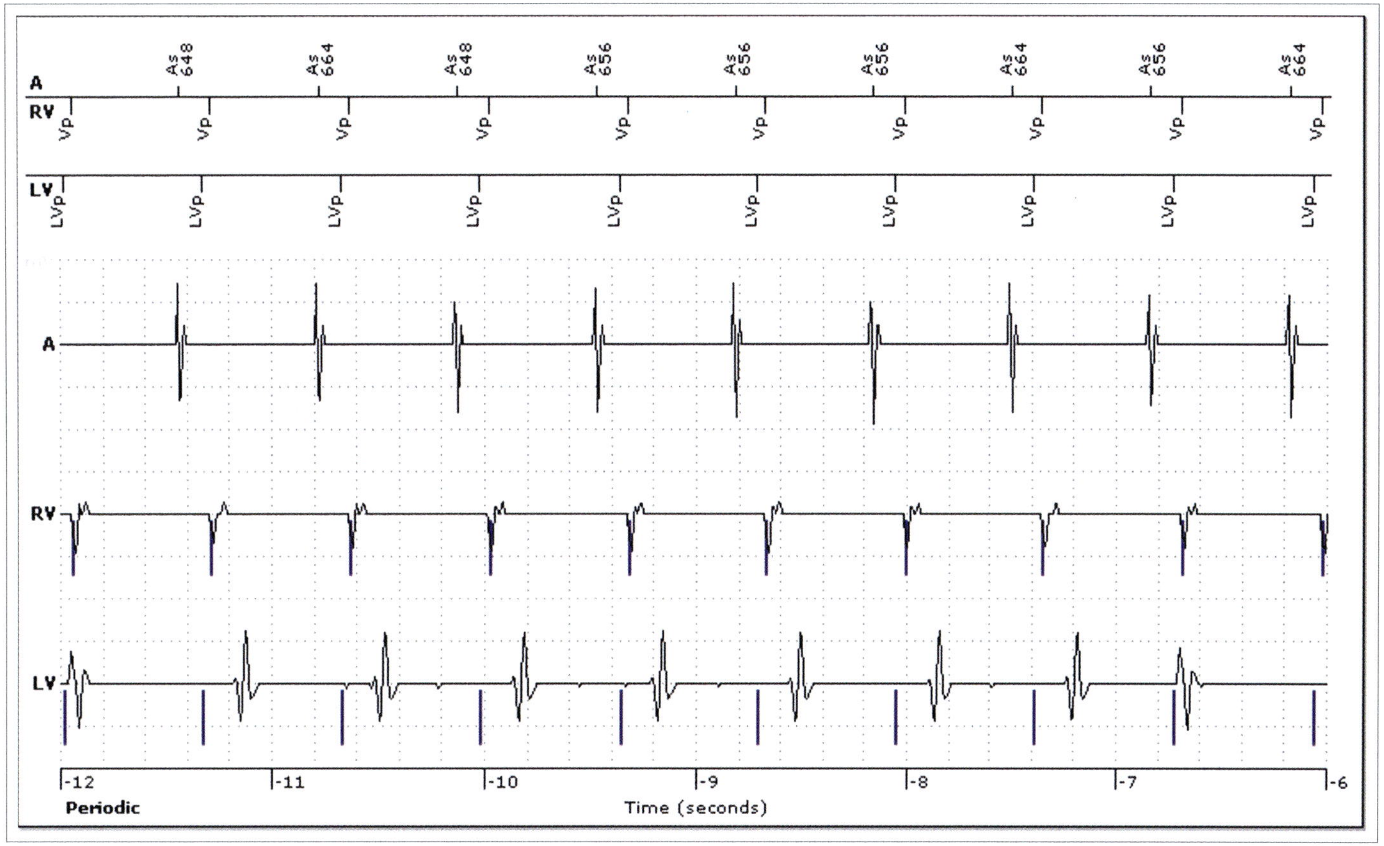

Courtesy of Mr T Bruggemann

What can be observed?

A Loss of RV pacing

B Loss of LV capture

C AV delay programmed too long

D Ventricular safety pacing

Answer

B Loss of LV capture

Figure 57.2 Annotated periodic real-time EGM obtained by remote transmission

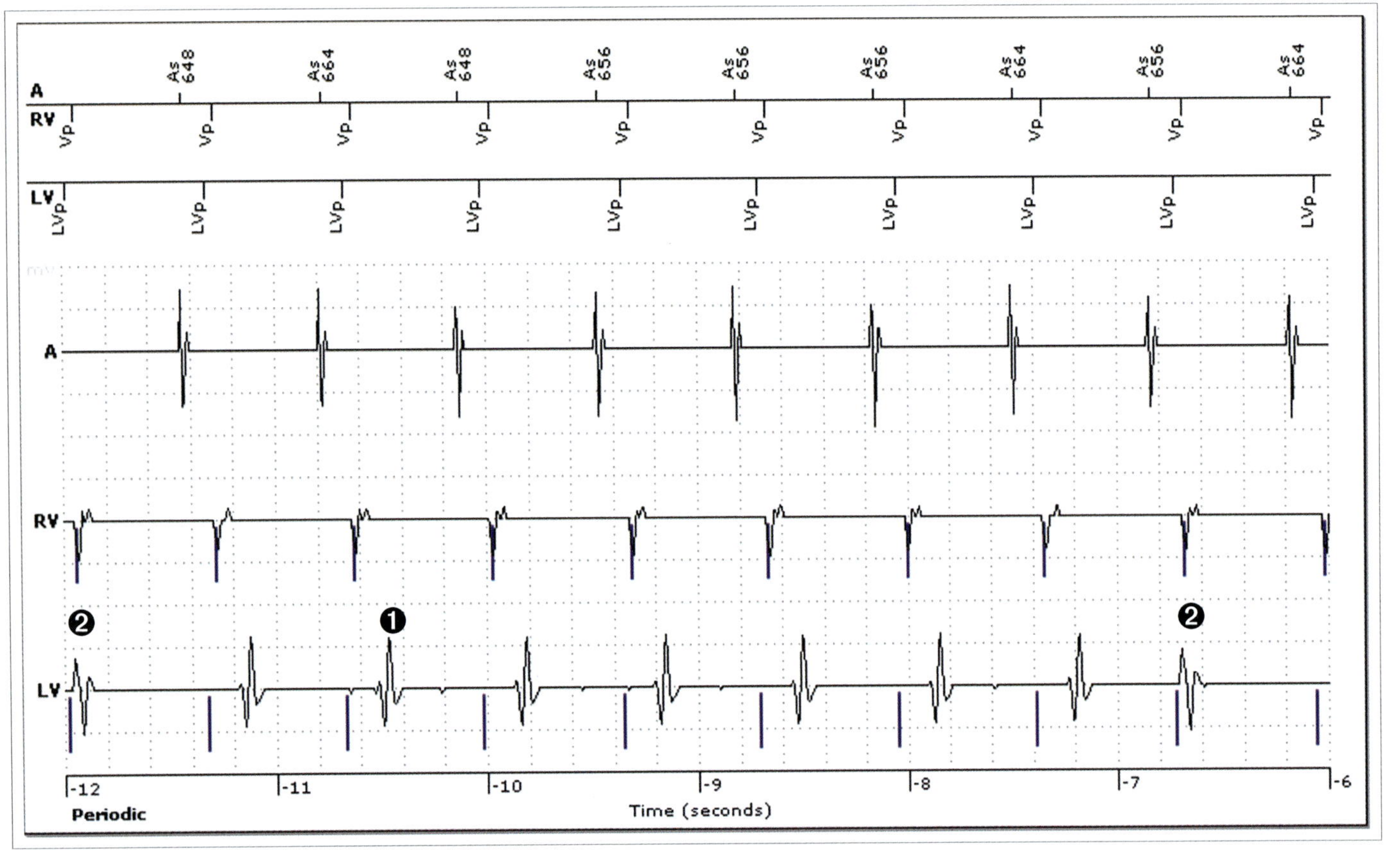

Courtesy of Mr T Bruggemann

❶ The LV EGM shows the absence of LV capture (Figure 57.2). There is a delay between pacing (indicated by the blue line) and the ventricular potential in this channel. This delay corresponds to the interval between the RV capture (that can be seen in the RV channel) and interventricular conduction. The LV events are not sensed, due to the interventricular refractory period.

❷ These two cycles show evidence of LV capture (the ventricular potential is seen directly after the spike, with a different morphology, compared to the other cycles without LV capture).

Comments

Loss of left ventricular capture

Loss of LV capture occurs in approximately 10% of patients with CRT, due to a rise in LV threshold, lead dislodgement, or lead failure.[1] This will result in RV capture only, which may be detrimental in patients with impaired LV function (and may be worse than no pacing at all).

Capture thresholds are often higher for the LV than in the RV, possibly due to less intimate contact of the lead with the myocardium. Day-to-day fluctuations of the LV threshold are also higher, particularly in patients who have a high LV threshold.[2] A sufficient safety margin must therefore be programmed, in order to ensure consistent LV capture. This may, however, compromise battery longevity or may lead to phrenic nerve capture. Automatic LV threshold algorithms are particularly useful, as they may allow reducing the pacing output.

References

1. Knight BP, Desai A, Coman J, Faddis M, Yong P. Long-term retention of cardiac resynchronization therapy. *J Am Coll Cardiol* 2004; **44**: 72–7.
2. Burri H, Gerritse B, Davenport L, Demas M, Sticherling C. Fluctuation of left ventricular thresholds and required safety margin for left ventricular pacing with cardiac resynchronization therapy. *Europace* 2009; **11**: 931–6.

CASE 58

Introduction to the case

A patient, who had been implanted 2 months ago with a CRT-D, was admitted for decompensated heart failure. A rhythm strip of the limb leads was recorded and is shown in Figure 58.1.

Question

Figure 58.1 ECG strip

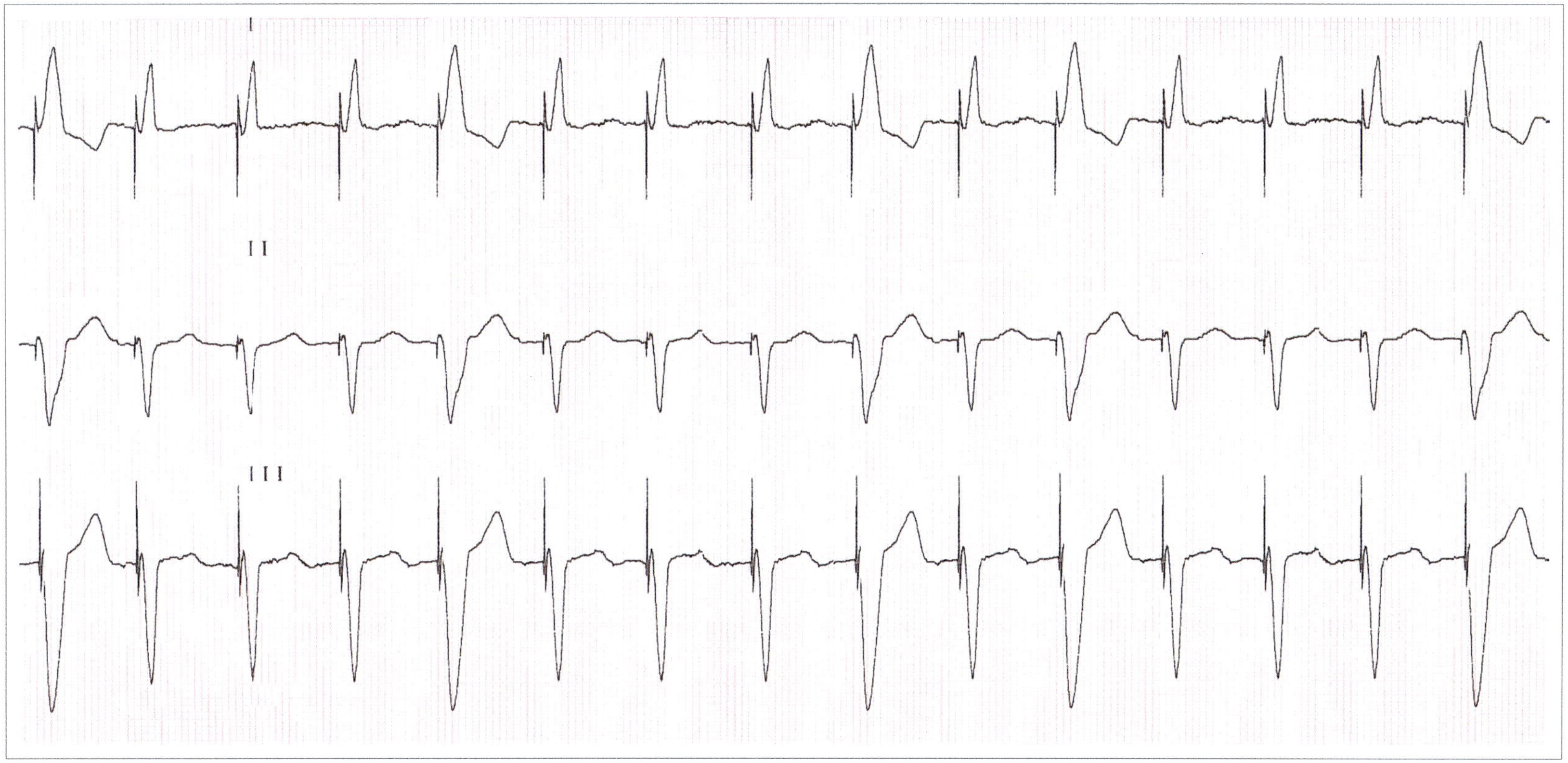

What is your diagnosis?

A Intermittent loss of RV capture

B Intermittent loss of LV capture

C Intermittent RV non-pacing

D Intermittent LV non-pacing

Answer

B Intermittent loss of LV capture

Figure 58.2 Annotated ECG strip

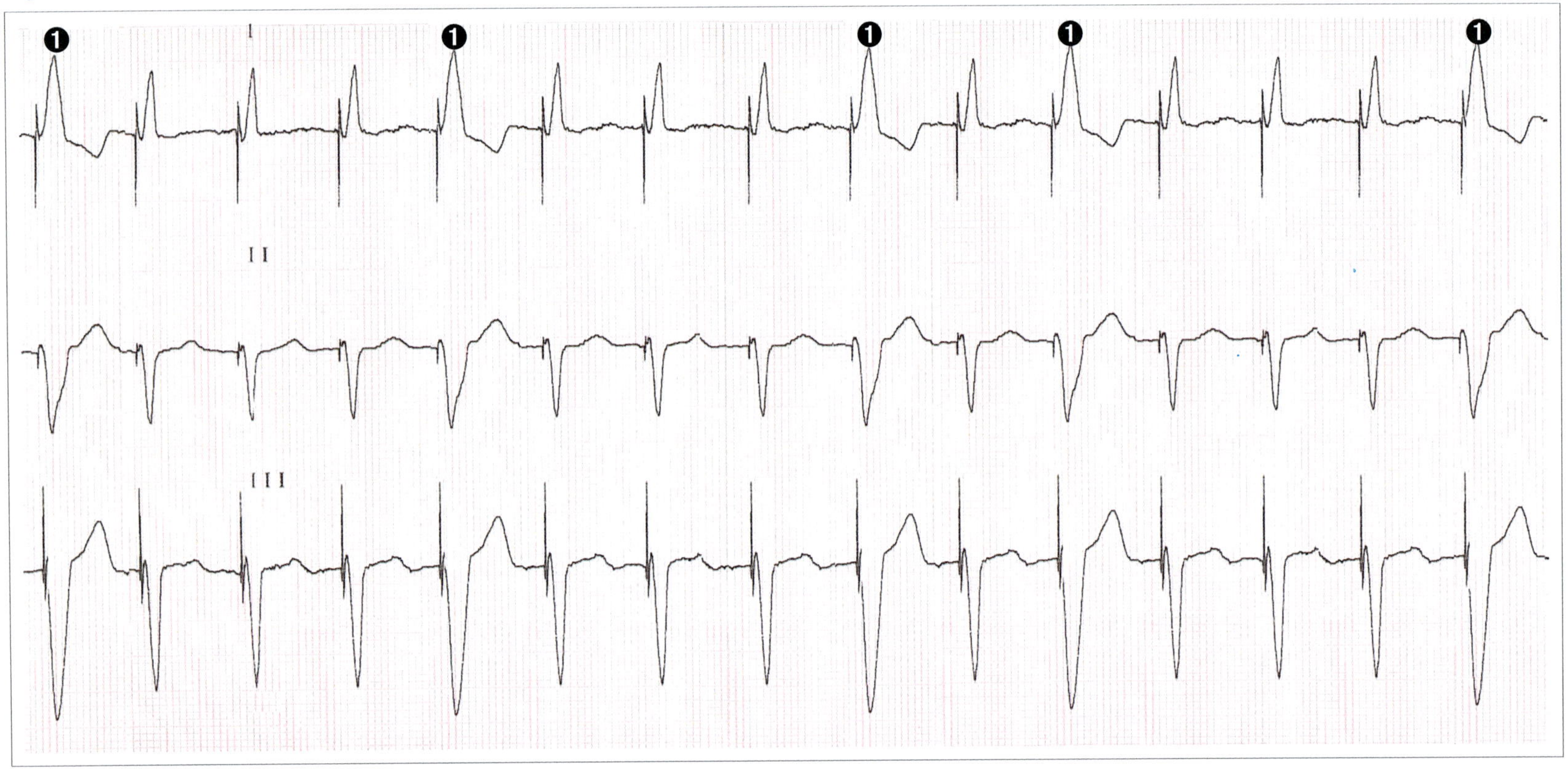

The ECG (Figure 58.2) shows two paced QRS morphologies.

❶ A wider QRS implies univentricular capture. The fact that this QRS complex is more positive in lead I than during biventricular capture implies that this is RV capture only (i.e. the right-to-left electrical forces are more dominant).

The pacing artefacts are of high amplitude in all the cycles, implying that LV pacing (which was programmed to an extended bipolar LV tip–RV coil configuration) was delivered each time. In this case, the pacing artefacts are not reconstructed by the electrocardiograph (this feature is available on some models to assist interpretation); otherwise, they would have been of identical amplitude in all ECG channels (and are smaller in lead II, due to this lead being perpendicular to the pacing vector).

Intermittent non-pacing due to interventricular crosstalk is rare, because of VRPs or because the LV channel is not used for sensing in most devices. Intermittent RV non-pacing is not compatible with the ECG changes (Figure 58.3). Intermittent LV non-pacing would have been accompanied by a change in the pacing spike amplitude.

Comments

Identifying intermittent loss of ventricular capture of cardiac resynchronization therapy by the surface electrocardiogram

The surface ECG may be useful to identify intermittent loss of RV or LV capture (due to an increase in LV threshold in this patient). Frontal QRS axes during different ventricular pacing configurations are shown in Figure 58.3 (data shown as mean ± 95th confidence interval). A simple algorithm has been described[1] (Figure 58.3) which evaluates the QRS width (a narrower QRS indicating biventricular capture), with increasing negativity (which is synonymous with decreasing positivity) in lead I indicating increasing contribution of LV capture.

Another useful lead is V1, which shows increasing positivity of the QRS complex with greater participation of LV capture (Figure 58.3). This holds true for an LV lead implanted in a (postero-) lateral position; however, the QRS complex will be negative in lead V1 in the case of an anterior LV lead.[1]

Figure 58.3 ECG changes with different pacing configurations of CRT

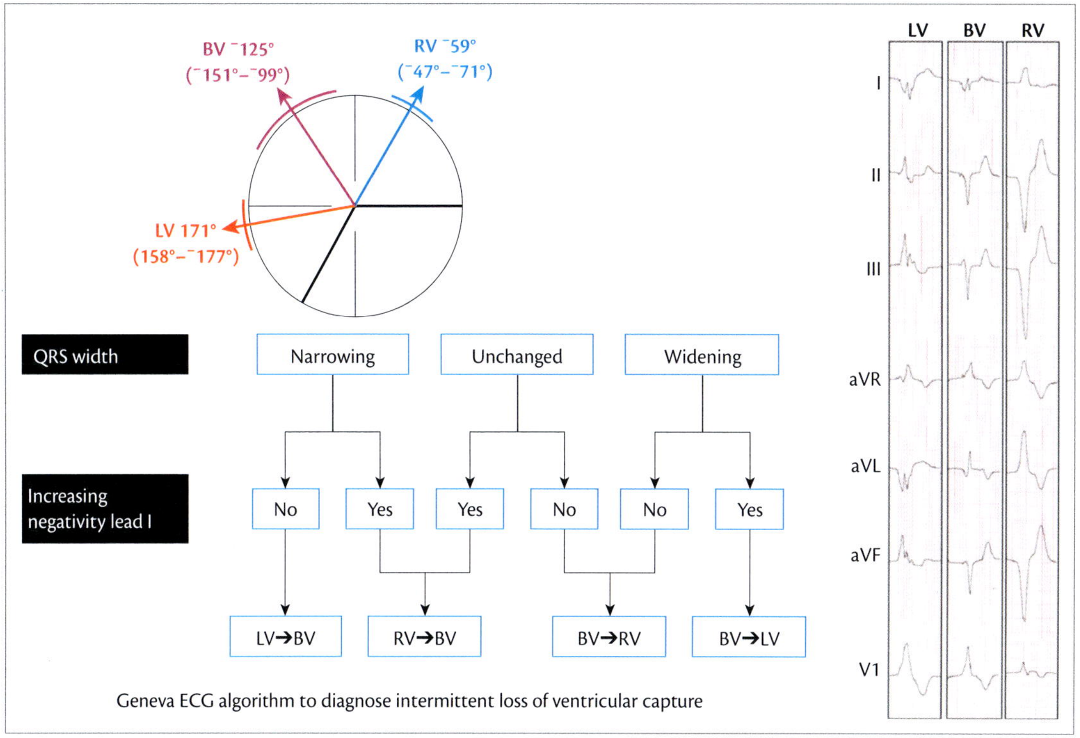

Reproduced with permission from Ganière *et al. Europace* 2013.[1]

Reference

1. Ganière V, Domenichini G, Niculescu V, Cassagneau R, Defaye P, Burri H. A new electrocardiogram algorithm for diagnosing loss of ventricular capture during cardiac resynchronisation therapy. *Europace* 2013; **15**: 376–81.

Introduction to the case

A patient, implanted with a biventricular pacemaker, was seen at follow-up. She complained of breathlessness. The device settings are shown in Table 59.1, and a rhythm strip with biventricular pacing temporarily inactivated on the right of Figure 59.1.

Table 59.1 Device settings

Pacing mode	DDD
Lower rate	50bpm
Upper rate	140bpm
AV delay (paced/sensed)	120ms/60ms
VV delay	20ms (LV first)
Atrial output	2.5V@0.4ms
RV output (bipolar)	2.5V@0.4ms
LV output (extended bipolar)	2.5V@0.4ms
Atrial sensitivity (bipolar)	0.3mV
RV sensitivity (bipolar)	2.0mV

Question

Figure 59.1 Rhythm strip with biventricular pacing, and temporary inactivation of pacing (last three cycles)

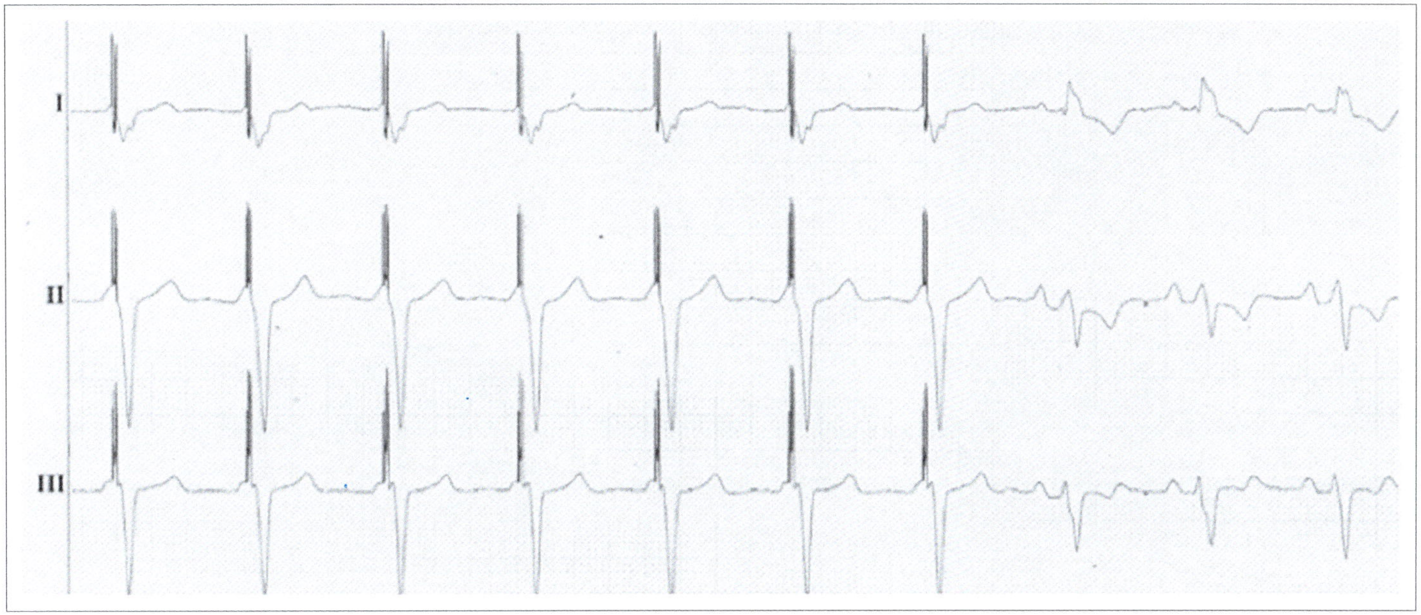

Which of the following statements is most likely to be true?

A The LV pacing ouput needs to be increased

B The VV delay needs to be decreased

C The atrial sensitivity needs to be increased

D The AV delay needs to be increased

Answer

D The AV delay need to be increased

Figure 59.2 Annotation of rhythm strip with biventricular pacing, and temporary inactivation of pacing (last three cycles)

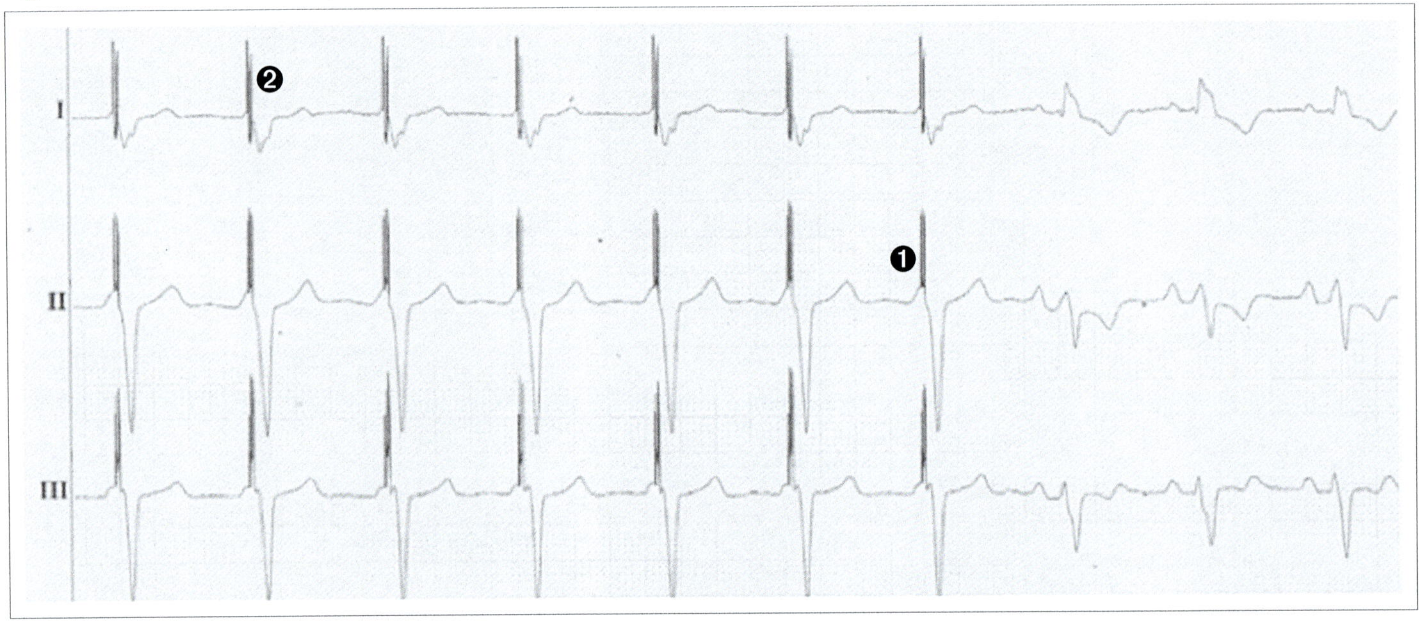

This example (Figure 59.2) shows how the surface ECG may indicate inadequate programming of the AV delay.

❶ The ventricular spikes fall on the peak of the P-waves, implying that the AV delay is likely to be programmed too short.

❷ The paced QRS complex is negative in lead I and narrower than in intrinsic rhythm, indicating biventricular capture. There is therefore no need to increase the ventricular output.

Comments

Recognizing a suboptimal atrioventricular delay using the surface electrocardiogram (1)

It is important that the AV delay is programmed adequately, as, if it is too short, ventricular filling may be compromised, and, if it is too long, ventricular pseudofusion may occur. A previous study has shown that ventricular pacing should occur at approximately 40ms after the end of the intrinsic P-wave.[1]

Another point that can be discussed in this case is that a negative paced QRS in lead I implies LV capture.[2] One should nevertheless be cautious regarding this observation, as a negative QRS in this lead may also be observed with RV capture only.[3,4,5]

References

1. Jones RC, Svinarich T, Rubin A, *et al.* Optimal atrioventricular delay in CRT patients can be approximated using surface electrocardiography and device electrograms. *J Cardiovasc Electrophysiol* 2010: **21**: 1226–32.
2. Ammann P, Sticherling C, Kalusche D, *et al.* An electrocardiogram-based algorithm to detect loss of left ventricular capture during cardiac resynchronization therapy. *Ann Intern Med* 2005; **142**: 968–73.
3. Burri H, Park C, Zimmermann M, *et al.* Utility of the surface electrocardiogram for confirming right ventricular septal pacing: validation using electroanatomical mapping. *Europace* 2011; **13**: 82–6.
4. Balt JC, van Hemel NM, Wellens HJ, de Voogt WG.Radiological and electrocardiographic characterization of right ventricular outflow tract pacing. *Europace* 2010; **12**: 1739–44.
5. Ganière V, Domenichini G, Niculescu V, *et al.* A new electrocardiogram algorithm for diagnosing loss of ventricular capture during cardiac resynchronisation therapy. *Europace* 2013; **15**: 376–81.

Introduction to the case

A patient was seen at 1-month follow-up after CRT implantation, complaining of worsening of dyspnoea since the procedure. Device follow-up showed normal thresholds. The device settings are shown in Table 60.1. Because there were no clues from the device interrogation as to the reason for worsening of the patient's symptoms, a transthoracic echocardiogram was performed. The transmitral pulsed-wave Doppler flow is shown on Figure 60.1.

Table 60.1 Device settings

Pacing mode	DDDR
Lower rate	60bpm
Upper rate	140bpm
AV delay (paced/sensed)	140/100ms
Atrial output	2.5V@0.4ms
RV output (bipolar)	2.5V@0.4ms
LV output (bipolar)	2.5V@0.4ms
Atrial sensitivity (bipolar)	0.3mV
RV sensitivity (bipolar)	0.4mV
LV sensitivity (bipolar)	2.5mV

Question

Figure 60.1 Pulsed-wave Doppler of transmitral flow

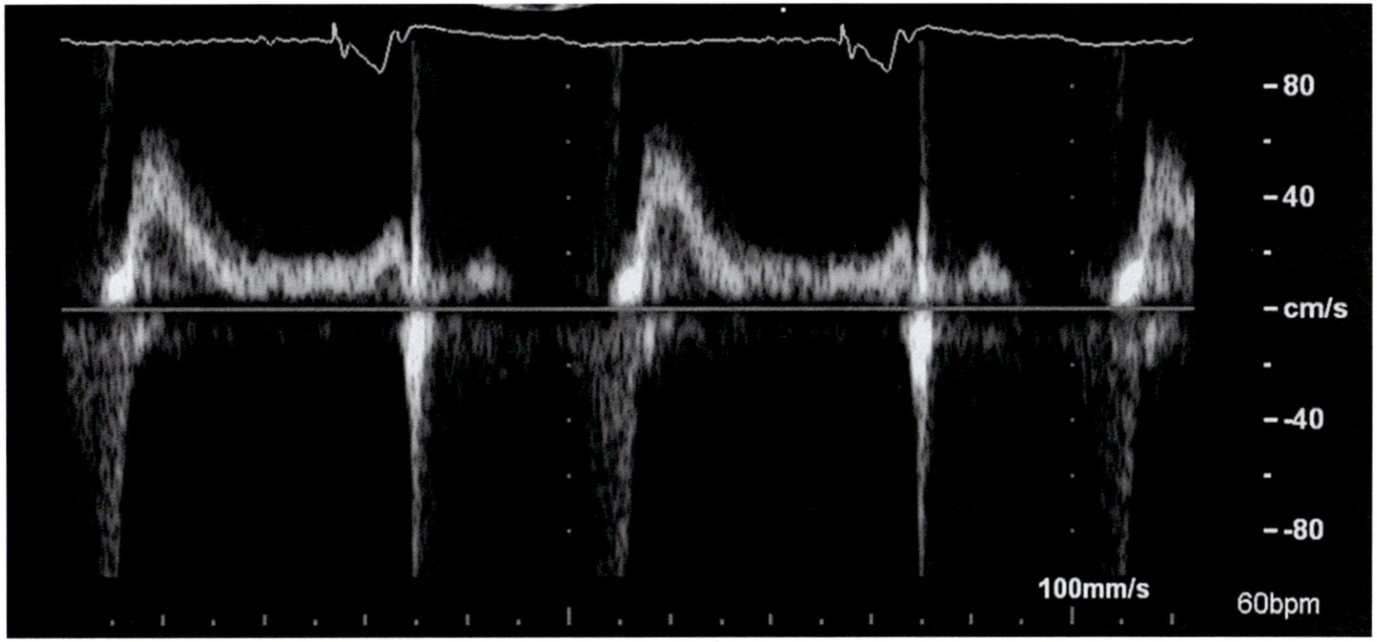

Based upon the transmitral Doppler flow, what should be done?

A Increase the AVI

B Decrease the AVI

C Increase the VV interval

D Decrease the VV interval

Answer

A Increase the AVI

Figure 60.2 Annotated pulsed-wave Doppler of transmitral flow

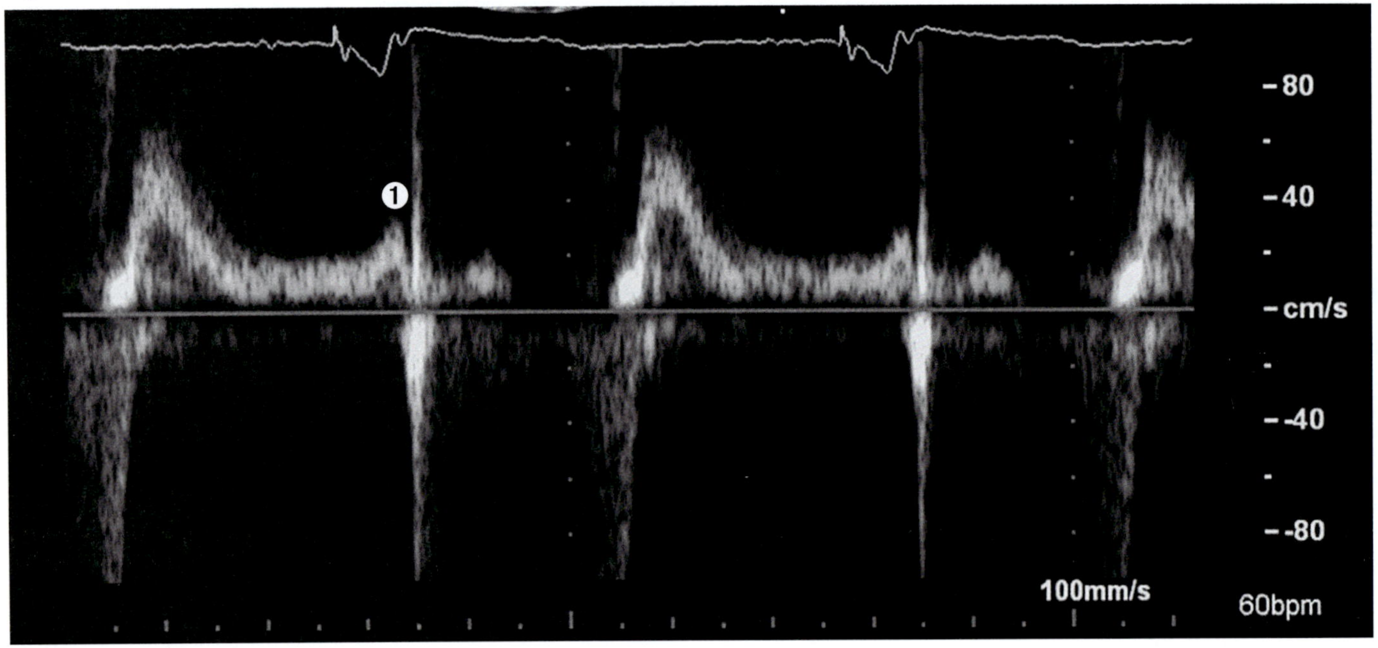

The transmitral flow was recorded during AV pacing at the out-of-the box AVI of 140ms (Figure 60.2).

❶ The A-wave is of low amplitude and seems truncated, and ventricular pacing occurs much earlier than the A-wave. This suggests that the AVI needs to be lengthened. The transmitral flow does not give any information on whether the VV interval needs to be adjusted.

Comments

Optimizing atrioventricular delays using echocardiography

There are a number of different techniques for AV optimization by echocardiography,[1] the simplest, and probably most robust one being the iterative method. The transmitral flow during AAI pacing is shown in Figure 60.3a; a large A-wave can be seen that contributes to about a third of ventricular filling. The patient's intrinsic AP–VS delay was measured at 340ms, so the AVI was programmed to 300ms and decremented by 20ms steps, with recording the transmitral flow at each step until A-wave truncation was apparent at a programmed AV delay of 240ms (Figure 60.3b). The AVI was finally programmed at 260ms (Figure 60.3c), which avoided A-wave truncation, while still resulting in biventricular capture (note that the ECG on the rhythm strip is different compared to that with AAI pacing) and was later confirmed by recording a 12-lead ECG.

The patient improved remarkably thereafter.

As it is impractical to perform AV optimization routinely, it may be useful to perform screening of the transmitral flow after device implantation and to limit optimization to those patients who have evidence of A-wave truncation.[2,3]

References

1. Burri H, Sunthorn H, Shah D, Lerch R. Optimization of device programming for cardiac resynchronization therapy. *Pacing Clin Electrophysiol* 2006; **29**: 1416–25.
2. Gorcsan J 3rd, Abraham T, Agler DA, *et al*. Echocardiography for cardiac resynchronization therapy: recommendations for performance and reporting—a report from the American Society of Echocardiography Dyssynchrony Writing Group endorsed by the Heart Rhythm Society. *J Am Soc Echocardiogr* 2008; **21**: 191–213.
3. Daubert J-C., Saxon L, Adamson PB, *et al*. 2012 EHRA/HRS expert consensus statement on cardiac resynchronization therapy in heart failure: implant and follow-up recommendations and management. *Europace* 2012; **14**: 1236–86.

Figure 60.3 Transmitral pulsed-wave Doppler during different settings

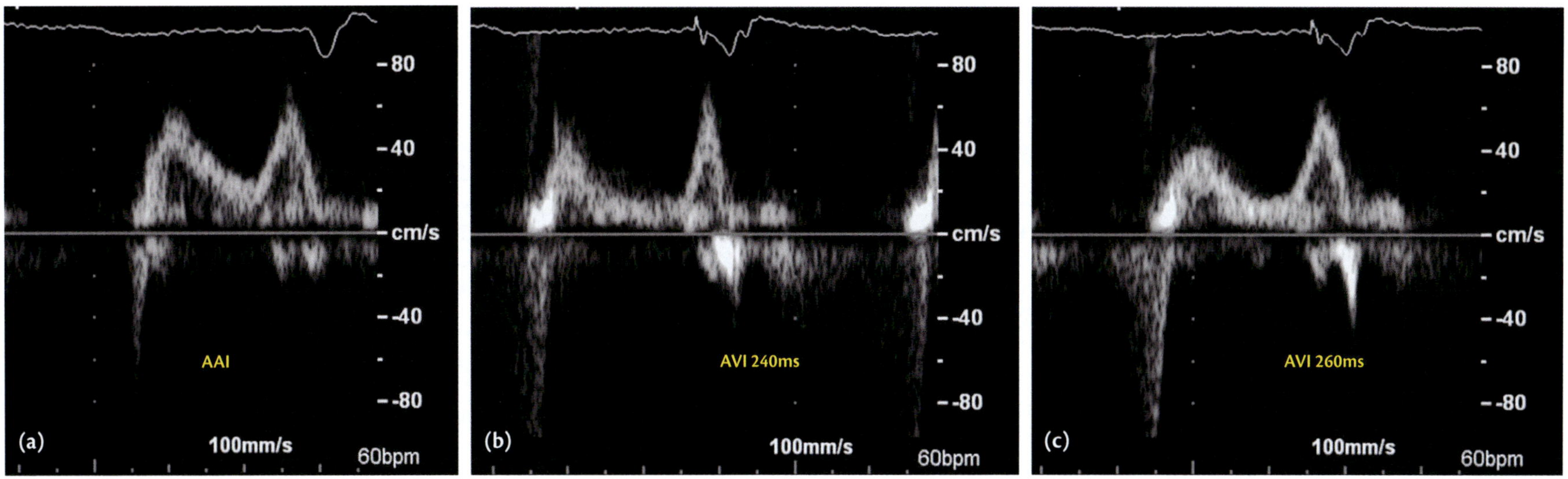

Introduction to the case

A patient implanted with a CRT-D was followed up at the device clinic, complaining of breathlessness. The device counters revealed 19% AP and 83% RV/LV pacing. The rate histograms are shown in Figure 61.1. The surface ECG during biventricular pacing and temporary inactivation of pacing is shown on Figure 61.2.

Figure 61.1 Rate histograms

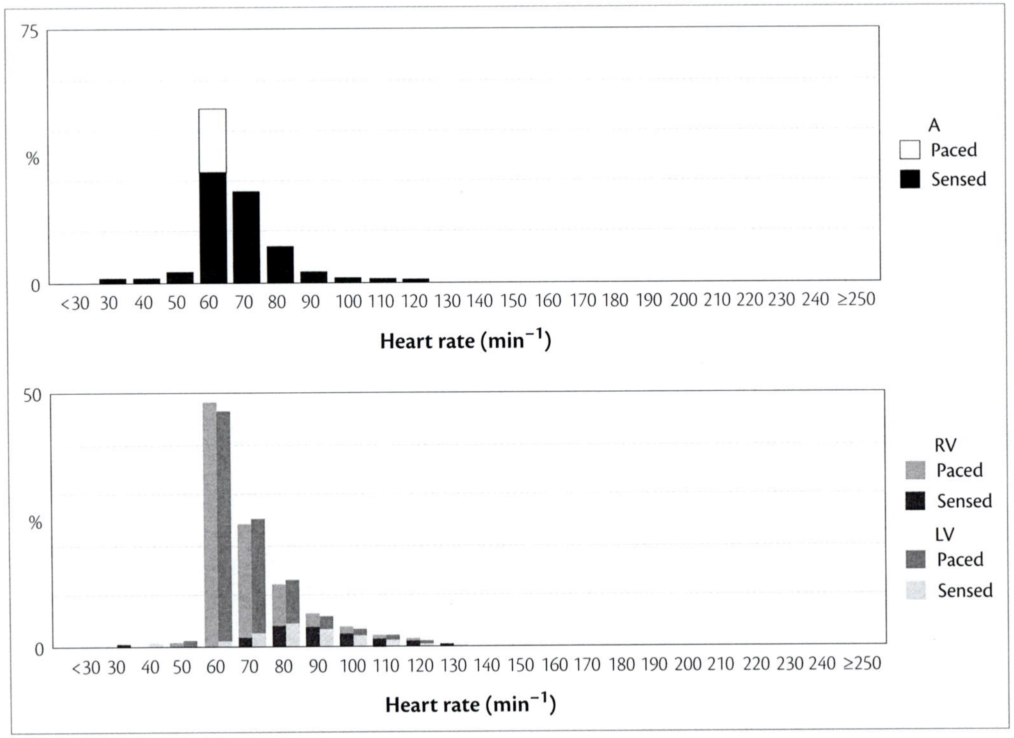

Question

Figure 61.2 ECG recorded during biventricular pacing (left) and after temporary inactivation of pacing (arrow)

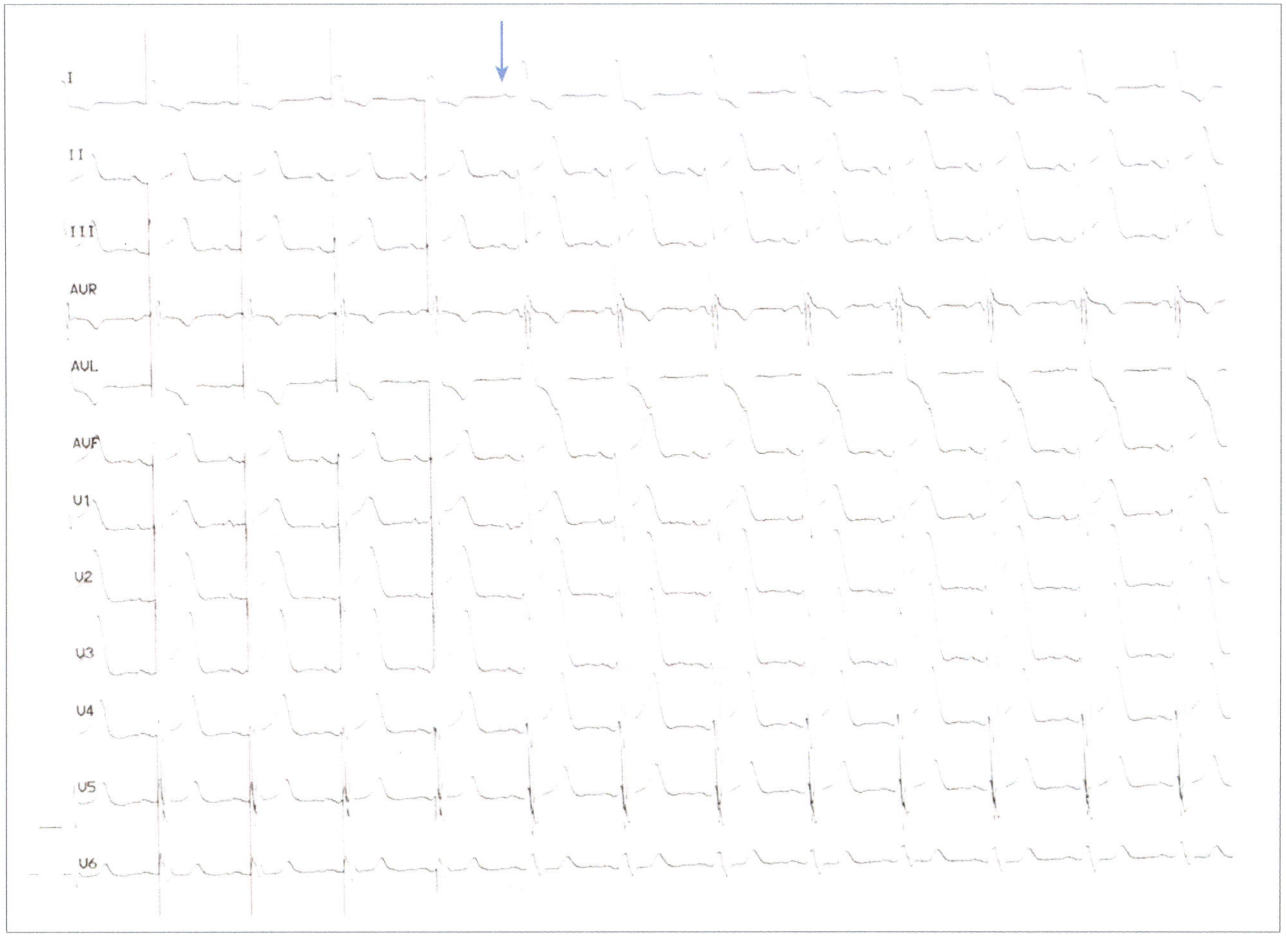

Based upon the information provided, what do you think should be modified in the device settings?

A Decrease the programmed AVI

B Increase the programmed AVI

C Increase the RV output

D Increase the LV output

Answer

A **Decrease the programmed AVI**

Figure 61.3 Annotated ECG recorded during biventricular pacing (left) and after temporary inactivation of pacing (arrow)

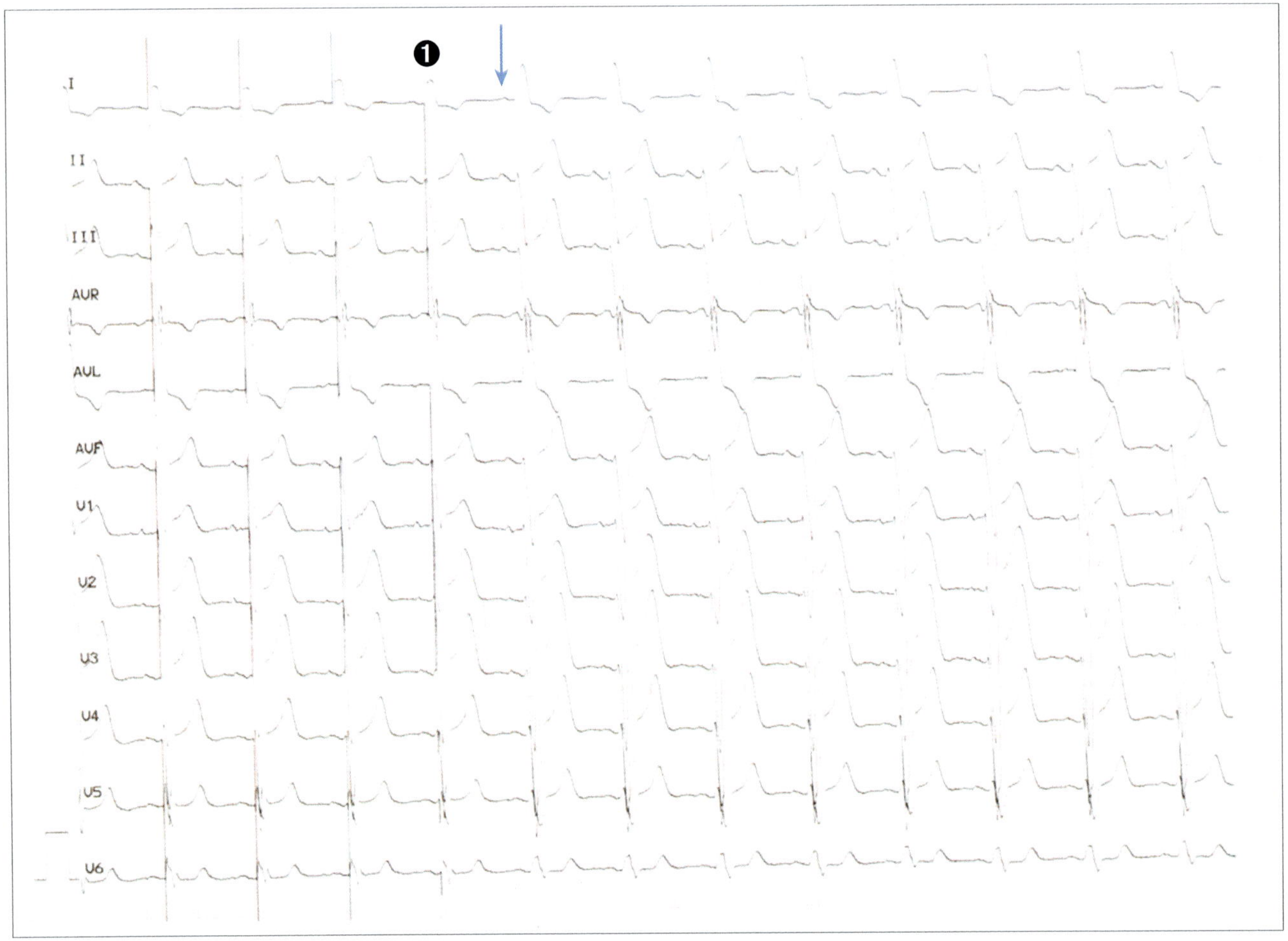

❶ The paced QRS complexes are only slightly different in morphology, compared to those in intrinsic rhythm. This indicates that there is fusion, but with little contribution of biventricular capture. The slight narrowing of the QRS complex during pacing, compared to intrinsic rhythm (that shows left bundle branch block), implies that there is LV capture (there is therefore no need to increase the LV output) (Figure 61.3).

Comments

Recognizing a suboptimal atrioventricular interval using the surface electrocardiogram (2)

This example illustrates how the surface ECG may be used to evaluate pseudofusion or fusion with little contribution of ventricular capture. The AVI was shortened from 140ms to 100ms under echocardiographic guidance, using the iterative method, which yielded a narrower QRS with a greater degree of contribution of biventricular capture to the fused QRS complex (Figure 61.4).

An alternative to shortening the AV delay would have been to programme rate-adaptive AVIs, as the rate histogram showed that intrinsic AV conduction occurred more frequently at higher heart rates (Figure 61.1). The rate adaptation of AVIs varies, however, between different device manufacturers, and a potential risk is truncation of the A-wave in case the interval is too short at higher heart rates.

Figure 61.4 ECG with biventricular pacing after shortening of the AV delay

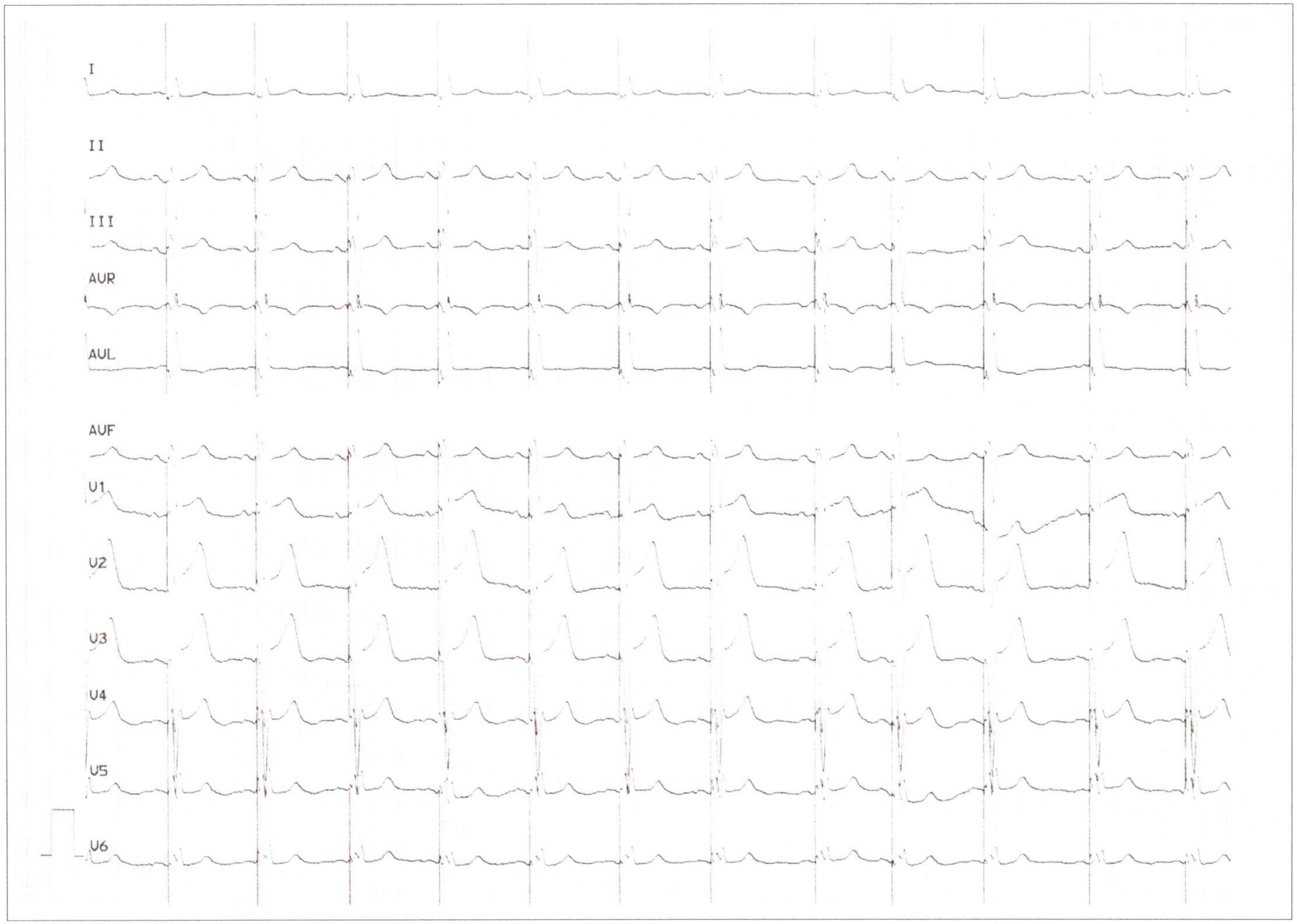

Introduction to the case

A patient implanted with a CRT-D for non-ischaemic heart disease was admitted for decompensated heart failure. A device follow-up was performed and showed normal parameters (RV threshold was 1.1 V@0.4ms, and LV capture threshold was 0.8V@0.4ms). A 12-lead ECG was recorded during simultaneous biventricular pacing (BiV0) and uni-ventricular RV and LV pacing (Figure 62.1).

Question

Figure 62.1 ECG with different pacing configurations

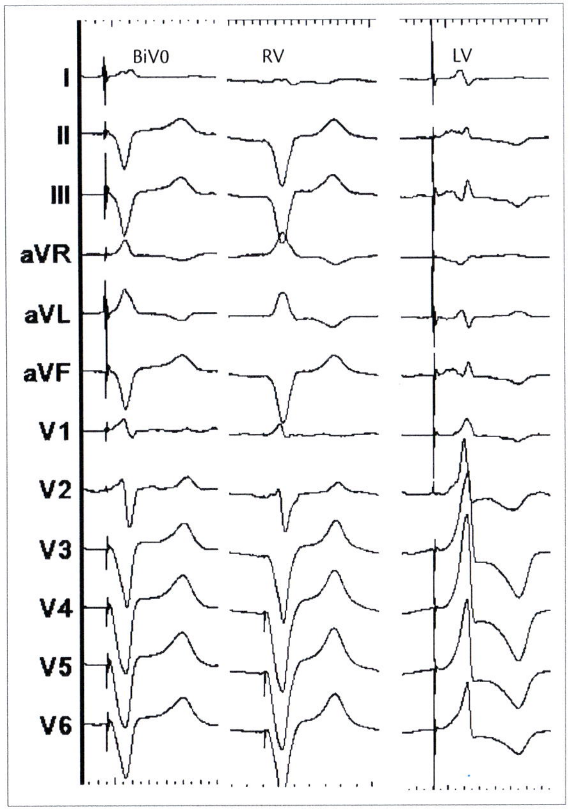

How may one explain the very similar ECG morphology between biventricular pacing and RV pacing?

A LV latency

B RV anodal capture

C LV anodal capture

D Increase in LV threshold

Answer

A LV latency

Figure 62.2 Annotated ECG with different pacing configurations

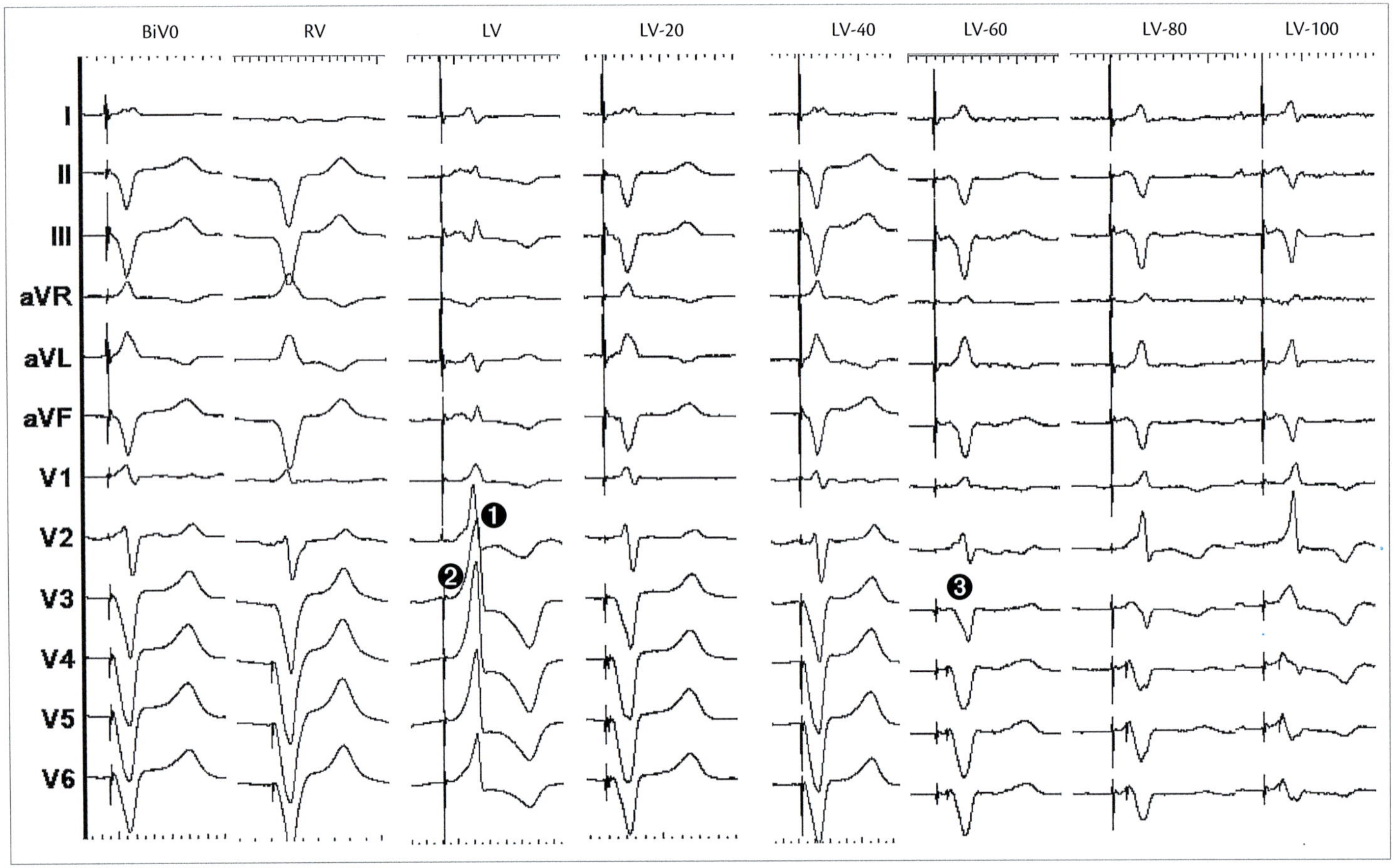

In addition to BiV0 and RV and LV pacing, different sequential biventricular pacing configurations with LV pre-excitation are shown in Figure 62.2.

❶ LV capture is evident during LV pacing alone, with a QRS morphology indicating a postero-lateral lead (positive QRS in the right precordial leads, relatively isoelectric QRS in the inferior leads).

❷ There is an isoelectric interval between the LV pacing spike and onset of the QRS complex, indicating latency.

❸ During sequential BiV pacing with increasing LV pre-excitation, increasing contribution of the LV vector is observed and is best appreciated in the precordial leads.

Comments

Left ventricular latency

A delay between the pacing spike and ventricular depolarization is known as latency and may result from myocardial ischaemia, anti-arrhythmic drugs, hyperkalaemia, and pacing at a site of scar.[1] A delay of <40ms to the rapid deflection of the QRS complex may be observed when pacing from a CS tributary, probably due to a delay of activation of the Purkinje fibres. If the LV pacing lead overlies scar tissue, an initial isoelectric interval in all 12 leads may be observed. This is an issue with CRT, as contribution of ventricular activation from the LV lead will be reduced, as in the present example, and may be corrected by programming sequential biventricular pacing with LV pre-excitation. LV latency was measured at 84ms in this patient (Figure 62.3; recorded at 100mm/s during LV pacing).

Sequential CRT with LV pre-excitation by 80ms was programmed, with remarkable improvement in the patient's symptoms thereafter.

This example illustrates the importance of systematically evaluating ECGs in patients with CRT.

Reference

1. Barold SS, Herweg B. Usefulness of the 12-lead electrocardiogram in the follow-up of patients with cardiac resynchronization devices. Part II. *Cardiol J* 2011; **18**: 610–24.

Figure 62.3 ECG (recorded at 100mm/s) during LV pacing showing evidence of latency

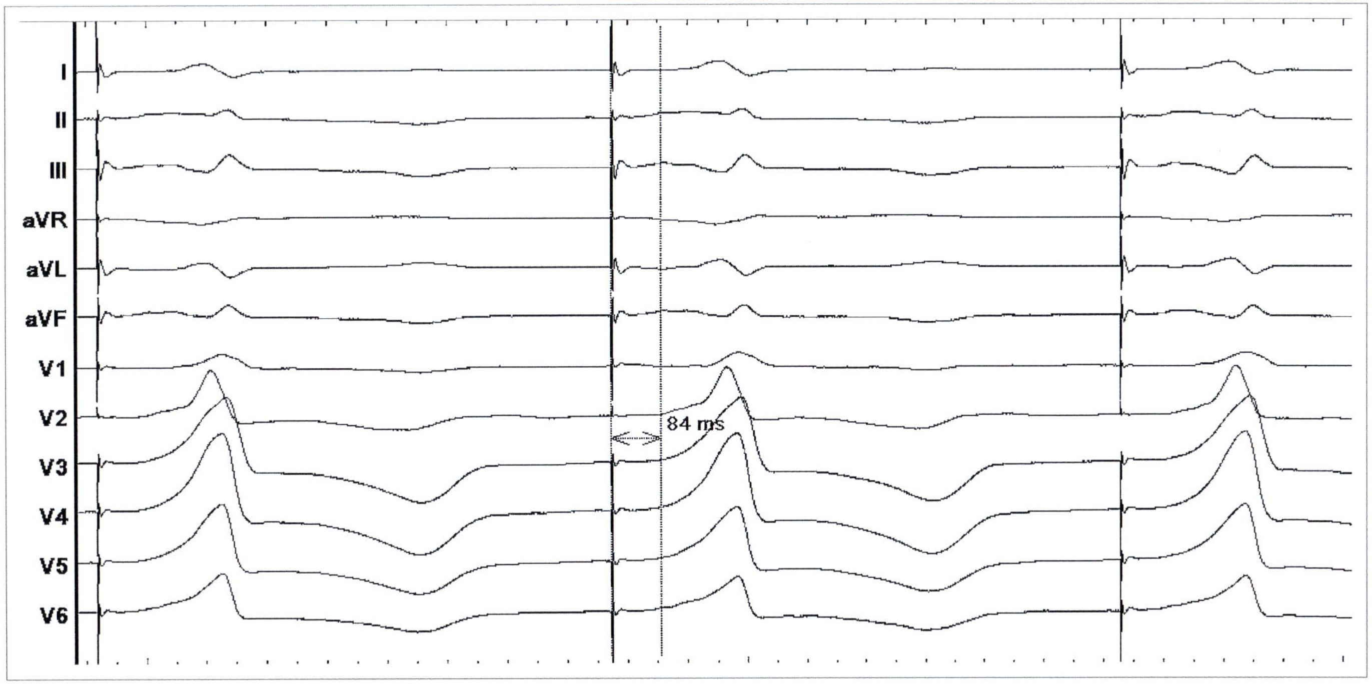

Introduction to the case

Follow-up was performed in a patient implanted with a CRT-D who was complaining of shortness of breath. A real-time EGM strip was recorded and is shown in Figure 63.1. Device settings are shown in Table 63.1.

Table 63.1 Device settings

Pacing mode	DDDR
Lower rate	60bpm
Upper rate	140bpm
AV delay—fixed (paced/sensed)	250ms/200ms
Atrial output	2.5V@0.4ms
RV output (bipolar)	2.5V@0.4ms
LV output (extended bipolar)	2.5V@0.4ms
Atrial sensitivity (bipolar)	0.3mV
RV sensitivity (dedicated bipolar)	0.4mV

Question

Figure 63.1 Real-time EGM strip recorded during follow-up

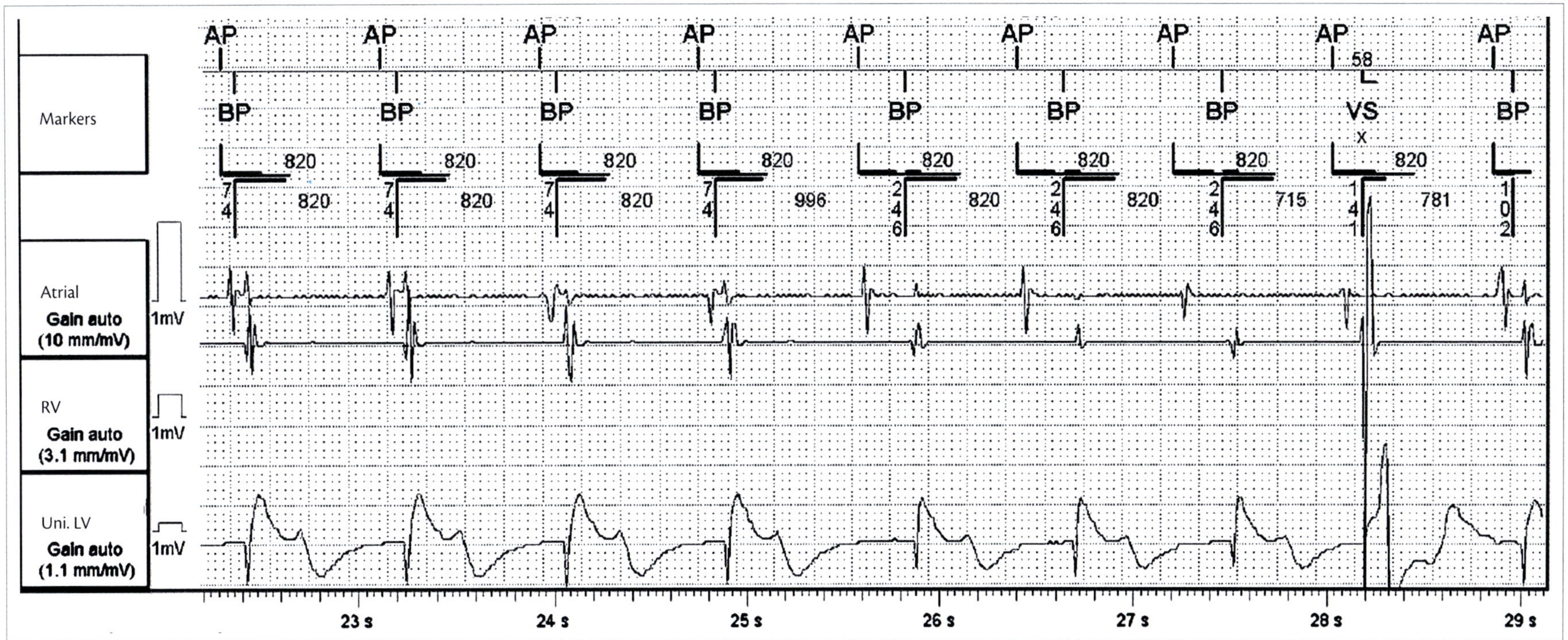

How do you explain the variable AVIs?

A Rate-adaptive AV delays

B Negative AV hysteresis

C Ventricular safety pacing

D Triggered ventricular pacing (VVT mode)

Answer

B Negative AV hysteresis

Figure 63.2 Annotated real-time EGM strip recorded during follow-up

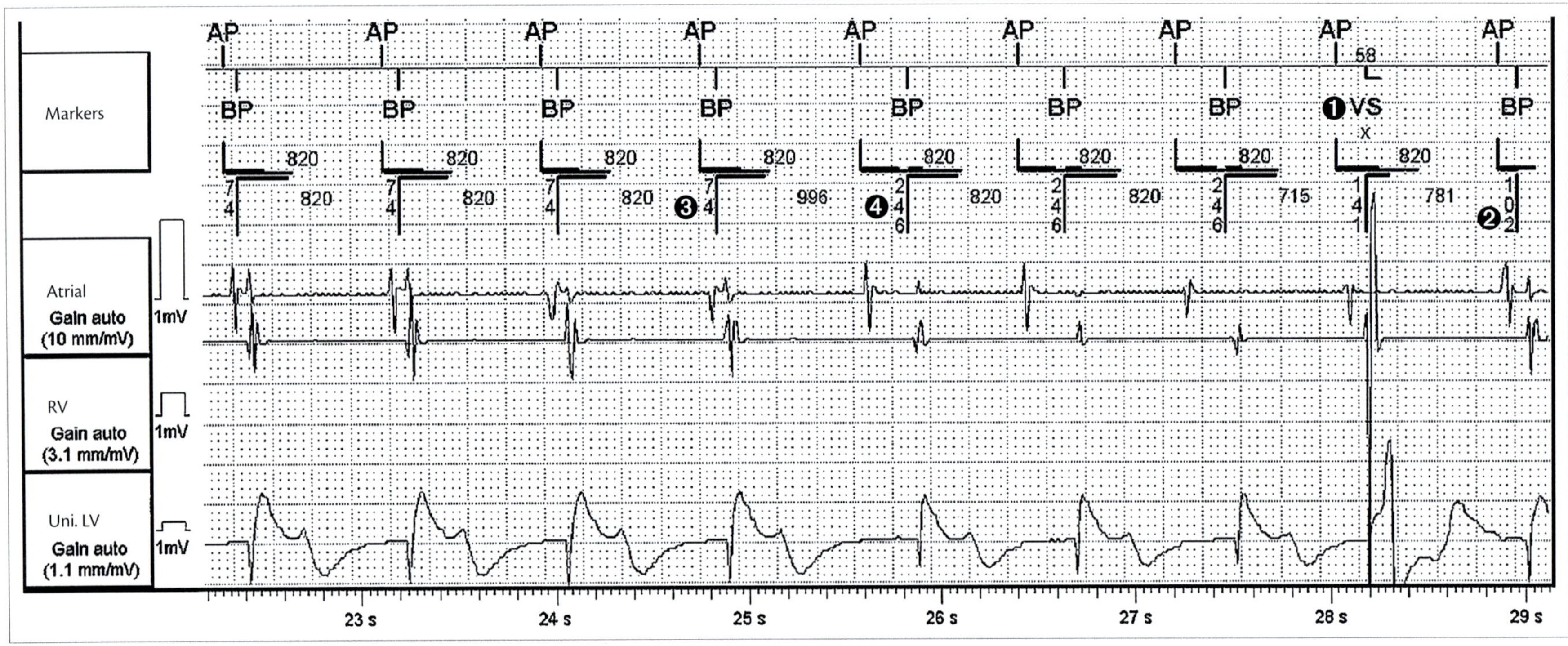

This patient had frequent VPBs, which led to variable AVIs due to the negative AV hysteresis algorithm (Figure 63.2).

❶ A VPB falls in the AVI (at 141ms after AP and after the end of the ventricular safety pacing window). Note that the morphology algorithm shows a mismatch with the stored template (labelled 'X', with 58% similarity).

❷ Negative AV hysteresis (set here at a value of –40ms) reprogrammes the AVI to 102ms.

❸ The AVI at the beginning of the tracing is only 74ms, due to a previous VPB (falling at 114ms after AP).

❹ Periodic extensions of the AVIs occur to the default value and, if VP occurs, are maintained at this value until the next Ax–VS event.

Comments

Negative atrioventricular hysteresis

This feature is designed to respond to events with intrinsic AV conduction and to maximize ventricular pacing. It was introduced initially in the era when RV pacing was believed to be useful in the setting of hypertrophic obstructive cardiomyopathy and is now mainly used in CRT devices. As AV conduction properties are variable during the 24-hour period, loss of CRT may be avoided in situations where AV conduction is facilitated (e.g. during exercise). However, as illustrated in this case, VPBs falling during the AVI may be interpreted as intrinsic conduction and unduly shorten this parameter. This may lead to reduced ventricular filling (due to A-wave truncation), with unfavourable haemodynamic consequences.

The feature was inactivated in this patient, with improvement in symptoms.

Introduction to the case

A patient implanted with a CRT-D presented for follow-up. He complained of dyspnoea and palpitations. A surface ECG was recorded and is shown in Figure 64.1.

Question

Figure 64.1 Presenting ECG recorded at follow-up

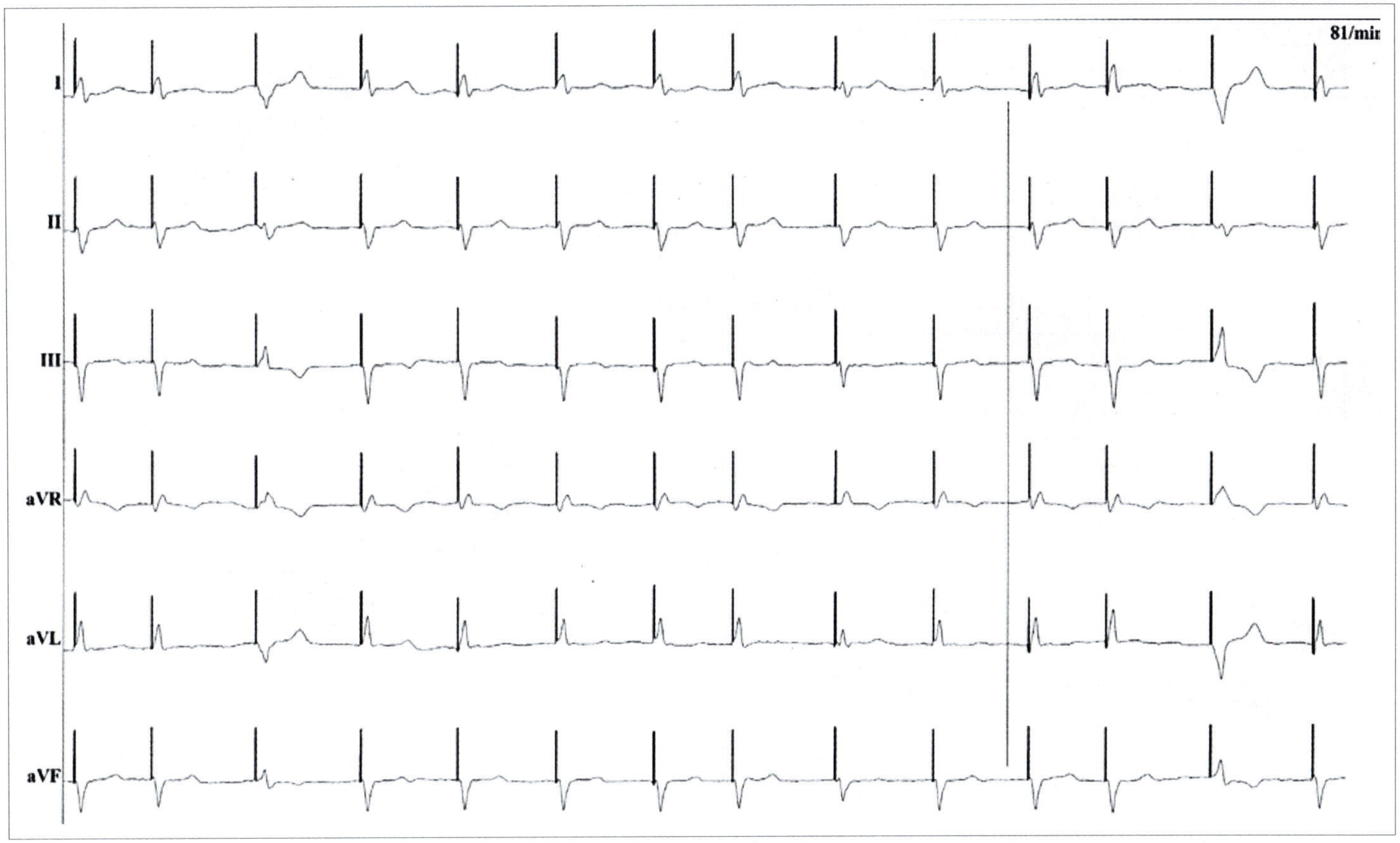

What do you observe?

A Rate-responsive pacing

B Intermittent atrial undersensing of AF

C Intermittent RV non-capture

D Triggered ventricular pacing (VVT mode)

Answer

D **Triggered ventricular pacing (VVT mode)**

Figure 64.2 Annotated presenting ECG recorded at follow-up

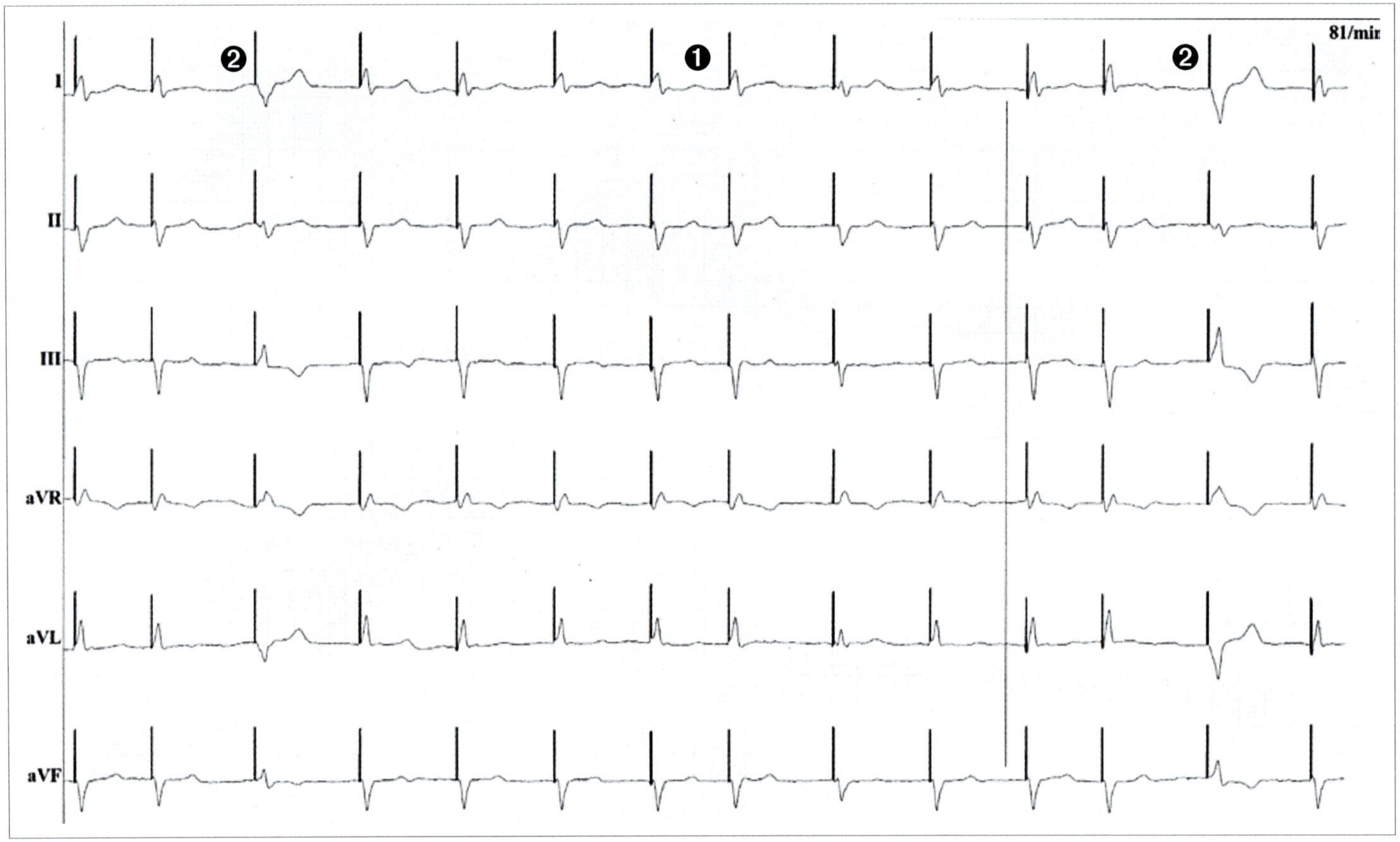

The baseline rhythm is AF with intrinsic AV conduction and irregular RR intervals; the device has a VS response algorithm that triggers LV pacing (VVT mode) as soon as an RV sensed event occurs, with a pacing spike at the beginning of each QRS complex (Figure 64.2).

❶ The narrower QRS complexes correspond to fusion between intrinsic AV conduction and triggered LV pacing.

❷ The wider QRS complexes occur at longer RR intervals and correspond to biventricular capture at the lower rate interval (and not to triggered LV pacing), explaining the greater contribution of LV capture to the QRS complex (with negativity in lead I). Note that the first of these two QRS complexes has a slight degree of fusion with intrinsic AV conduction (the QRS complex is less negative in lead I).

Ventricular pacing at an irregular rate is always due to tracking (in this case, of the ventricle). Intermittent atrial undersensing of AF may indeed also lead to an irregular paced ventricular rhythm (see Case 25) but does not explain the different QRS morphologies.

Comments

Algorithms for enhancing cardiac resynchronization therapy delivery during atrial fibrillation

Triggered LV pacing occurs during RV sensed events in AF (and, in some devices, also in sinus rhythm) as an attempt to maintain CRT, despite intrinsic AV conduction. If the patient has a left bundle branch block, with a wide QRS complex, this may indeed lead to fusion pacing, which may have some favourable haemodynamic effect. However, in patients with a narrower QRS or RBBB (in which case ventricular sensing by the RV lead is delayed with respect to the QRS onset), triggered LV pacing occurs too late to result in meaningful capture. The algorithm was inactivated temporarily and showed that there was some LV capture (the QRS complex with VVT pacing is slightly narrower, with less positivity in lead I; Figure 64.3).

The patient's symptoms were due to recent onset of AF (and not the VVT algorithm), which was subsequently cardioverted electrically.

Another algorithm featured on some devices reacts to conducted AF by increasing the baseline rate temporarily to override the intrinsic AV conduction.

Figure 64.3 Temporary inactivation of triggered ventricular pacing

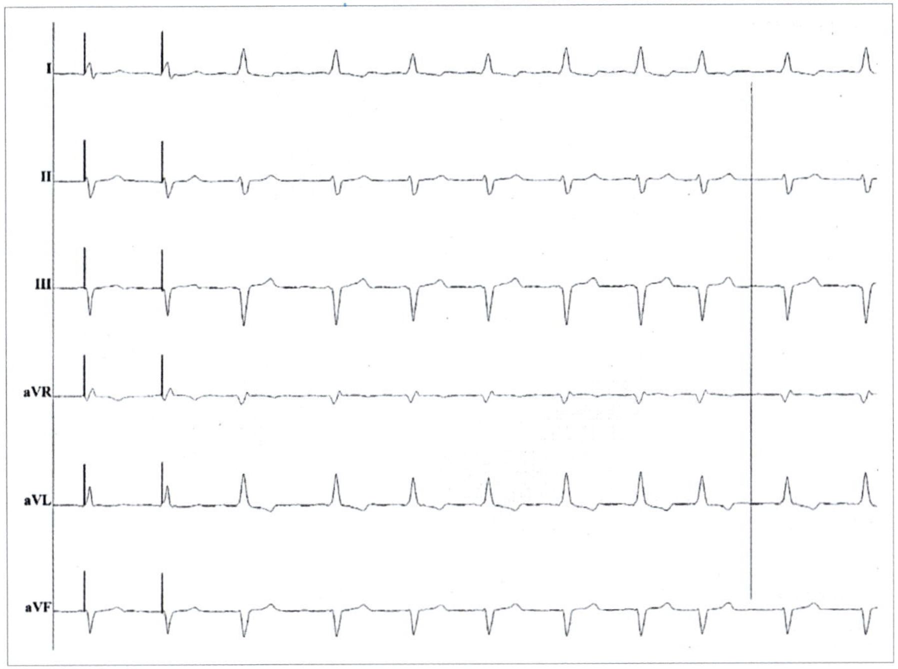

Introduction to the case

A patient implanted with a CRT pacemaker presented for follow-up, without complaints. The counters revealed 100% of RV sensing and 100% of LV pacing. The device settings are shown in Table 65.1, and a real-time EGM is shown in Figure 65.1.

Table 65.1 Device settings

Pacing mode	DDD
Lower rate	50bpm
Upper rate	140bpm
AV delay (paced/sensed)	220ms/180ms
VV delay	0ms
Atrial output	2.5V@0.4ms
RV output (bipolar)	2.5V@0.4ms
LV output (unipolar)	2.5V@0.4ms
Atrial sensitivity (bipolar)	0.3mV
RV sensitivity (integrated bipolar)	0.4mV
LV sensitivity (bipolar)	2.5mV

Question

Figure 65.1 Real-time EGM at follow-up

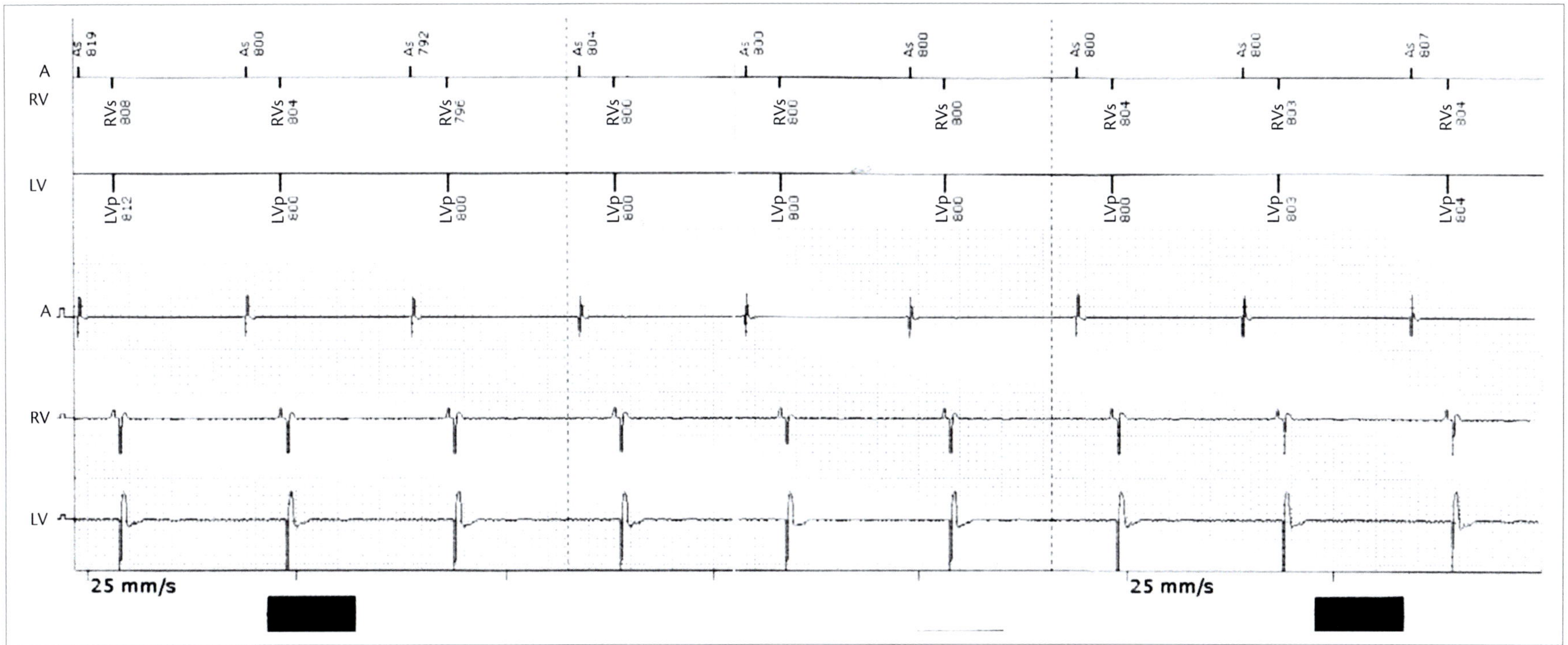

What do you observe?

A Ventricular safety pacing

B Triggered LV pacing (VVT pacing)

C Negative AV hysteresis

D Programmed LV pacing only

Answer

B Triggered LV pacing (VVT pacing)

Figure 65.2 Annotated real-time EGM at follow-up

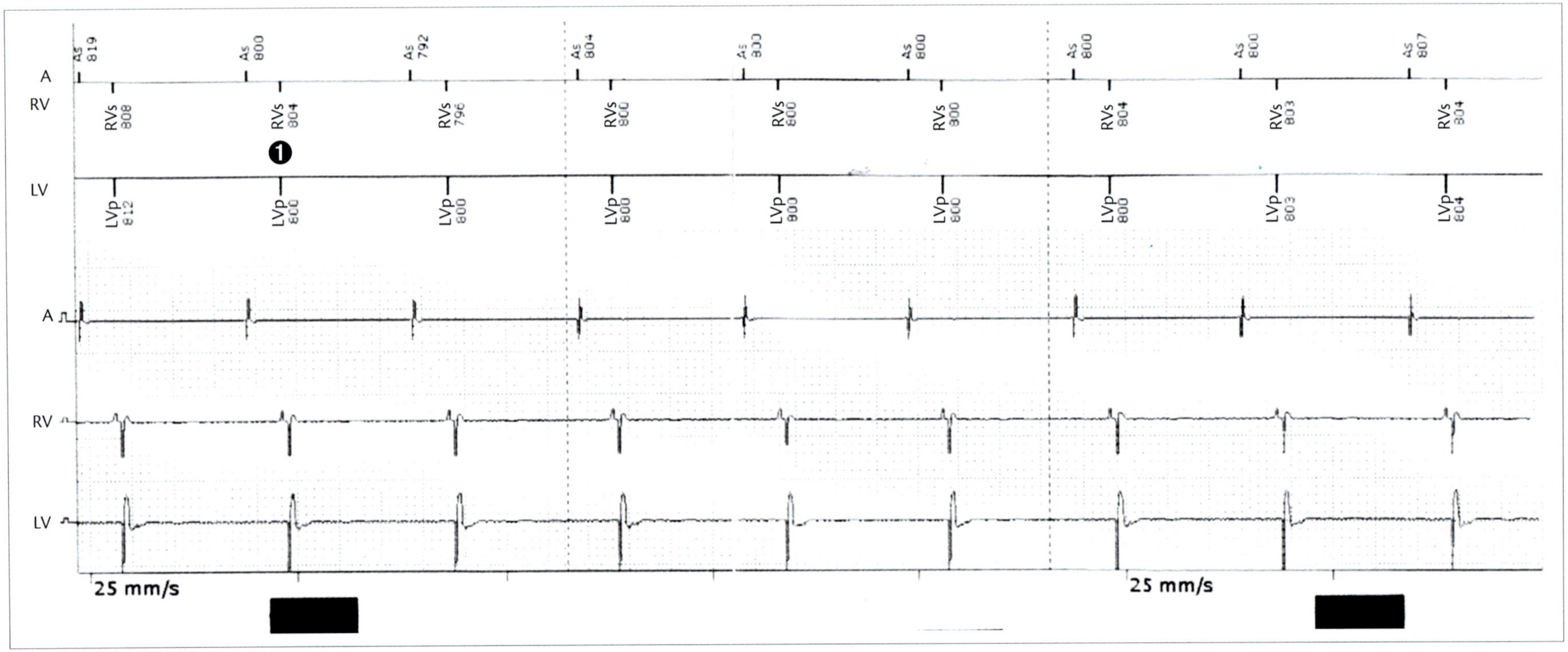

❶ RV sensing occurs, due to intrinsic AV conduction. This triggers LV pacing (VVT pacing). The 4ms difference in RV and LV timing of the first cycle is due to inaccuracy of the device clock (Figure 65.2).

Ventricular safety pacing only occurs after AP events and would have been timed at an AVI of 100ms in this device. Negative AV hysteresis would have led to shortening of the AVI with biventricular pacing. As shown in Table 65.1, the device was programmed to simultaneous biventricular pacing.

Comments

Triggered left ventricular pacing

Triggered LV pacing in this case led to fusion with intrinsic AV conduction and substantial LV capture, as evidenced by narrowing of the QRS complex and increasing negativity in lead I (Figure 65.3).

Fusion pacing was intentional in this patient, in order to allow the longest possible AV delay to avoid A-wave truncation of the transmitral flow (which was tolerated poorly). This was due to interatrial conduction delay, as can been appreciated by the notched and prolonged (140ms) P-wave (best seen in lead II on the right panel of Figure 65.3).

Figure 65.3 Effect of triggered LV pacing with ventricular capture and narrowing of the QRS

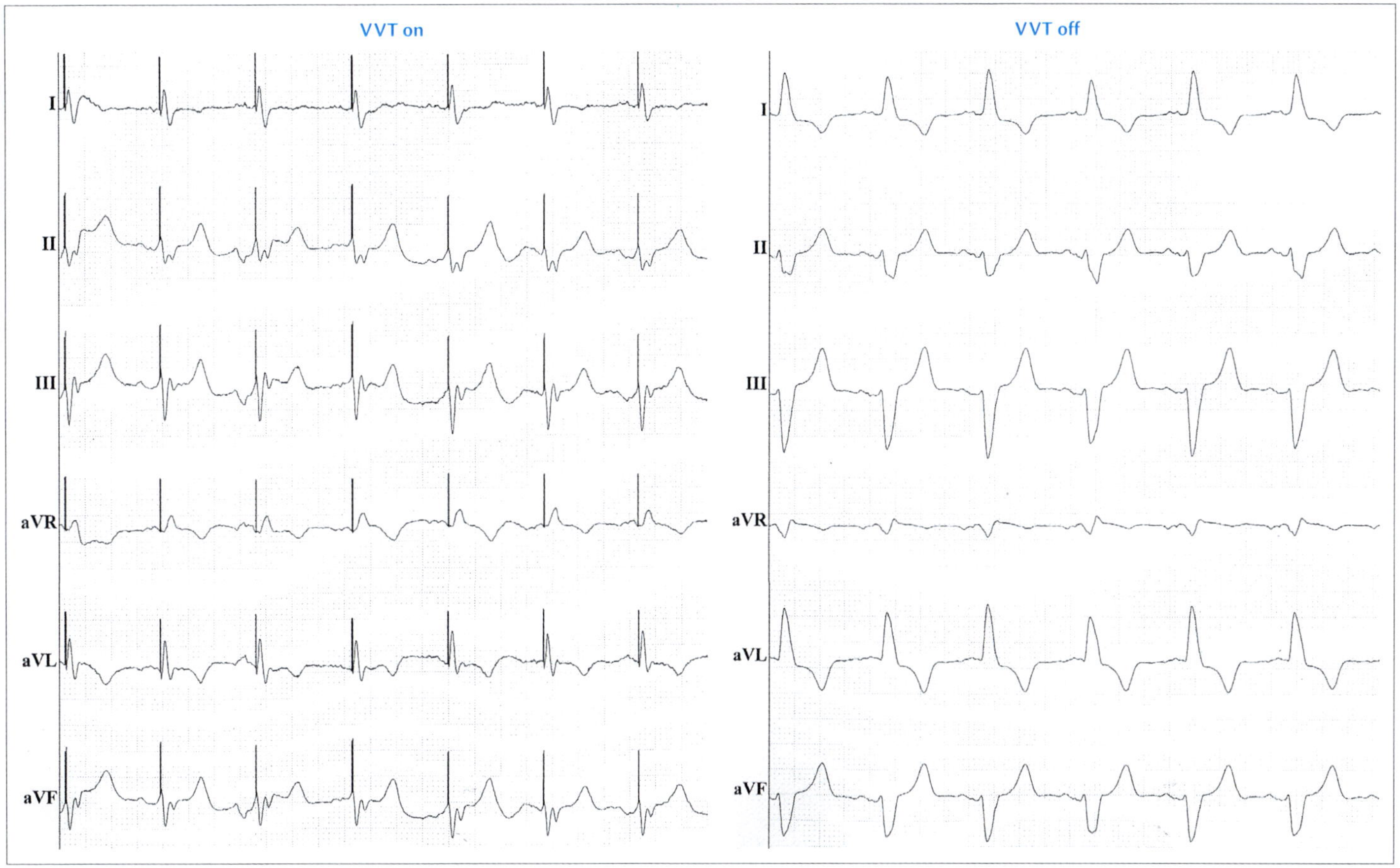

Introduction to the case

A patient was implanted with a CRT-D, with an LV lead in the anterior cardiac vein (Figure 66.1a), and consulted after 3 weeks due to breathlessness. The device counters showed 100% RV pacing and 100% LV sensing (Figure 66.1b). The programmed settings are shown in Table 66.1. A real-time EGM is shown in Figure 66.2.

Figure 66.1 Postero-anterior fluoroscopic view showing the LV lead in the anterior cardiac vein (a) and the rate histograms (b)

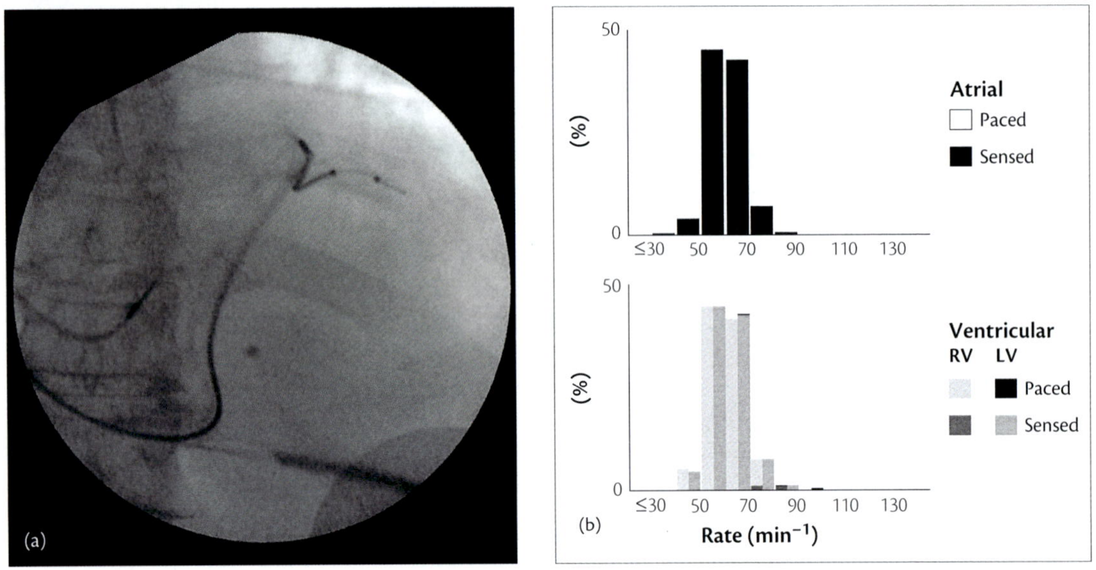

Table 66.1 Device settings

Pacing mode	DDD
Lower rate	50bpm
Upper rate	140bpm
AV delay (paced/sensed)	140/120ms
Atrial output	2.5V@0.4ms
RV output (bipolar)	2.5V@0.4ms
LV output (extended bipolar)	2.5V@0.4ms
Atrial sensitivity (bipolar)	0.3mV
RV sensitivity (integrated bipolar)	0.4mV
LV sensitivity (bipolar)	2.5mV

Question

Figure 66.2 Real-time EGM

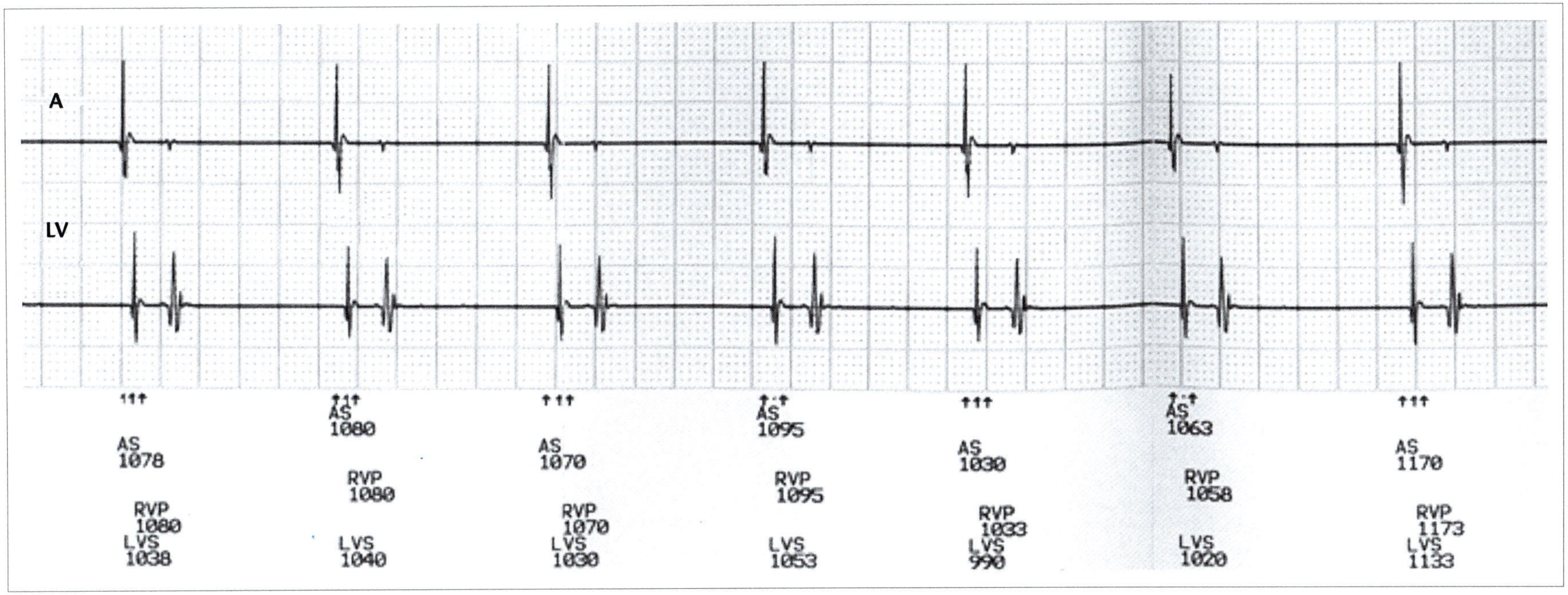

What is the cause for the lack of LV pacing?

A Far-field P-wave oversensing

B FFRW oversensing

C R-wave double-counting

D T-wave oversensing

Answer

A Far-field P-wave oversensing

Figure 66.3 Annotated real-time EGM

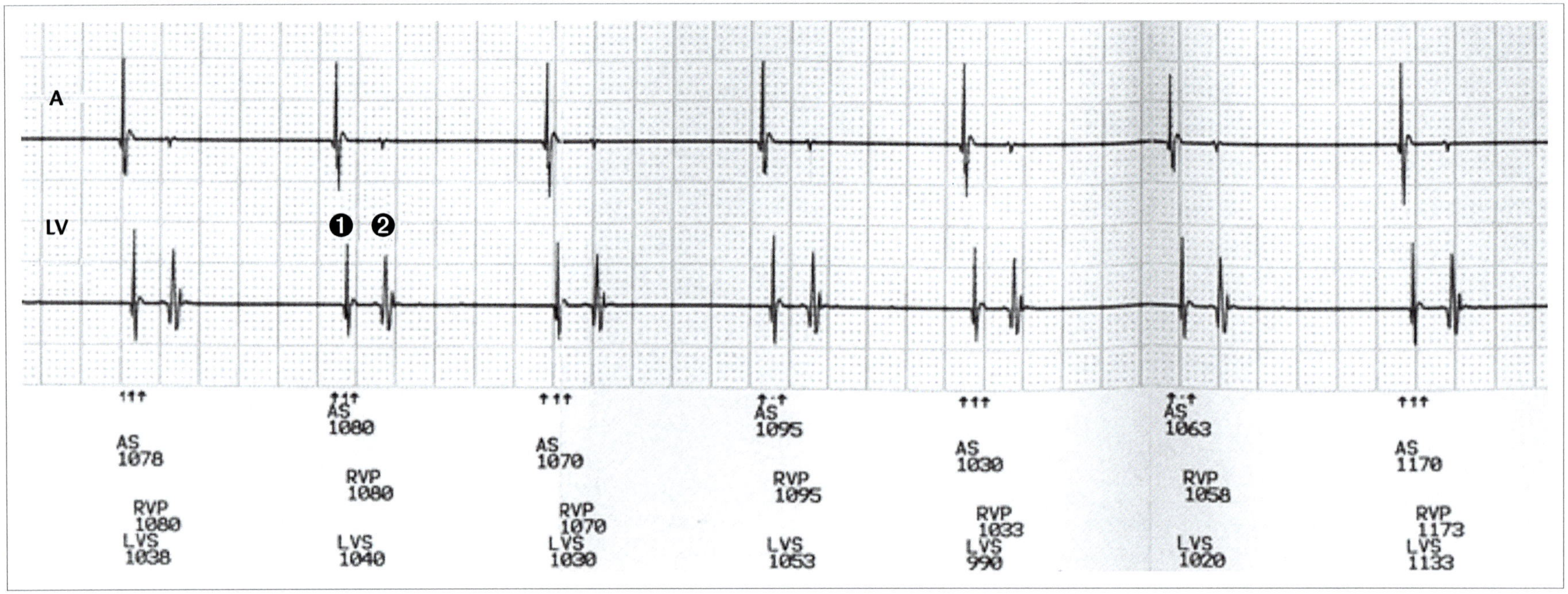

The far-field P-wave oversensing of the LV lead was due to its basal position in the CS tributary (Figure 66.3). Dislodgment of the lead into the CS would also result in a similar EGM.

❶ The 1st potential on the LV EGM corresponds to left atrial activity (and follows too shortly after right atrial sensing to correspond to AV conduction). The LVS event inhibits LV pacing but does not reset the timers in this device. RV pacing therefore occurs at the end of the programmed AVI.

❷ The 2nd potential on the LV EGM corresponds to local ventricular activity.

Comments

Far-field P-wave oversensing of the LV lead

The proximal pole of the LV lead was picking up atrial signals, due to its basal location. Extending the PAVB would not be useful, as this period is only activated after AP. Decreasing the sensitivity levels would also not be a solution, as the far-field P-wave is of greater amplitude than the R-wave. The problem was resolved by eliminating the LV proximal electrode from the sensing circuit and programming an extended bipolar configuration (LV tip to RV coil), without any far-field P-wave signal (Figure 66.4).

Figure 66.4 LV EGM after programming sensing to extended bipolar

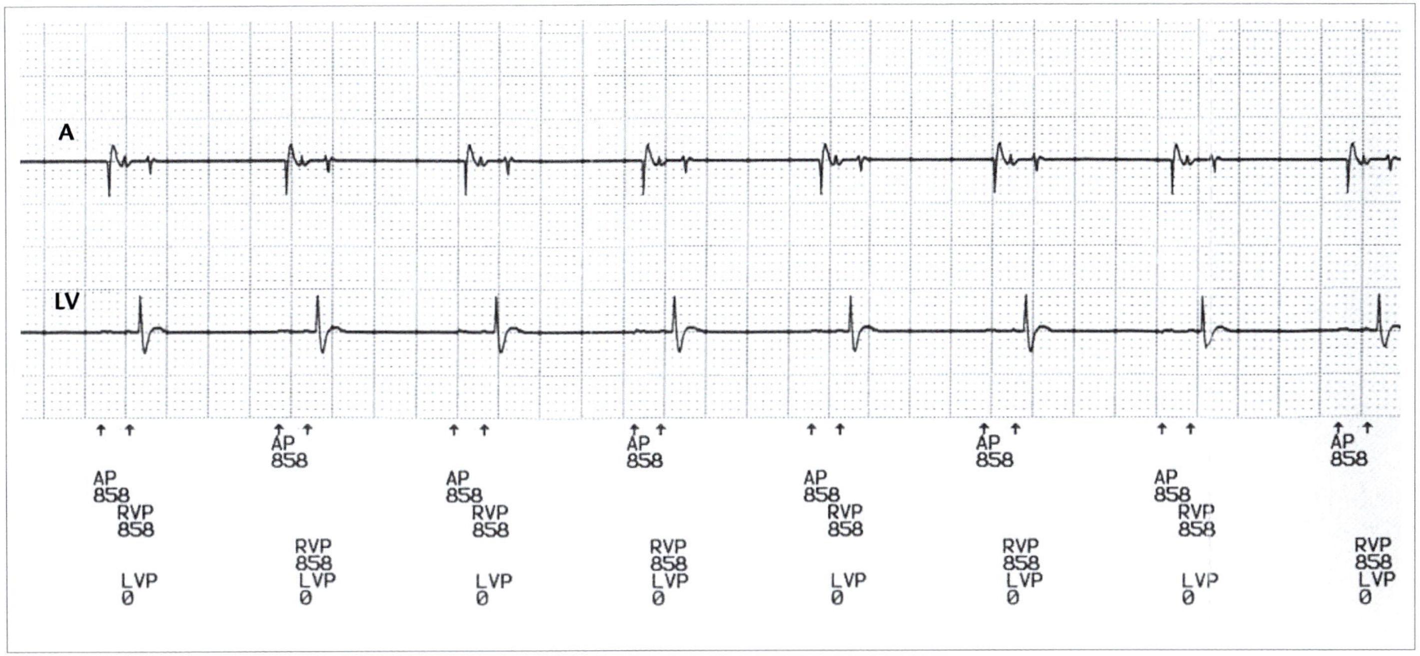

Introduction to the case

A patient implanted with a CRT-D was seen at 2 months' follow-up, without any improvement in symptoms. An LV threshold test was performed at 0.4ms pulse width (with bipolar pacing) and is shown in Figure 67.1.

Question

Figure 67.1 EGM recorded during the LV threshold test

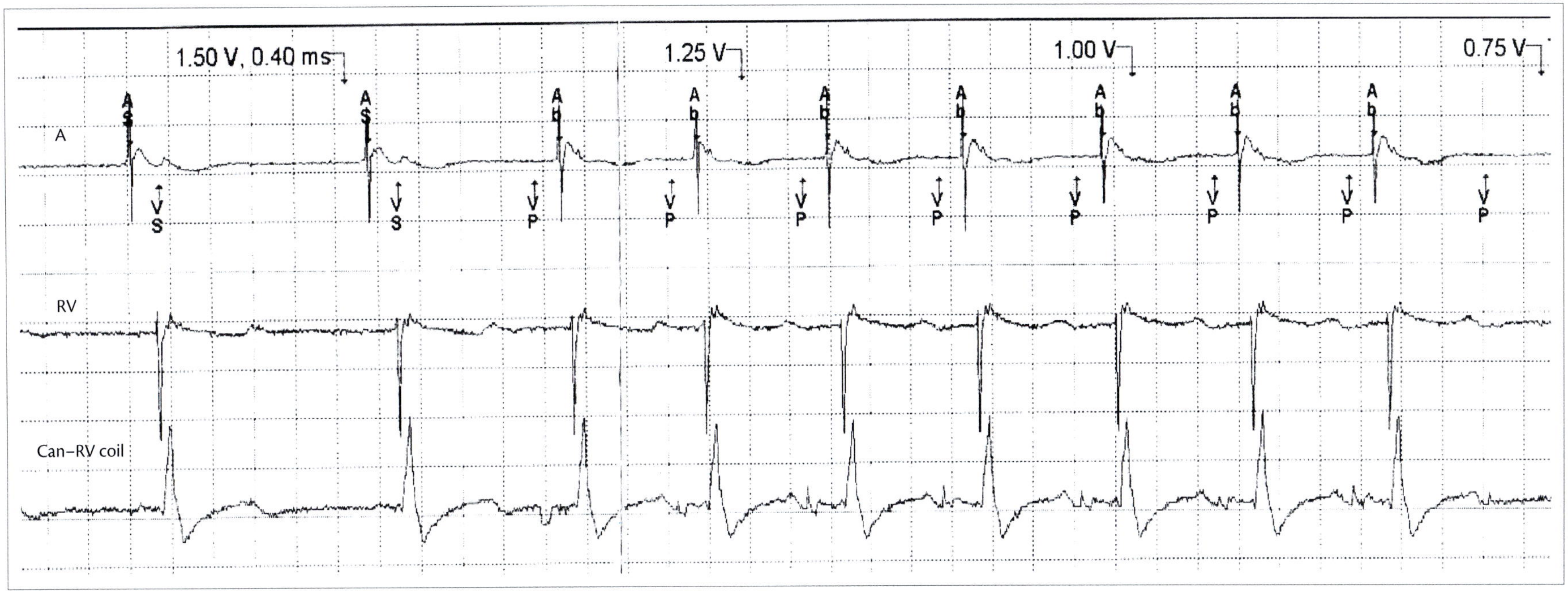

What is the LV capture threshold amplitude?

A 0.75V

B 1.00V

C 1.25V

D Some other value

Answer

D **Some other value**

Figure 67.2 Annotated EGM recorded during the LV threshold test

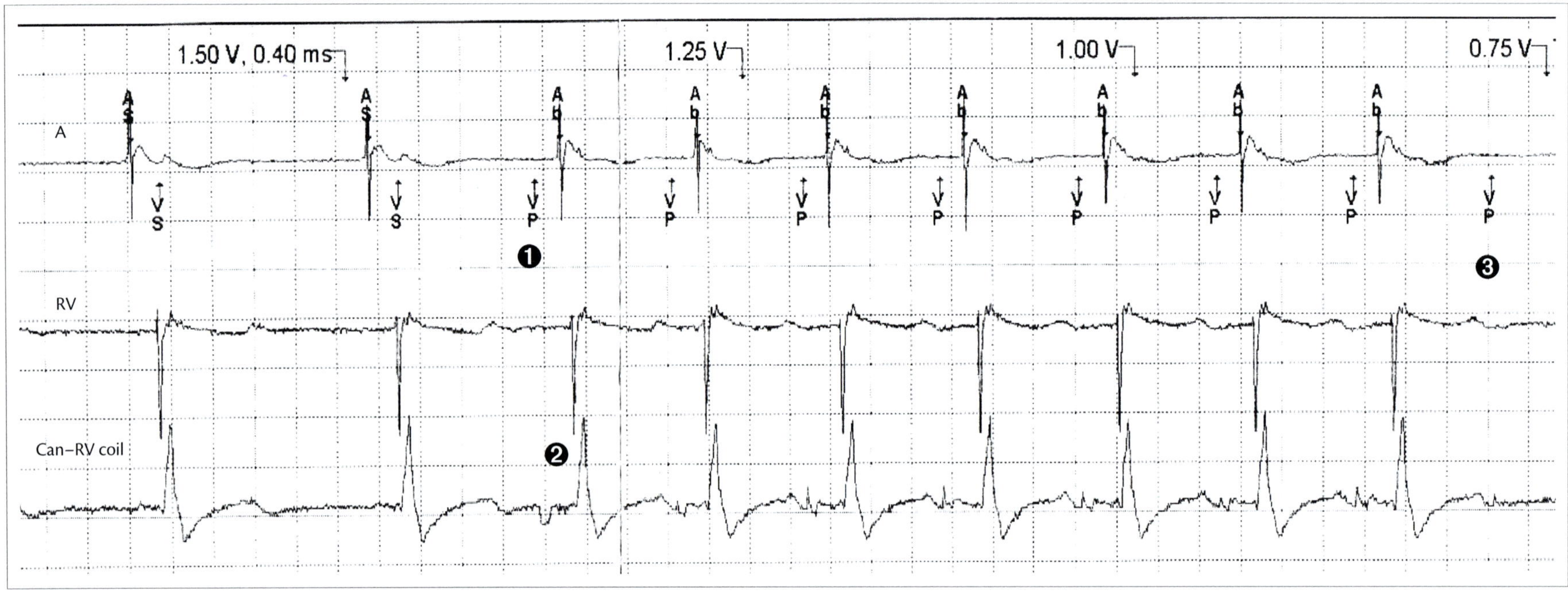

The patient had left atrial capture during the LV threshold test, due to a dislodged LV lead (Figure 67.2).

❶ The LV threshold test is initiated with pacing at 1.5V/0.4ms. There is a delay between LV pacing and the atrial event labelled as Ab (falling in the atrial blanking period). However, this delay is slightly shorter than that of the event in the RV channel, which is unusual (one would expect the interval of retrograde VA conduction to be longer than that of interventricular conduction). Also, the RV EGM morphology is identical during LV pacing compared to during intrinsic rhythm, which points against ventricular capture.

❷ The far-field EGM shows that LV pacing results in atrial capture. Also, the QRS morphology is identical during ventricular pacing and intrinsic rhythm (i.e. the two previous cycles).

❸ This cycle corresponds to loss of left atrial capture.

Comments

Left ventricular lead dislodgement with left atrial pacing

This is an example that illustrates the utility of recording a surface ECG during threshold tests, as issues may be identified more readily than by evaluating the near- or far-field EGMs.

The LV lead had dislodged to the proximal CS due to Twiddler's syndrome (Figure 67.3), and the patient admitted to having flipped the generator in the pocket several times.

Pacing from this lead resulted in left atrial capture during the threshold test. New leads were implanted due to possible damage, the generator was fixated in a retropectoral pocket, and the patient was instructed not to manipulate the region anymore.

Figure 67.3 Chest X-ray showing the LV lead dislodged to the proximal coronary sinus, with twisted leads in the device pocket due to Twiddler's syndrome

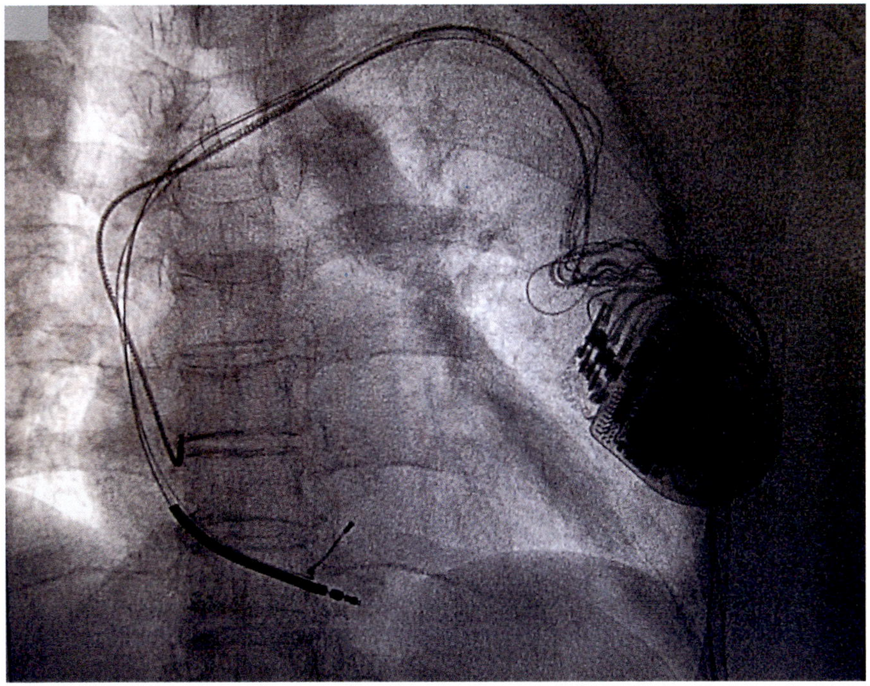

Introduction to the case

A patient equipped with a CRT-D was followed up at 6 months after device implantation. The LV threshold had been measured at 2.7V/0.8ms at the 2-month visit. The device settings are shown in Table 68.1, and the LV threshold test performed at a pulse width of 0.8ms is shown in Figure 68.1.

Table 68.1 Device settings

Pacing mode	DDD
Lower rate	50bpm
Upper rate	140bpm
AV delay (paced/sensed)	160/140ms
Atrial output	2.5V@0.4ms
RV output (bipolar)	2.5V@0.4ms
LV output (LV tip–RV coil)	5.0V@0.8ms
Atrial sensitivity (bipolar)	0.3mV
RV sensitivity (bipolar)	2.5mV
LV sensitivity (LV tip–RV coil)	2.5mV

Question

Figure 68.1 Real-time EGM during the LV threshold test

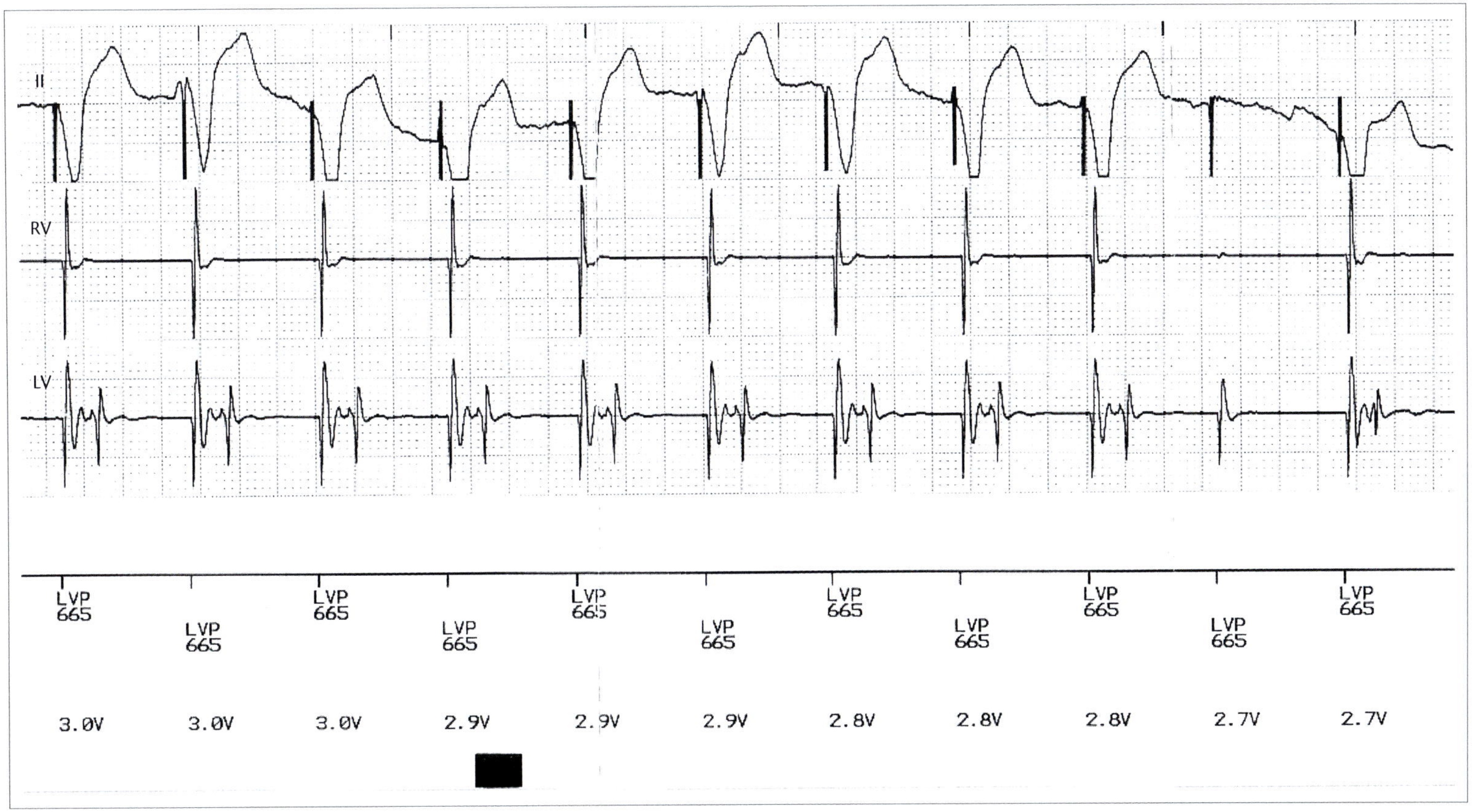

What is the LV capture threshold?

A 2.7V

B 2.8V

C 2.9V

D Some other value

Answer

D **Some other value**

Figure 68.2 Annotated real-time EGM during the LV threshold test

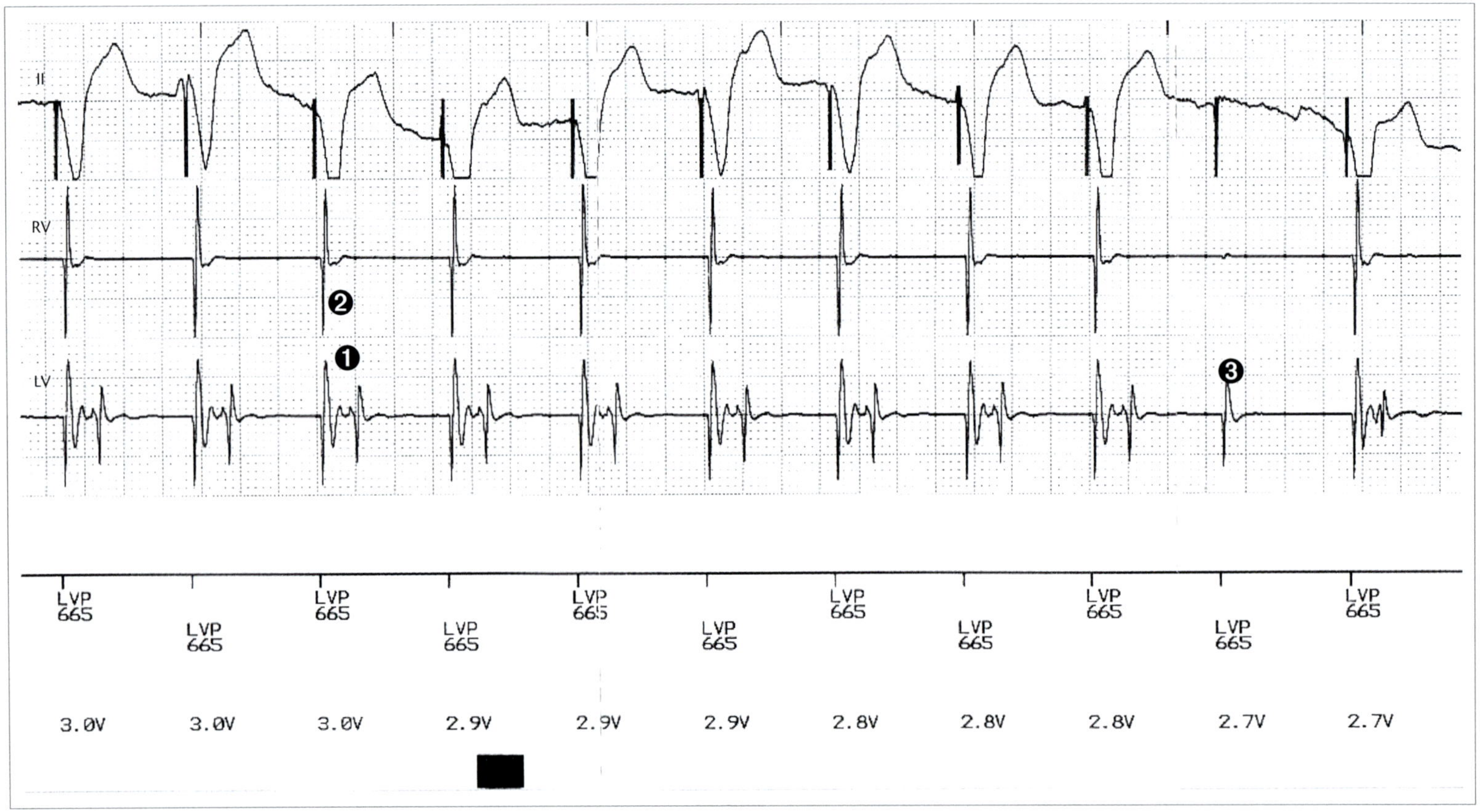

The LV lead had dislodged, but RV anodal capture resulted from the LV tip–RV coil (extended bipolar) pacing configuration (Figure 68.4).

❶ The LV EGM shows two distinct potentials (Figure 68.2). The 1st potential corresponds to RV anodal capture, which is visible because sensing is programmed in the LV tip to RV coil configuration. The 2nd potential is the local LV depolarization that occurred with interventricular conduction.

❷ The RV EGM shows evidence of RV capture (note the negative deflection).

❸ There is loss of RV anodal capture at 2.7V/0.8ms. The deflection on the LV EGM that occurs directly after the pacing spike is due to tissue polarization (after-potential) and is different in morphology, compared to the 1st potential of the previous complexes (which are recorded during capture). Note that the RV EGM also shows the absence of capture.

Comments

Anodal capture

Total loss of LV capture was confirmed in this patient by performing the threshold test in a unipolar (LV tip to can) pacing configuration (Figure 68.3).

Anodal capture may occur due to a 'virtual cathode' of negatively charged tissue surrounding the anode (with higher thresholds, compared to cathodal capture). In CRT, it occurs when the LV pacing configuration is programmed to an extended bipolar configuration (see Figure 68.4 relating to an LV threshold test in a different patient). It occurs more commonly with CRT pacemakers than CRT-D, as the RV ring electrode has a smaller surface area than the RV ICD coil with higher current density (although as illustrated by the present case, anodal capture with the RV coil is possible).

The consequences of anodal capture in CRT include:

- erroneous LV capture thresholds (as in the present example). The pacing output may be programmed consequently to a subthreshold value in the LV, resulting in loss of CRT
- simultaneous biventricular capture despite programming of sequential CRT pacing with LV pre-excitation
- maintenance of biventricular capture in case the RV lead output is programmed to subthreshold values.

Figure 68.3 LV threshold test with unipolar pacing, showing absence of capture (VPBs are annotated by an *)

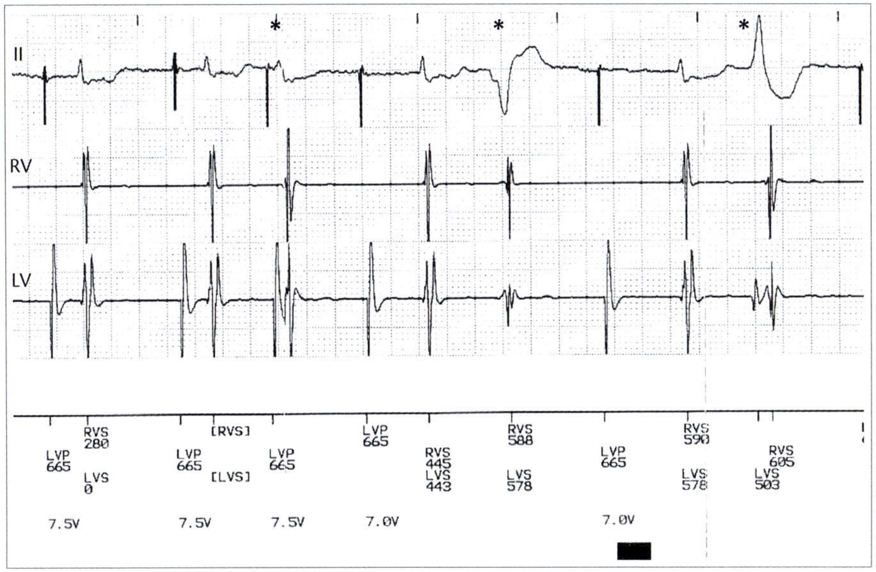

Figure 68.4 Extended bipolar LV configuration (a), and ECG recorded during an LV threshold test showing initial biventricular capture due to LV plus RV anodal capture, followed by LV capture only (b)

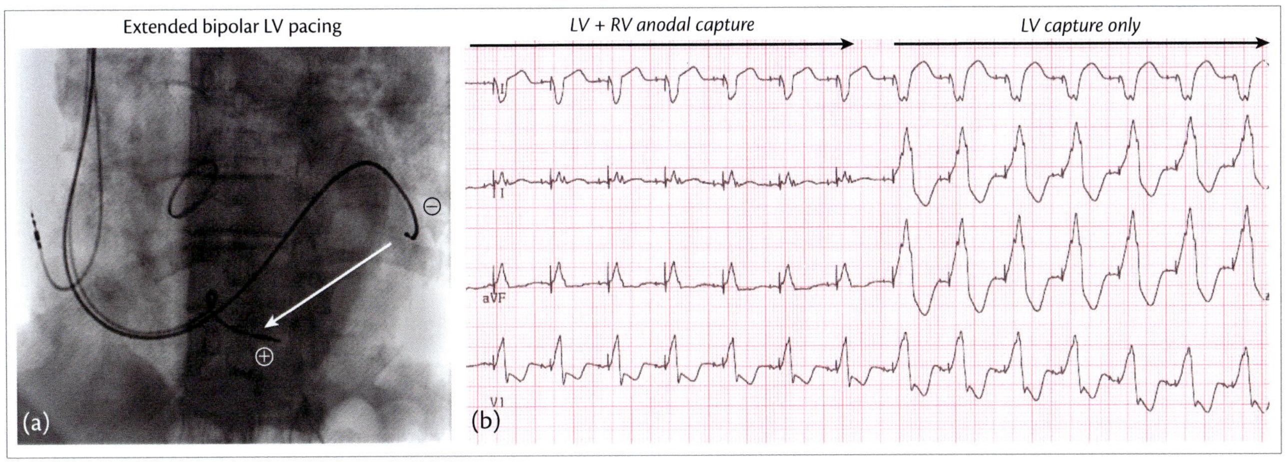

Introduction to the case

During CRT-D implantation, a change in rhythm was observed on the monitor. The real-time EGM recorded with wireless telemetry is shown in Figure 69.1.

Question

Figure 69.1 Real-time EGM recorded by wireless telemetry during CRT implantation

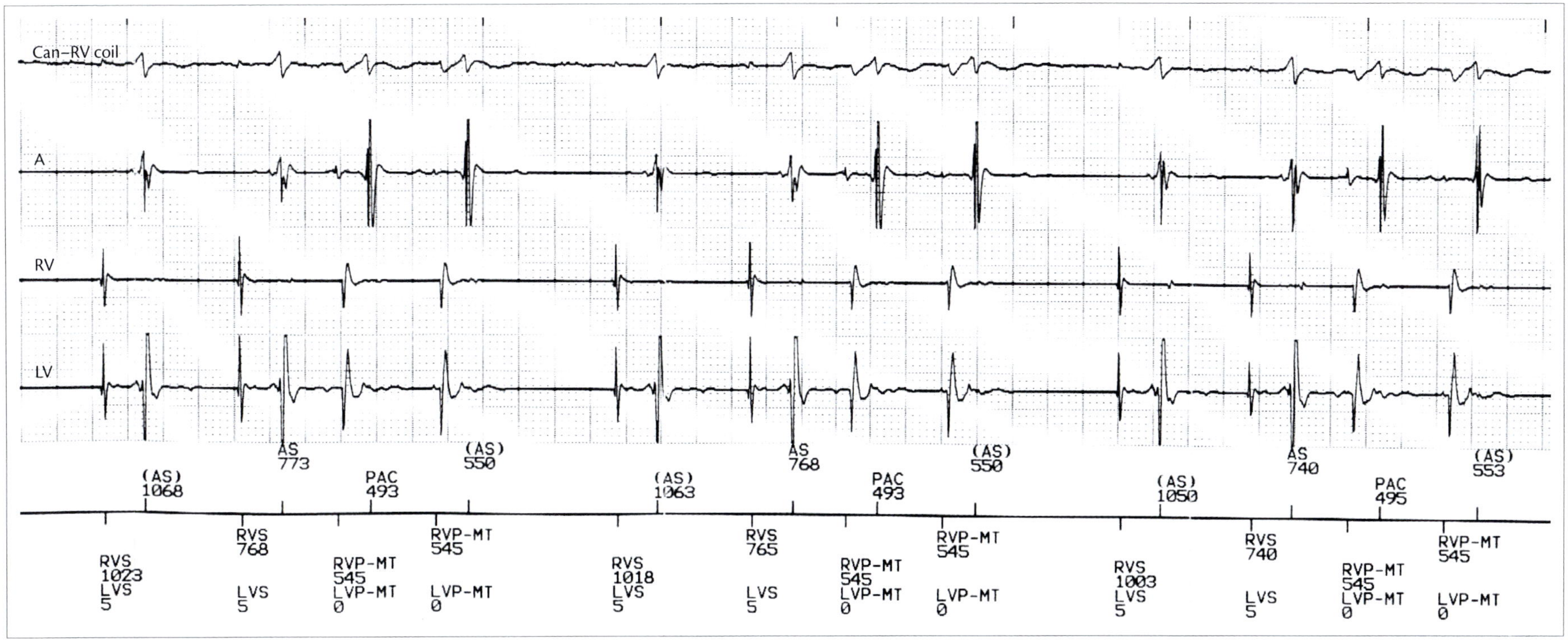

What is the problem?

A VPBs

B Switching of the RV and LV leads

C Switching of the A and RV leads

D Switching of the A and LV leads

Answer

C Switching of the A and RV leads

Figure 69.2 Annotated real-time EGM recorded by wireless telemetry during CRT implantation

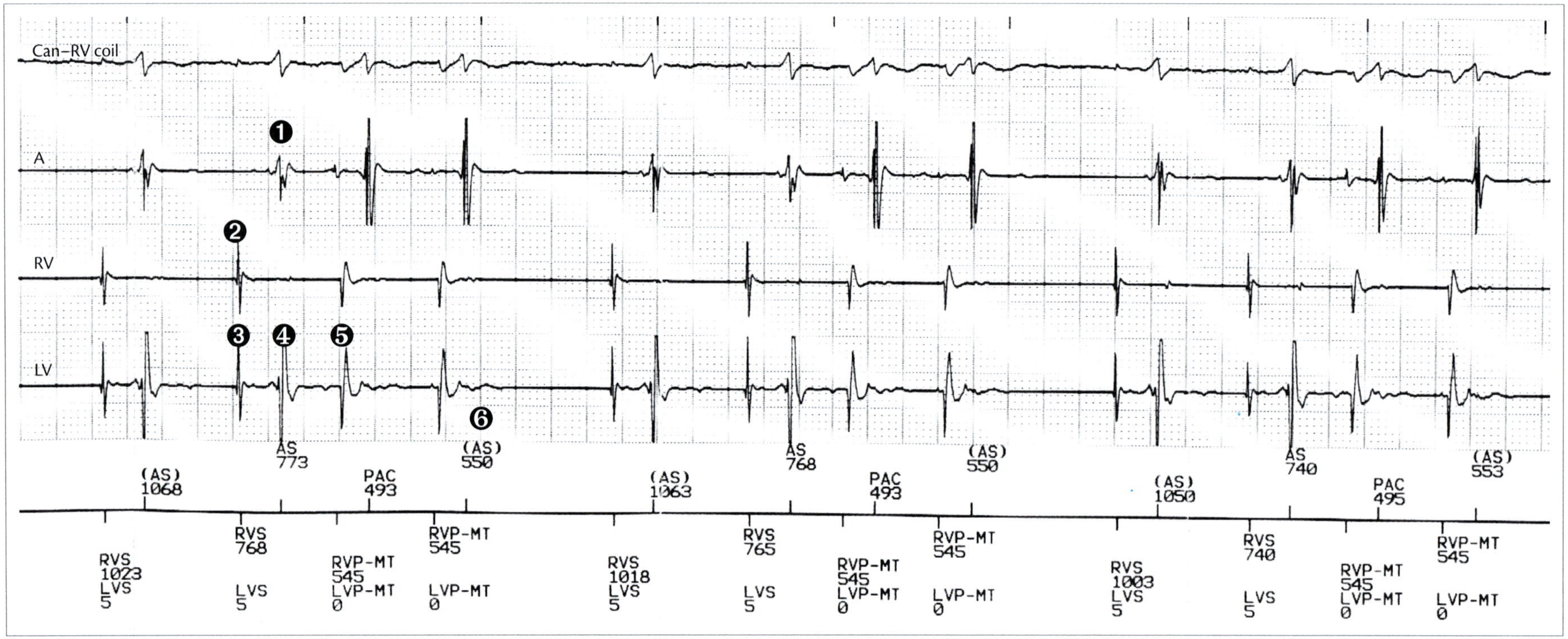

Inadvertent insertion of the A lead into the RV connector, and vice versa, was identified and corrected immediately during the procedure (Figure 69.2).

❶ The atrial EGM signal is synchronous with the QRS complex visible on the far-field (can–RV coil) channel, implying that the atrial port is connected to one of the ventricular leads.

❷ The RV EGM signal is synchronous with the P-wave, implying that the atrial lead is connected to this port.

❸ An atrial signal is visible on the LV EGM. This is because LV sensing is programmed to an extended bipolar configuration (i.e. there is an internal connection in the generator between the LV and RV channels. As the atrial lead is connected to the RV port, an atrial EGM is visible).

❹ The 2nd signal on the LV EGM corresponds to the LV signal. It is not sensed by the device, due to the VRP.

❺ Ventricular pacing occurs at the UTR, due to tracking of the preceding AS event.

❻ This AS event falls in the PVARP and therefore is not tracked. The sequences repeat themselves, leading to grouped beating.

Comments

Lead switch

Another example of A/V lead switch on the header occurring during implantation was shown in Case 19. The present case illustrates again the importance of verifying the rhythm after connecting the leads at device implantation. It also shows the utility of wireless telemetry for rapidly identifying the problem.

With ICDs, another potential mistake is to switch the DF-1 connectors, as shown in Case 53. Yet another possible error with CRT devices is to switch the RV and LV leads. This may not need to be corrected, unless the LV dislodges or if sensing issues, such as far-field P-wave oversensing of the LV lead, occurs (see Case 6). The recent advent of IS-4 leads will avoid switches with an IS-1 RV lead, but there is the potential for switching IS-4 and DF-4 leads. These two standards, however, have slightly different designs, as the IS-4 pin is larger than the DF-4 pin and will not fit fully into the header (Figure 69.3). The error can be identified by measuring high HV impedances at implantation, as there is no electrical connection between the DF-4 header and the IS-4 pin.

Figure 69.3 Differences between DF-4 and IS-4 pins and connectors

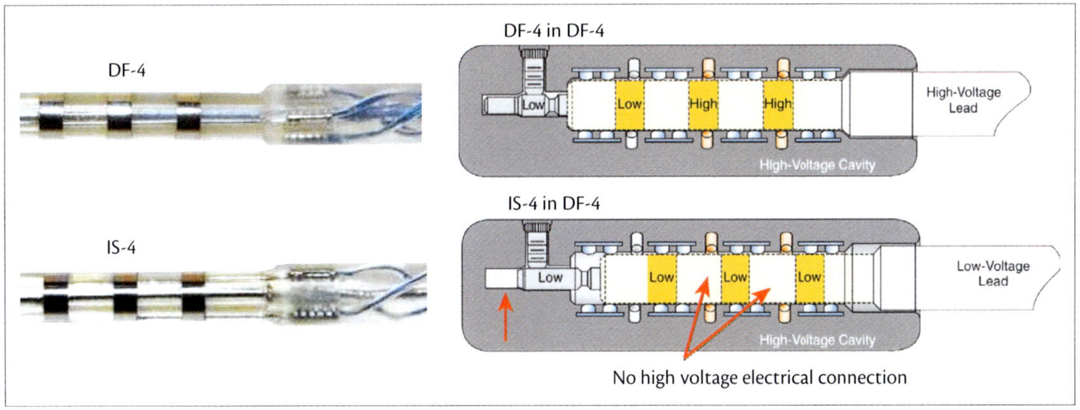

Courtesy of Mr H Leersen

Introduction to the case

A Holter test was performed in a patient implanted with a CRT-D, due to palpitations without any recorded arrhythmias. The test revealed periods with frequent VPBs that coincided with the patient's symptoms. In addition, an event was recorded while the patient was sleeping, and is shown in Figure 70.1. The device settings are shown in Table 70.1.

Table 70.1 Device settings

Pacing mode	DDD
Lower rate	50bpm
Upper rate	140bpm
AV delay (paced/sensed)	140/100ms
VV delay	LV −4ms
Atrial output	Auto@0.4ms
RV output (bipolar)	Auto@0.4ms
LV output (extended bipolar)	Auto@0.4ms
Atrial sensitivity (bipolar)	0.3mV
RV sensitivity (true bipolar)	0.45mV
LV sensitivity	Not available

Question

Figure 70.1 Holter recording

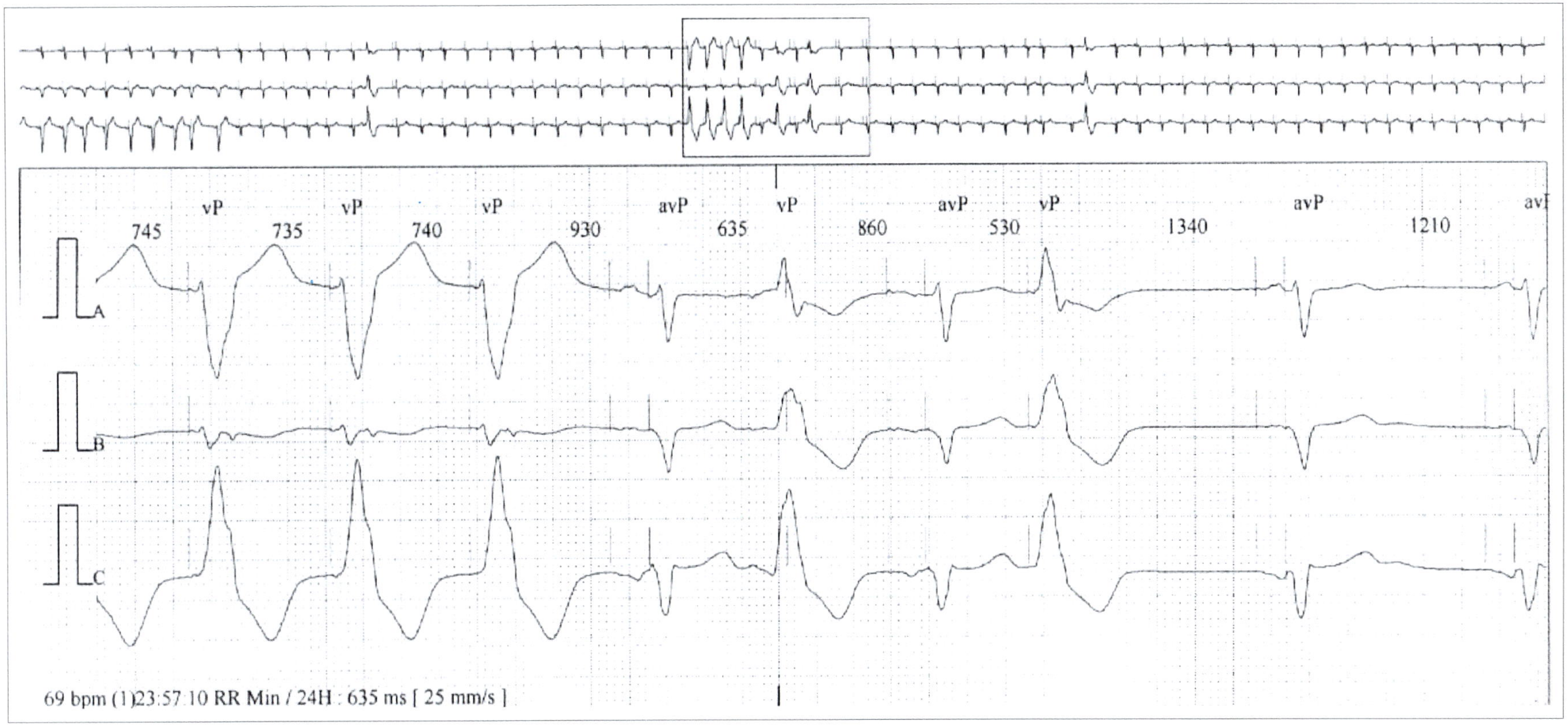

How can one explain the device behaviour?

A Ventricular safety pacing

B Automatic sensing algorithm

C Automatic atrial threshold test

D Automatic ventricular threshold test

Answer

D Automatic ventricular threshold test

Figure 70.2 Annotated Holter recording

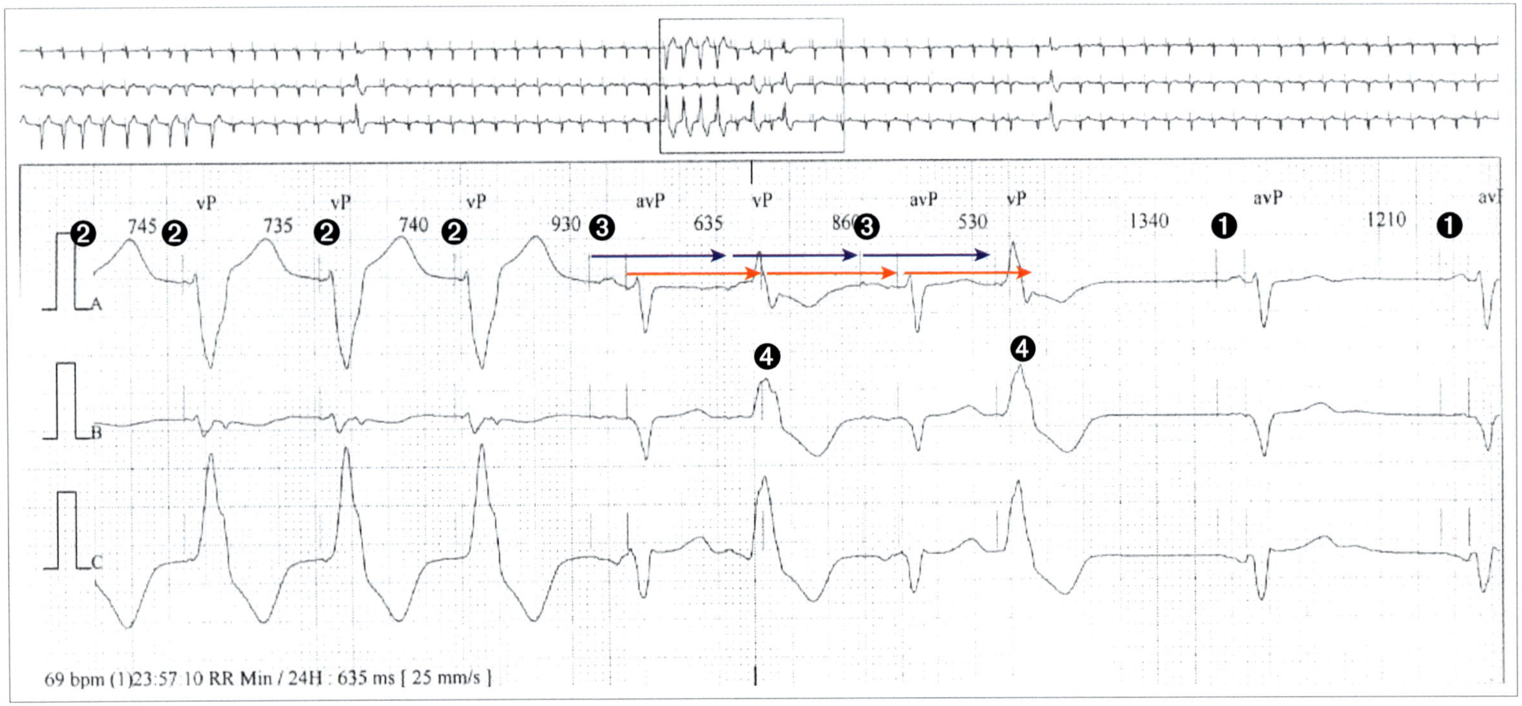

The Holter recording (Figure 70.2) shows an automatic LV threshold test being initiated and then aborted due to VPBs.

❶ These two complexes show biventricular pacing (narrow paced QRS) with the programmed device settings (at 50bpm and a paced AV delay of 140ms).

❷ The four initial beats show a very wide paced QRS complex at intervals of 740ms. Theses cycles are AV pacing with an interval of 30ms (the ventricular spike is not reconstructed by the Holter) with univentricular LV pacing for the interventricular conduction test (Figure 70.3). Pacing at a faster rate is not observed with options A and B.

❸ These two cycles show biventricular pacing at 740ms with a longer AV delay, corresponding to the AV conduction test (Figure 70.3).

❹ VPBs are observed. The 1st beat is not detected by the device, as a ventricular spike can be seen (if the premature beat originates in the LV, detection may be delayed in the RV lead, and this device does not have LV sensing). The 2nd premature beat is probably detected, as the coupling interval is slightly shorter. As there is an AP–VS event during the AV conduction test, the automatic LV threshold test is aborted (Figure 70.3).

The blue arrows correspond to AP–AP interval timing during the test. Note that no spike is visible at the end of the 1st arrow, either because of an intrinsic P-wave or because the atrial spike is not detected and reconstructed by the Holter. The red arrows correspond to VP–VP interval timing.

Comments

Automatic LV threshold test

Unexpected device behaviour may be explained sometimes by automatic threshold tests (such as seen in Case 33). The details of the function of these algorithms vary between manufacturers and are almost impossible to remember, but they can be consulted on technical manuals or online resources (e.g. <http://www.medtronicfeatures.com>).

In this case, the device was a Medtronic model that was performing the LV capture management algorithm. The function of this algorithm is detailed as follows.

The algorithm functions on the principle that the interventricular interval tends to be shorter than the intrinsic AVI. A captured LV test pace will therefore be sensed in the RV earlier than the conducted VS of a non-captured test pace. The device first evaluates the interventricular conduction (LVP–RVS interval) and ascertains that AV conduction is sufficiently longer than the interventricular delay (Figure 70.3). If the criteria are fulfilled, a threshold test is performed, with loss of capture being defined as an RVS event that occurs >50 ms after the maximum LVP–RVS interval.

The test is usually performed at 1 a.m. and was done at around midnight in this patient, due to the device being set to winter time.

Figure 70.3 Initiation of the automatic LV threshold test

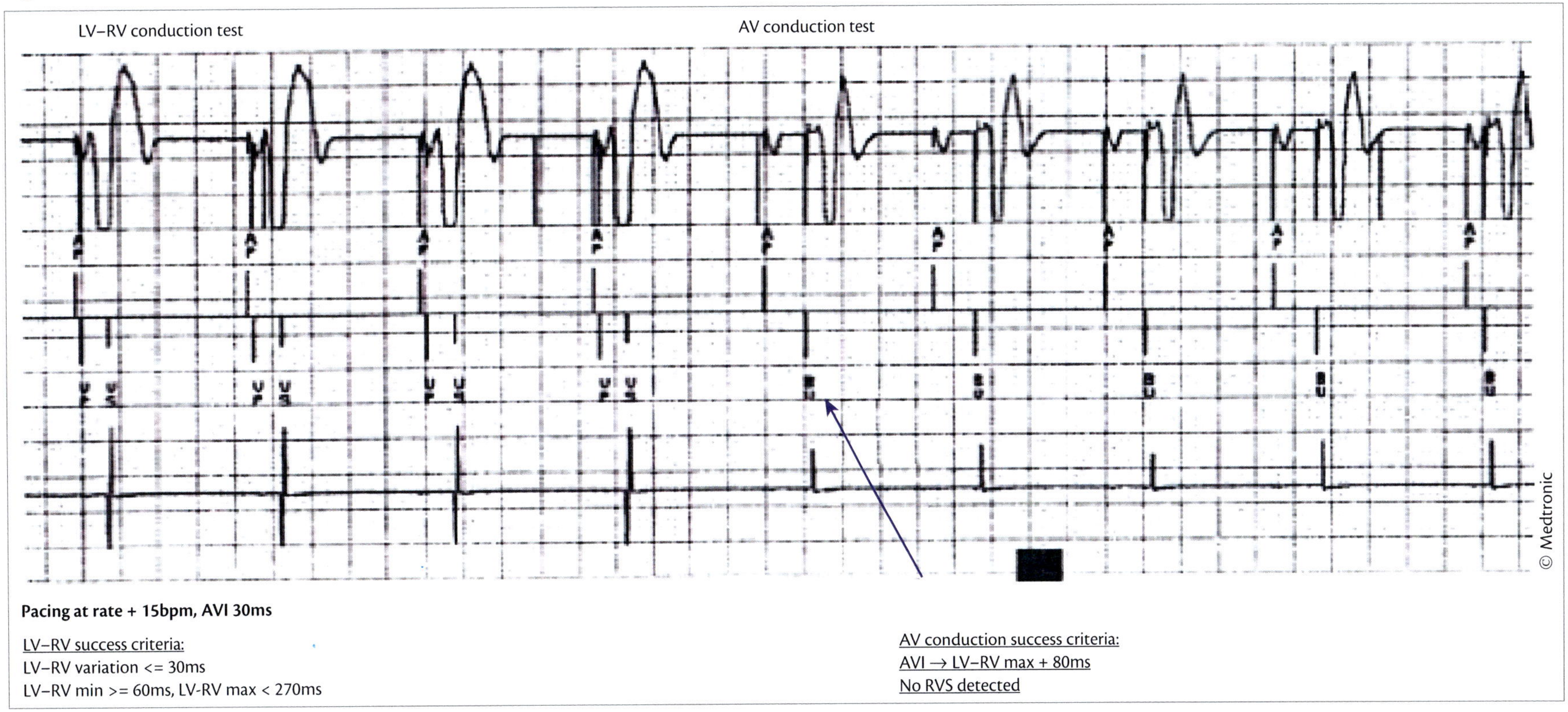

Index

D

E

F

G

H

I

L

U

V

W

INDEX

The manufacturer's authorised representative in the EU for product safety is Oxford University Press España S.A. of El Parque Empresarial San Fernando de Henares, Avenida de Castilla, 2 – 28830 Madrid (www.oup.es/en or product.safety@oup.com). OUP España S.A. also acts as importer into Spain of products made by the manufacturer.

Printed in the USA/Agawam, MA
April 14, 2026

903556.122